WOMEN'S

A Guide to Symptoms, Illness, Surgery,
Medical Tests & Procedures

H. Winter Griffith, M.D.
with Hugh S. Miller, M.D.

Surgical Illustrations by Mark Pederson

PERIGEE

A Perigee Book
Published by The Berkley Publishing Group
A division of Penguin Putnam Inc.
375 Hudson Street
New York, New York 10014

First edition: August 1999

Published simultaneously in Canada.

The Penguin Putnam Inc. World Wide Web site address is
http://www.penguinputnam.com

Library of Congress Cataloging-in-Publication Data

Griffith, H. Winter (Henry Winter), 1926–1993
    Women's health : a guide to symptoms, illness, surgery, medical
  tests & procedures / H. Winter Griffith, with Hugh S. Miller ;
  surgical illustrations by Mark Pederson.
        p.   cm.
    Includes index.
    ISBN 0-399-52518-1
    1. Women—Health and hygiene. 2. Women—Diseases.   I. Miller,
  Hugh S. (Hugh Stephen) II. Title.
  RA777.8.G75   1999
  613'.04244—dc21   99-18380
                                             CIP

Printed in United States of America
10 9 8 7 6 5 4 3 2 1

Contents

About the Authors

H. Winter Griffith, M.D., authored many medical books, including the best-selling *Complete Guide to Prescription & Nonprescription Drugs; Complete Guide to Symptoms, Illness & Surgery for People Over 50; Complete Guide to Sports Injuries* and *Complete Guide to Pediatric Symptoms, Illness & Medications*, all from The Body Press. Others include *Instructions for Patients; Drug Information for Pediatric Patients; Vitamins, Minerals and Supplements* and *Medical Tests—Doctor-Ordered and Do-It-Yourself*.

Dr. Griffith received his medical degree from Emory University in 1953. After 20 years in private practice, he established a basic medical-science program at Florida State University. He subsequently became an Associate Professor of Family and Community Medicine at the University of Arizona College of Medicine. Until his death in 1993, Dr. Griffith lived in Tucson, Arizona.

Hugh S. Miller, M.D., is clinical Associate Professor in the Division of Maternal-Fetal Medicine, Department of Obstetrics and Gynecology, University of Arizona College of Medicine, Tucson, Arizona.

A Woman's Responsibility

The person primarily responsible for your health is not your doctor—it is you. But where does a woman go to become an informed advocate for her own health care? This book is a good place to start.

For over twenty years, Dr. H. Winter Griffith worked to fulfill a personal goal to translate complicated, technical medical information into up-to-date, easily understood information that anyone could use. The *Complete Guide to Prescription and Nonprescription Drugs* was his first major step toward that goal. The public's response to that effort has been overwhelmingly positive, and millions of people now rely on that book as a medical reference in their homes.

This book is another major step toward Dr. Griffith's goal. It has evolved out of more than 25 years of work as a family doctor, an author and a teacher answering questions of patients and medical students. This is the first book by Dr. Griffith that is written completely for a woman. Like his other works, it offers the most comprehensive medical information available—information you can use to become an informed advocate for your own health.

Your role in your health care

Armed with knowledge about medical conditions and surgical procedures discussed in this book, you are better able to become an advocate for your own health because
• You can better understand the nature of your illness.
• You can more easily recognize circumstances when a doctor's help is necessary.
• You can learn useful facts about how to prevent disease and injury.
• You can confirm, refresh your memory about, and help your family learn and understand the facts regarding your illness or condition.

• You can discuss issues with your doctor if treatment steps outlined in the book differ from what your doctor advises. Doctors do not always agree on the best course of treatment for a particular illness. When information from different medical sources has varied, this book has tried to provide the general, up-to-date medical consensus.

If your doctor's recommendations differ from those of this book, remember that they may still be valid. However, equipped with the information in this book, you can intelligently explore your options with your doctor. Your physician should welcome and answer your questions. If your physician does not welcome your questions, consider consulting another doctor.

By being educated about her health, recognizing that she is primarily responsible for her own well-being, and becoming an active participant in her health-care team, a woman has the best chance of achieving and maintaining good health throughout her life.

This book's role in your health care

This book provides easy-to-understand information about various women's health topics. Each topic is in a chart format that allows you to quickly read through the entire topic or find the answers to specific questions (e.g., I am having pain in my legs after abdominal surgery. Is this a side effect of the surgery, or is it unrelated? Is it something I need to deal with now, or can it wait until my next doctor appointment?).

By providing the reader with a way to educate herself and find quick answers to questions, this book removes many of the "road blocks" that have kept women from being fully participatory in their own health care.

Another major role of this book is as a back-up for the information that your caregiver provides. Even when information is competently conveyed to the patient, a woman often has no follow-up written reminder to reinforce what she has learned. This book is intended to supplement the information you have received from your doctor. With the hectic nature of the modern woman's lifestyle, the "dos" and "don'ts" that are so clearly understood in the doctor's office are often forgotten when she hurries on her way. In addition to providing a reminder of your doctor's instructions, this book can help you avoid unnecessary worry over details of your doctor's instructions that you may have forgotten.

What information is in this book?

This book contains several sections: Symptoms, Breasts, Gynecology, Contraception, Pregnancy, Infertility and General Health. Within each section, topics are presented in an easy-to-use one- or two-page chart format. (There are a few rare exceptions when, because of the vast amount of information about a particular topic, the chart may be three or more pages.) The chart format varies depending on whether the topic involves a surgery or procedure, an illness or disorder, or just symptoms. Each format is explained in detail in the following pages.

There are a number of topics that do not fit into any of the three chart formats used throughout the book. These topics include instructions for breast self-examinations, information on condom usage to prevent sexually transmitted diseases, a comparison of contraceptive methods, and others. In these cases, the chart format varies slightly from the rest of the book, but the information is still presented in a concise, easy-to-use manner.

A special feature of the book is a list of resources for additional information. If you want more in-depth information about symptoms, illnesses, surgeries or other medical problems, the list provides a starting place to find that type of information. The resource list contains names, addresses and telephone numbers of organizations and government health agencies devoted to specific disorders. Many of these agencies and organizations also have websites where you can obtain additional information; website addresses are given when available.

A glossary section includes definitions of medical tests and medical terms that are used throughout the book. In addition, it will give a brief description of some rare illnesses and disorders that are not covered in the other sections due to lack of space.

With all of this information, why see a doctor?

It is very important to note that, while this book contains a great deal of information about women's health, it represents only a fraction of the knowledge doctors have acquired from their medical education and experience in treating patients.

Condensing the available mass of medical and surgical knowledge into one volume has required much simplification. This book attempts to cover major facts and concepts, but out of necessity, many details have been left out.

It is impossible to include all the factors and circumstances that affect each individual's health. Thus, your doctor may take into account other factors not included here when making a precise diagnosis and recommending treatment for you.

Only your doctor knows your medical history and special circumstances about your health. Only you know the intensity and exact quality of your symptoms. The printed page cannot capture or convey the feelings that accompany illness. While this book can be a valuable resource to you, it is not intended as a substitute for good communication between you and your doctor.

Guide to Symptom Charts

The symptom charts are designed to suggest one or more illnesses and disorders that a specific symptom might indicate. Each chart focuses on one common symptom as shown on the list at the beginning of the section.

These charts do not include every possible *sign* or *symptom* the human body can exhibit, but they represent the most familiar and easily recognizable ones. *Signs* are observed. *Symptoms* are felt or experienced. A sign may be observed by the patient or by someone else. Symptoms are feelings only the patient can describe.

The charts provide a guide for how serious symptoms are. They give you clues as to what symptoms can mean. They refer you to other sections of the book for further information. *However, they are not intended as self-diagnosis charts.* No book should replace a competent doctor's diagnosis! The charts are only to help you decide how to proceed when you or someone else develops symptoms.

Refer to the numbers on the sample chart on page ix for an explanation of each heading described below.

1—Symptom Name

Charts are titled and arranged alphabetically by the name that is most common or that best describes the symptom **(Menstrual Periods, Late or Absent)**.

If you can't find your symptom under its own name, refer to the list at the start of the section and check alphabetically for the main part of the body it affects.

2—Symptoms & Factors

The main symptom is grouped in the first column with other symptoms or factors that frequently accompany it. Each group represents one or more separate illnesses or disorders that the symptom can indicate.

For instance, rash with fever can mean many things, depending on what other symptoms appear with it. When accompanied by a painful red blister and general ill feeling, rash with fever can be a sign of genital herpes. When accompanied instead by rapid heartbeat, fatigue and weakness, and excessive thirst, it can be a strong indication of toxic shock syndrome or a serious bacterial infection.

Often, none of the symptom groups will match your present problem. Your doctor knows your medical history and can perform a physical examination and use laboratory tests to diagnose your condition.

3—Possible Problem

The center column provides a short description of what a symptom group can indicate and may briefly define the illness or disorder to which you are referred in the third column.

In some cases, a group of symptoms can indicate more than one illness—sometimes they are totally unrelated. In that event, each description is listed next to an editor's bullet. In other cases, a possible diagnosis not necessarily appropriate for a women's medical book (i.e., cold, flu, etc.) may be enclosed in parentheses. In these cases, you will normally be directed to consult your doctor in the third column, "What to Do."

No attempt has been made to include every possible illness or disorder signaled by a symptom group. The identifications are based on illnesses that are *more obvious, most common or most serious.* For similar reasons, some rare illnesses described on illness charts in this book may not be referred to on symptom charts.

4—What to Do

The more serious medical problems that require immediate help are usually preceded by directions to call your doctor *now*. Below that, you will often be directed to the illness chart in this book that explains the problem. For instance, one entry has the instructions:

- Call doctor now.
- See Toxic Shock Syndrome.

All "See . . ." instructions refer to illness charts. Exceptions to this rule will be noted on the symptom chart.

If the chart says "Call doctor now," don't waste precious time looking up the illness in this book. Wait to read more about it when the crisis has passed. Call your doctor immediately!

If anyone develops dramatic symptoms that you think represent life-threatening danger, call for *emergency help*. Dial 911 or 0 for the operator and report your address or location (with directions).

In extreme situations, render what first aid you can, such as giving cardiopulmonary resuscitation (CPR). Yell for help from anyone within range.

Additional emergency information appears on the pages just before the index.

Menstrual Periods, Late or Absent

SYMPTOMS & FACTORS	POSSIBLE PROBLEM	WHAT TO DO
• Menstrual periods absent, plus 1 or more of following: • Unexplained weight gain. • Masculine voice. • Abnormal hairiness.	Hormone imbalance.	• Consult doctor. • See Hirsutism.
Menstrual periods absent in woman over age 38.	Normal menstrual irregularities at this age.	See Menopause.
• Menstrual periods absent. • Recent quick weight loss from drastic dieting. OR • Current participation in strenuous exercise program. OR • Recent illness. OR • Tension or worry. OR • Change in lifestyle such as new job or new home. OR • Menstrual periods absent since discontinuing use of oral contraceptives.	• Hormone changes. • Effect of stress. • Hormone changes caused by discontinuing pill.	See Amenorrhea.
• Menstrual periods absent. • Use of prescription drug.	Adverse reaction or side effect of drug.	• Consult doctor. • See Amenorrhea (all charts).
• Menstrual period late by 2 or more weeks. • Sexual intercourse within last month.	Pregnancy.	• Consult doctor to confirm pregnancy. • Take home-pregnancy test.
Menstrual periods absent since delivery of baby.	Normal occurrence caused by hormone changes following childbirth.	• If bottle-feeding, consult doctor if periods do not resume within 8 weeks after delivery. • If breast-feeding, consult doctor if periods do not resume within 4 weeks after weaning.
Menstrual periods have never started.	Hormone changes of puberty have not occurred.	• Consult doctor if older than 16. • See Amenorrhea, Primary.
• Irregular menstrual periods. • Gastrointestinal upsets. • Discomfort or pain in lower abdomen.	• Cyst. • Cancer.	• See Polycystic Ovarian Syndrome. • See Ovarian Cancer.

Guide to Illness & Disorder Charts

The information about illnesses and disorders is organized in condensed, easy-to-read charts. These charts are intermixed with charts about surgeries and medical procedures (see page xvi).

Each one is described in an easy-to-use format shown in the sample chart on page xiii, **Vaginitis, Bacterial.**

Major sections of the chart format are numbered and explained in the next few pages.

Most of the charts in this section refer to an illness. In some cases, however, charts refer to conditions, disorders or problems that are not really illnesses. The chart **Menopause**, for example, is not about a disease—or even a disorder. It deals with a normal process that all women experience. It would be a disorder only if it did not occur.

1—Chart Name

Charts are arranged alphabetically, within the appropriate section of the book, by the most common name for the illness, disorder or medical problem. Other names or terms for these appear in parentheses below the main heading. For example, bacterial vaginitis may also be referred to as *nonspecific vaginitis.*

Sometimes names for various medical problems vary in different geographic regions. All names in this book, including alternate names, are cross-referenced in the index.

To find information about a medical problem, check the index. You may also look up its major symptom in the symptom charts. If you can't find the illness chart you want, ask your doctor or nurse for alternate names by which the disorder is known.

2—General Information

This section includes seven topics: *Definition; Signs and Symptoms; Causes;*
Risk Increases With; How to Prevent; Probable Outcome and *Possible Complications.* Each is discussed separately.

3—Definition

A short definition of the problem or disease is provided. Sometimes the definition may include information from other categories, such as causes. The definition may also include information of general interest, such as how common a disease is, or whether it is contagious, cancerous or inherited.

The definition may include a list of specific body parts or organs, such as bones, skin or liver. Sometimes general body systems, such as central nervous system, genitourinary system or gastrointestinal system, will be listed. The list usually includes body parts affected at the beginning of the disease, as many diseases spread to other body parts as they progress.

This section may also list the age group usually affected. These are generalizations, and variations can occur with specific individuals.

Sometimes labels, such as "newborns" or "adolescents," are used to describe age ranges. These labels are arbitrary names for specific ages, but they are commonly used in medical texts. Following are the age classifications:
- Newborns (0 to 2 weeks)
- Infants (2 weeks to 1 year)
- Young children (1 to 5 years)
- Older children (5 to 12 years)
- Adolescents (12 to 20 years)
- Young adults (20 to 40 years)
- Middle-aged adults (40 to 60 years)
- Older adults (over 60 years).

4—Signs & Symptoms

Signs are observed. *Symptoms* are felt or experienced.

A sign may be observed by the patient

or by someone else, or it may represent physical findings determined by laboratory tests, x-rays and other diagnostic measures. Symptoms are feelings only the patient can describe.

Refer to the sample chart, **Vaginitis, Bacterial**. The first item under this heading—thin, gray-white vaginal discharge—is a sign. It can be observed by the patient and others around her. The second item—genital swelling, burning, and itching—is a sign *and* a symptom. It can be observed by others and felt by the patient. The third—vaginal discomfort—is a symptom that only the patient can feel and describe.

Signs and symptoms are listed together in this book; no attempt is made to separate the two. On most charts, a wide range of possible signs and symptoms are listed. *It is unlikely that any patient will have all, or even most, of the possible signs and symptoms.* The presence or absence of signs and symptoms may vary according to:
• The age and sex of the patient.
• Extent of the illness.
• The stage of the illness.
• Medical and family history.
• Current state of health.

5—Causes
Many times the cause of a disorder is unknown. Causes for most medical problems include the following:
• Inherited (congenital) defects.
• Infections from bacteria, viruses, parasites, yeasts or fungi. All of these are sometimes referred to as "germs," but most people associate "germs" with bacteria only.
• Physical injury.
• Toxins (poisons) from a wide range of sources, such as contaminated food, environmental pollution or bites from poisonous snakes or insects.
• Allergies.

• Tumors. These may be benign or malignant. Benign tumors do not spread to adjacent or distant organs and threaten life. Malignant (cancerous) tumors can.
• Endocrine disorders. This means too many or too few hormones are produced by the pituitary gland, thyroid gland, parathyroid gland, pancreas, adrenal glands, ovaries, testicles or thymus gland.
• Mental or emotional disorders, such as anxiety, depression or schizophrenia.
• Diseases caused by defects in the body's immune system. These include disorders of hypersensitivity, such as rheumatic fever, rheumatoid arthritis, systemic lupus erythematosus and many others.

6—Risk Increases With
Many disorders have known risk factors that can trigger the problem, make it more likely to occur or increase its duration and intensity. The most common risk factors include:
• Age, especially older persons or newborns and infants.
• Stress—either physical or emotional.
• Anxiety, depression and other mental or emotional problems.
• Fatigue or overwork.
• Poor nutrition due to improper diet or disease.
• Obesity.
• Recent or chronic illness that can lower resistance to other diseases.
• Recent surgery or injury.
• Genetic factors, such as family or ethnic tendency toward a disease.
• Use of drugs, such as alcohol, tobacco, caffeine, narcotics, psychedelics, hallucinogens, marijuana, sedatives, hypnotics or cocaine.
• Use of medications, whether prescription or nonprescription. Even necessary drugs cause adverse reactions and side effects that can complicate treatment and outcome of medical

problems.
- Exposure to allergens, environmental pollutants or poisons.
- Certain geographic areas.
- Crowded or unsanitary living conditions.
- Socioeconomic factors.
- Unprotected sexual activity.
- History of sexually transmitted diseases.

7—How to Prevent

Prevention can be of two types—prevention of the initial disease or prevention of a relapse or recurrence after recovery.

Prevention of any medical problem is the *best treatment*. Researchers continue to discover ways to prevent, delay or diminish some illnesses, pain, disability and untimely deaths. These ways are included whenever available.

The causes and risk factors for a disease often provide the best clues for prevention. Many diseases, however, cannot be prevented at present.

8—Probable Outcome

A very important concern with any illness is the patient's question, "What is going to happen to me? How will this disease or injury affect my life?"

No one can completely predict the outcome of an accident or illness. The predictions in this section are guesses based on averages.

Patients and doctors work toward optimal results, but medicine is an inexact science. Response to treatment depends on many variables, and there are many unanswered questions about health and disease.

Some illnesses are considered incurable at present. The term "incurable" is a general one that includes everything from insignificant conditions that are mere annoyances to fatal diseases that bring certain death in a short time. For that reason, additional information about life expectancy is usually included for incurable illnesses. Again, individual variations are common, but the predictions are an attempt to answer a patient's most important questions. They help you adopt optimistic but realistic expectations.

In almost all cases—no matter how serious the illness—symptoms can be relieved or controlled to minimize pain and discomfort.

9—Possible Complications

Complications are additional medical problems triggered by or as a result of the original illness. Complications sometimes occur, despite accurate diagnosis and competent treatment. Some are preventable, a few are inevitable—but most are rare.

In addition, even the simplest medical problems sometimes develop complications and require a doctor's care. In those cases, a doctor's treatment can be appropriate even though it applies to a small fraction of cases.

Find a competent personal physician who communicates well with you and with whom you can establish a good rapport and mutual respect.

Psychotherapy, counseling or biofeedback training may be the only useful health care for a medical problem caused mainly by stress or emotional problems.

Counseling and therapy are also helpful in providing personal and family support, especially with illnesses that are terminal or represent major lifestyle adjustments.

Rehabilitation is often helpful for illnesses or injuries that cause temporary or permanent disability. Rehabilitation may be provided by trained physical therapists or physiatrists (medical doctors who

Vaginitis, Bacterial (Gardnerella Vaginitis; Nonspecific Vaginitis; Bacterial Vaginosis)

👤 GENERAL INFORMATION

DEFINITION—Vaginitis means infection or inflammation of the vagina. Nonspecific vaginitis (bacterial vaginosis) implies that any of several infecting germs, including Gardnerella, Escherichia coli, Mycoplasma, streptococci or staphylococci, have caused the infection. These infections are contagious and may be sexually transmitted. Vaginitis can affect all ages, but most often occurs during reproductive years.

SIGNS & SYMPTOMS—Severity of the following symptoms varies among women and from time to time in the same woman.
- Thin, gray-white (sometimes profuse) vaginal discharge that has an unpleasant odor.
- Genital swelling, burning and itching.
- Vaginal discomfort.
- Painful urination.
- Change in vaginal color from pale pink to red.
- Discomfort during sexual intercourse.

CAUSES—The germs normally present in the vagina can multiply and cause infection when the pH and hormone balance of the vagina and surrounding tissue are disturbed. E. coli bacteria normally inhabit the rectum and can cause infection if spread to the vagina. The following conditions increase the likelihood of infections:
- General poor health.
- Allergies to soaps, detergents, bubble bath, feminine deodorant spray or douches.
- Hot weather, nonventilating clothing (especially underwear) or any other condition that increases genital moisture, warmth and darkness. These foster the growth of germs.
- Poor hygiene (sometimes).

RISK INCREASES WITH
- Diabetes mellitus.
- Menopause.
- Illness that has lowered resistance.
- Multiple sexual partners.
- Use of an intrauterine device (IUD).
- HIV infection.

HOW TO PREVENT
- Keep the genital area clean. Use plain unscented soap.
- Use latex condoms during sexual intercourse.
- Take showers rather than tub baths.
- Wear cotton underpants or pantyhose with a cotton crotch.
- Don't sit around in wet clothing, especially a wet bathing suit.
- After urination or bowel movements, cleanse by wiping or washing from front to back (vagina to anus).
- Lose weight if you are obese.
- Avoid vaginal douches, deodorants and bubble baths.
- If you have diabetes, adhere strictly to your treatment program.
- Change tampons or pads frequently.

PROBABLE OUTCOME—Usually curable in 2 weeks with treatment.

POSSIBLE COMPLICATIONS
- Discomfort and decreased pleasure with sexual activity.
- Pelvic inflammatory disease (PID).
- Nonspecific vaginitis in pregnant women has been associated with preterm birth. The disorder should be carefully evaluated and treated when it occurs in pregnancy.

⚕ HOW TO TREAT

GENERAL MEASURES
- Diagnostic tests may include laboratory studies of vaginal discharge, Pap smear and pelvic examination.
- Drug therapy will be directed to the specific organism. Your sexual partner may need treatment also. It is best not to do self-treatment for the disorder until the specific cause is determined.
- Don't douche unless prescribed for you.
- If urinating causes burning, urinate through a a toilet-paper roll or plastic cup with the bottom cut out, or pour a cup of warm water over the genital area while you urinate.

MEDICATION
- Antibiotics or antifungals to treat the infection; these are usually vaginal, rather than oral, medications. Metronidazole (Flagyl) is often used for treatment of bacterial vaginosis. Don't drink alcohol or use vinegar when you take metronidazole. Alcohol or vinegar combined with metronidazole causes a violent reaction with nausea, vomiting, weakness and sweating.
- Soothing vaginal creams or lotions for nonspecific forms of vaginitis may be recommended.

ACTIVITY—Avoid overexertion, heat and excessive sweating. Delay sexual relations until after treatment.

DIET—No special diet instructions except those involving alcohol or vinegar (see Medication).

☎ CALL YOUR DOCTOR IF

- You or a family member has symptoms of vaginitis.
- Symptoms persist longer than 1 week or worsen, despite treatment.
- Unusual vaginal bleeding or swelling develops.

specialize in physical therapy). If rehabilitation is mentioned as appropriate health care, ask your doctor for information specific to your disability.

10—How to Treat

This section reminds you of instructions your doctor has given you. The information should not replace your doctor's instructions, because treatments vary a great deal between individuals.

If the instructions don't seem to fit your problem, ask your doctor or nurse for answers that apply uniquely to you.

The four major headings include *General Measures; Medication; Activity* and *Diet.*

11—General Measures

The information under this heading includes diagnostic measures and appropriate health-care steps.

Your own observation of symptoms is usually the first—and often, most important—diagnostic measure. It is the first step toward medical treatment. For that reason, it is listed under this heading on many of the illness charts.

A medical history and physical exam by a doctor are also almost universal requirements before treatment for any disorder can begin. Even if a medical problem is usually treated at home, a history and exam will be necessary if complications develop that require medical treatment.

Additional diagnostic measures include laboratory studies and other medical tests. Some common diagnostic measures include:
• Studies of body fluids, such as blood, serum, plasma or spinal fluid.
• Microscopic and chemical examination of excreted material, such as urine or stools.
• CAT (computerized axial tomography)

scans or x-rays of the affected body part.
• Ultrasound imaging of affected body parts or organs.
• Surgical examinations such as laparoscopy, hysteroscopy, biopsy, colposcopy and others.
• Therapeutic trial of medication. This is used sometimes for a critically ill patient without a specific diagnosis while awaiting laboratory results.

You may not undergo every diagnostic test listed on the chart, and conversely, you may undergo tests not listed. Some tests are performed only if previous tests have not provided enough information. Others are performed only when complications develop. All medical diagnostic tests mentioned in this book are defined in the Glossary.

Self-care or home-care methods are sometimes listed as the first form of appropriate health care. It is an important part of care for almost all disorders. Sometimes total self-care suffices if you have previous experience with a medical problem and a source to review important points in treatment.

Usually, however, a medical problem should be diagnosed by a doctor before you attempt self-care. Once your doctor diagnoses an illness and outlines a treatment program, self-care or home care is often important. Treatment measures outlined in this book are designed to guide you, whether you are caring for yourself or taking care of someone else.

Effective self-care includes maintaining a positive attitude about yourself and being determined to improve or heal. During illness, a sense of humor and a positive outlook are just as helpful as medication or other treatments.

A doctor's care is often necessary, not only to diagnose and prescribe treatment for a medical problem, but to supervise self-care (or hospitalization, when necessary) and to provide additional medical treatment such as surgery.

Other common measures for self-care include soaks for skin problems or pain, appropriate clothing, bandages or bathing.

Also included may be an instruction to "See the Resource section of this book for additional information." This refers to the pages titled Resources for Additional Information, where you will find a list of support groups and organizations that can provide you with additional education or support regarding a particular illness or condition.

These instructions are not complete and may not apply to everybody, but they provide a good review of general measures helpful for most patients.

12—Medication

Information under this heading is generally of two types—drugs your doctor may prescribe and nonprescription drugs you can take safely.

Prescription drugs are named by generic name or drug class. A brief description of a drug's purpose and effect is usually given.

For more information about drugs that are listed, you may wish to refer to the *Complete Guide to Prescription and Nonprescription Drugs*, by H. Winter Griffith, M.D.

13—Activity

Patients are often confused about whether they must stay in bed during an illness. They are often concerned with returning to work or school, and whether activity will be restricted after recovery. These questions are answered under this heading.

In some topics, guidelines are given for resuming sexual relations—an important area that patients are sometimes reluctant to mention. If the illness has been life-threatening, or if it involves abdominal or genital organs, this is particularly pertinent information.

Exercise references are often included, and when not specified otherwise, references to regular physical exercise mean an *aerobic* exercise such as walking.

14—Diet

Diet information can vary from "no special diet" to references to specialized diets such as a weight loss diet.

For information on specialized diets, consult your doctor or a dietitian.

15—Call Your Doctor If

For most medical problems, a phone call or visit to your doctor is recommended to establish a diagnosis.

After diagnosis, when the course of an illness differs from what is expected, your doctor wants to know. Many developing complications can be averted with prompt medical treatment. Specific symptoms are usually listed that indicate complications.

Of course, if any other symptoms begin that you believe are related to your illness or the drugs you take, call your doctor about them, too.

Guide to Surgery & Procedure Charts

The information about common surgeries and medical procedures is organized in charts with a format similar to that for illness and disorder charts (see sample surgery chart on facing page).

Generally, procedures discussed in this section are those commonly performed as treatment for a disorder, such as cryosurgery, or as a diagnostic procedure, such as dilatation and curettage. The surgery topics may be about such minor procedures as a pelvic examination and Pap smear, or such major lifesaving procedures as a total mastectomy.

Sometimes a surgery is mentioned on an illness chart as part of treatment for that disorder. For instance, mastectomy is mentioned as a treatment on the chart for breast cancer.

Each major heading on the surgery and procedure charts is numbered in the sample chart, and the numbered sections are explained in the next few pages.

1—Name of Procedure

Charts are usually titled with the name that most simply describes the procedure. In some cases, medical professionals refer to the surgery or procedure by a more technical name. The technical name appears in parentheses below the main title.

Abdominal hysterectomy is usually understood by everyone, but your surgeon may refer to it as *salpingo-oophorectomy*. Both names are included on the chart, and the surgery appears in the index under both names.

2—General Information

This section contains six topics: *Definition*; *Reasons for Procedure*; *Risk Increases With*; *Description of Procedure*; *Probable Outcome* and *Possible Complications*. Each topic is discussed separately.

3—Definition

A short definition of the surgery may include information about how common the procedure is and whether or not the medical problem requiring surgery is caused by congenital defects or is the result of disease or injury.

4—Reasons for Procedure

This section lists the most common reasons for a surgery or procedure. (Of course, it cannot include *all* possible reasons.)

If the medical problems listed are unfamiliar to you, refer to the index. Some have separate illness charts, and the rest may be explained in the Glossary.

5—Risk Increases With

Risk factors make a surgery more complicated or delay healing. Following are common risk factors for most surgeries:
• Stress, anxiety, depression or other emotional problems.
• Poor nutrition from any cause.
• Chronic illness.
• Recent illness, surgery or injury.
• Genetic factors.
• Obesity.
• Smoking.
• Alcoholism.
• Age, especially newborns and infants or older adults.
• Use of drugs of abuse, such as narcotics, psychedelics, hallucinogens, marijuana, sedatives, hypnotics or cocaine.
• Use of some drugs or medications, whether prescription or nonprescription. Medicines most likely to increase surgical risk include antihypertensives, muscle relaxants, tranquilizers, sleep inducers, insulin, sedatives, cortisone, beta-adrenergic blockers, calcium channel blockers and antibiotics.

These same drugs, of course, are lifesaving for some serious illnesses, but

Hysterectomy, Abdominal (Salpingo-Oophorectomy)

GENERAL INFORMATION

DEFINITION—Removal of the uterus, cervix, and often the fallopian tubes and ovaries, through an incision in the abdomen. Be sure you understand all aspects of this surgical procedure, its risks and benefits and any possible alternative therapies. With removal of the ovaries, sudden surgical menopause occurs.

REASONS FOR PROCEDURE
• Uterus: Cancer or suspected cancer, fibroid tumors, chronic bleeding, prolapsed (dropped) uterus, endometriosis, chronic pelvic infection, severe menstrual pain or voluntary sterilization.
• Fallopian tubes and ovaries: Cancer or suspected cancer of the ovaries, precancerous or twisted ovarian cysts, ovarian pregnancy, ovarian abscess, damage to the ovaries from severe endometriosis.

RISK INCREASES WITH
• Obesity.
• Smoking.
• Conditions resulting in excessive estrogen exposure, such as estrogen drugs, delayed childbirth, chronic anovulation (see Glossary).
• Iron-deficiency anemia, heart or lung disease, or diabetes mellitus.
• Use of drugs such as cortisone, diuretics, antihypertensives or beta-adrenergic blockers.

DESCRIPTION OF PROCEDURE
• A general or regional anesthetic is given.
• A urinary catheter is placed.
• An incision is made in the abdomen (horizontal or vertical depending on the condition).
• The abdominal organs are examined.
• In a simple hysterectomy, only the uterus and cervix are removed along with visible tumors. In a total hysterectomy, the fallopian tubes and ovaries are cut free and removed as well (salpingo-oophorectomy).
• Any stretched ligaments are repaired.
• The vagina is often closed with sutures at its deeper end; the surgical wound is closed.
• The catheter may remain for hours to days.

PROBABLE OUTCOME
• Relief from symptoms caused by benign uterine conditions.
• Cancer prognosis is good when treated early.
• Expect permanent sterility (see Glossary).

POSSIBLE COMPLICATIONS
• Risk of infection or bleeding.
• Inadvertent injury to the bowel, bladder or ureters (see Glossary).
• Anesthetic problems.
• Urinary tract infection.
• Respiratory infection, particularly pneumonia.

FOLLOW-UP CARE

GENERAL MEASURES
• Hospital stay may be 2 to 5 days.
• To keep lungs clear, cough frequently while using appropriate support. Deep breathing aids are frequently available.
• Once home, someone should be available to help care for you for the first few days.
• Use an electric heating pad, a heat lamp or a warm compress to relieve incisional or gas pain.
• Shower as usual. You may wash the incision gently with mild unscented soap.
• Use sanitary napkins—not tampons—to absorb blood or drainage (discharge is normal but has an unpleasant odor).
• Surgery aftereffects may include constipation, fatigue, urinary symptoms and weight gain.
• The psychological aftermath of a hysterectomy will depend on the individual. Some women feel only relief, others experience frequent and unexpected crying episodes (may be due to hormonal changes) and a few suffer from depression. Seek help from your doctor and support from family and friends.

MEDICATION
• After surgery, medicines for pain, gas, nausea or constipation may be prescribed.
• Antibiotics if infection develops.
• Hormone replacement is recommended unless there are reasons why they should not be taken.

ACTIVITY
• To help recovery and aid your well-being, resume daily activities and work as soon as you are able. Recovery at home takes 1 to 3 weeks, with full activities resumed in 6 to 8 weeks.
• Resume driving 2 weeks after returning home.
• Sexual relations may be resumed in 4 to 6 weeks (or when advised). Most women experience no change in sexual function, some report improvement, while others have a worsening sexual function, specifically, loss of libido (sexual desire).

DIET—Clear liquid diet until the gastrointestinal tract functions again. Then eat a well-balanced diet to promote healing.

CALL YOUR DOCTOR IF

• Vaginal bleeding soaks more than 1 pad per hour.
• Frequent urge to urinate or excessive vaginal discharge persists longer than 1 month.
• You experience increased pain or swelling in the surgical area.
• You develop signs of infection: headache, muscle aches, dizziness or a general ill feeling and fever.

they can complicate treatment and the outcome of other medical or surgical problems.

6—Description of Procedure

This section may include information about diagnostic tests performed prior to surgery; who performs the procedure; where the surgery or procedure is performed; the type of anesthesia used; and a step-by-step description of the surgical procedure.

Diagnostic tests related to surgery can occur before, during or after the surgical procedure.

Laboratory studies are helpful in diagnosis and in providing necessary anatomical information prior to surgery. Many tests are the same as those discussed in the "How to Treat" section of the illness charts.

Some tests are especially useful in surgery. Examples include:
• Special x-ray studies of the gastrointestinal tract (upper GI series or lower GI series).
• Intravenous studies of the kidney and urinary tract (intravenous pyelogram and retrograde pyelogram).
• Biopsy (microscopic study of tissue) before surgery to establish a diagnosis prior to extensive surgery (usually for cancer) and biopsy afterward of tissue removed during the surgical procedure.

Surgery may be performed by a variety of different types of medical doctors. A routine surgery is often performed by a general surgeon or by a doctor who specializes in the body system involved. For instance, either a general surgeon or an obstetrician-gynecologist might remove an ovarian cyst.

Highly complicated surgeries, such as a heart transplant, are usually done by surgeons with additional specialized training.

We have included the type of surgeon most likely to perform the procedure, but variations can occur. In many communities general surgeons perform operations that are customarily performed elsewhere by a surgical subspecialist.

Your surgeon should not be uneasy about discussing with you before surgery his or her previous experience and education. Most competent surgeons welcome and sometimes recommend a second opinion when the surgery to be performed is elective rather than an emergency.

A surgical procedure may be performed in any of the following places:
• A doctor's office.
• An independent, outpatient surgical facility.
• A hospital outpatient surgical facility.
• The operating room of a hospital.
• An emergency room.

Anesthesia makes surgery possible without pain. Prior to giving anesthesia, many surgeons prescribe preoperative medications. These generally consist of:
• Tranquilizers or sedatives to help reduce apprehension.
• Pain relievers (frequently a narcotic drug such as morphine). This medication also reduces apprehension and decreases the amount of anesthesia needed.
• An anticholinergic drug, such as scopolamine or atropine, to decrease secretions from the nose, throat and lungs during the operation.

The type of anesthesia used depends on the surgical problem, the age and general condition of the patient and sometimes on the availability of personnel to administer the anesthesia.

If an operation can be performed with any of several types of anesthesia, you have a right to know the advantages and disadvantages of each. If you wish, you have the right to participate in the selection. Don't hesitate to ask questions.

Before you have any anesthesia, tell

your doctor about any allergic responses you have had to anesthesia in the past. Also inform him or her about any prescription or nonprescription drugs you take, and about any cardiovascular disease, heartbeat irregularities or peripheral vascular disease you have.

If a chart lists several anesthesia options for a surgery, you will have one of them, but not all.

The various types of anesthesia include:

Local Anesthesia—This is usually an injectable form of a drug ending in "caine," such as novocaine or lidocaine.

Local anesthesia is frequently injected into an injury site, such as a fracture, and bleeding from the injury disperses the anesthetic to all pain-sensitive parts of the injury. Local anesthesia blocks specific nerve bundles, allowing a pain-free procedure such as a cervical biopsy.

Regional Anesthesia—This is used when it is desirable for the patient to remain conscious during the operation. Regional anesthesia works only on the part of the body upon which surgery is performed. Types of regional anesthesia include spinal or epidural anesthesia.

Spinal anesthesia involves an injection of local anesthetic into the spinal canal, above the level of the surgery site. It relieves pain satisfactorily for many procedures below the waist, such as surgery of the rectum, genitourinary tract or lower extremities.

A special type of low-spinal anesthesia is called caudal anesthesia or "saddle block" (it affects the body area that comes into contact with a horse saddle).

Epidural anesthesia involves an injection of local anesthetic into the extradural (epidural) space in the lower back. It is used to block pain for the abdominal region.

General Anesthesia—This form of anesthesia is generally administered by inhalation or injection, or a combination of the two.

A short-acting hypnotic or sedative is injected into a vein, followed by a muscle relaxer. This quickly produces light sleep and allows placement of an airway tube (endotracheal tube) without discomfort. The tube is connected to hoses that lead to gas machines.

The anesthesiologist controls the flow of anesthesia gases and monitors many body functions, such as blood pressure, breathing rate, pulse and ECG, while the patient sleeps.

When you awaken, the endotracheal tube may still be in place, or it may have been removed. Unless your respiration needs continued machine support, the endotracheal tube is usually removed in the recovery room.

The tube will make your throat sore for about 24 hours. This is normal and requires no treatment.

The surgical procedure is described in brief, nontechnical terms. Individual surgeons may use slightly varying techniques, but the basic steps are included and only details vary.

If you want additional information, your surgeon can give more details or a librarian can suggest resource materials with fuller descriptions and explanations.

During some surgeries of the gastrointestinal tract, a hollow tube (Levin tube) is passed through your nose into your stomach after you are asleep. The tube will probably be in place when you awaken in the recovery room. The purpose of the tube is to keep the stomach empty to prevent vomiting or aspiration of material while you are asleep. It also keeps the stomach decompressed until normal muscular movement of the gastrointestinal tract can resume after surgery. An empty stomach is more comfortable and helps prevent complications that may arise if the stomach becomes distended with air or gas.

The average time in surgery and in the recovery room are usually left out because variations are too great. Factors that affect the time limits depend upon:
- The exact techniques chosen.
- The experience and preference of the surgeon.
- The availability and experience of assistants and operating room personnel.
- The presence or absence of complications during surgery.
- The age and condition of the patient prior to surgery.

Don't hesitate to ask your surgeon to estimate the time your operation will require.

7—Probable Outcome

This heading relates to the surgery's effect on the underlying disorder and the average length of time required to recover from surgery. Estimates are based on the assumption that complications do not occur and healing proceeds normally. Complications can alter the course of healing dramatically. A positive outlook following surgery is an important factor in good outcome and rapid healing.

8—Possible Complications

Complications are additional medical problems related to the surgery that occur during or after the procedure. They sometimes happen despite accurate diagnosis, skillful surgery, competent assistance and well-equipped operating rooms. Some complications are preventable, and some occur frequently—but most are rare.

9—Follow-Up Care

This section generally provides instructions for self-care during recuperation after hospitalization. It should serve as a reminder for instructions given you by your surgeon. It should not replace your doctor's instructions.

The section has four major topics: *General Measures; Medication; Activity* and *Diet.*

10—General Measures

Some questions are almost universal following surgery. Most patients are unsure how to care for a surgical wound. They have questions about pain, bathing, stitches, clothing and other matters. These questions are answered in this section.

Patients also want to know how long they can expect to be hospitalized following surgery. For some topics, an average hospital stay is given. This estimate is based on an average. It varies according to how healing and recuperation progress and whether complications develop before, during or after surgery. It is also influenced by the amount insurance companies will allow as reimbursement of specific procedures. Be sure to ask your doctor how long you will need to stay in the hospital.

11—Medication

Drugs usually prescribed after surgery are described; sometimes, brief instructions for their use are also described.

For more information about drugs that are listed, you may wish to refer to the *Complete Guide to Prescription and Nonprescription Drugs,* by H. Winter Griffith, M.D.

12—Activity

Resumption of activity is a strong area of concern for postsurgical patients. Guidelines are provided for when to return to school or work, when to resume driving, when to resume sexual relations and what types of exercise are appropriate. Again, it should serve as a reminder for instructions given you by your surgeon. It should not replace your doctor's instructions.

13—Diet

During surgery with general anesthesia, the gastrointestinal tract is kept empty. After the patient awakens, clear liquids are usually provided until the gastrointestinal tract begins to function again. When appropriate, this information is included in the surgery charts. For specialized diets, consult your doctor or a dietitian.

14—Call Your Doctor If

Call your doctor if healing and recuperation after surgery don't follow the usual course of events. Excessive bleeding and general or surgical-wound infection are common dangers after most surgical procedures, and these are always mentioned on surgery charts when appropriate.

Other reasons listed can serve as reminders of possible complications. If you develop symptoms you believe are related to your illness—even if they don't appear on the chart—call your doctor about them.

Symptoms

Symptom Charts

Find your main symptom on this list and then look at that chart for additional symptoms you may have.

Abdominal or Pelvic Pain
Abdominal Swelling
Anxiety and Nervousness
Appetite Loss
Backache
Behavioral or Emotional Changes
Breast Pain, Tenderness or Lumps
Depression
Diarrhea
Fatigue or Tiredness
Fever
Genital Sores, Blisters, Warts or Boils
Hair Growth in Women, Excessive
Headache
Heartbeat Irregularity
Itching
Menstrual Periods, Late or Absent
Menstrual Periods, Painful or Heavy
Rash with Fever
Rash without Fever
Sexual Intercourse, Painful
Sweating, Excessive
Swelling or Lump
Trembling or Twitching
Urination, Frequent
Urination, Lack of Control
Urination, Painful
Urine, Abnormal Color
Vaginal Bleeding, Unexpected
Vaginal Discharge, Abnormal
Vaginal Itching
Vomiting, Recurrent Attacks
Vomiting, Sudden Attack
Weight Gain
Weight Loss

Abdominal or Pelvic Pain (continued on next page)

SYMPTOMS & FACTORS	POSSIBLE PROBLEM	WHAT TO DO
Abdominal pain following excessive consumption of alcohol or food.	• Indigestion. • Gastritis.	Consult doctor.
• Abdominal pain. • Diarrhea. • Vomiting.	• Gastroenteritis. • Food poisoning. • Salmonella infection.	Consult doctor.
• Abdominal pain. • Diarrhea. • Flatulence and bloating.	Food allergy/intolerance.	Consult doctor.
• Abdominal pain that began in small of back, spreading to genital area. • Fever. • Frequent, painful, occasionally bloody urination.	• Cystitis. • Kidney infection.	Consult doctor.
• Mild pain in lower abdomen. • Constipation or gas. • Recent diet change, such as adding more fiber.	Intestinal disturbance caused by diet change.	Consult doctor if discomfort persists longer than 3 hours.
• Severe abdominal pain, plus any of following: • Temperature of 100F (37.8C) or higher. • Constipation. • Abdominal swelling. • Vomiting.	• Intestinal obstruction. • Appendicitis. • Aneurysm. • Peritonitis.	Call doctor now.
• Severe abdominal pain. • Menstrual period late 4 or more weeks. • Shoulder pain. • Abdominal pain that began in small of back, spreading to genital area. • No fever at onset of pain. • Smoky or bloody urine.	• Pregnancy developing outside uterus. • Kidney colic.	See Ectopic Pregnancy.
• Pain in lower abdomen. • Green-yellow, heavy or bad-smelling vaginal discharge.	Infection of reproductive organs.	• See Pelvic Inflammatory Disease. • See Ovarian Tumor, Benign.
• Burning pain of abdominal skin with tenderness along pain route. • Skin blisters.	Herpes zoster.	Consult doctor.
• Pain in upper right abdomen that may spread to chest, back or shoulders. • Nausea or vomiting.	• Gallstones. • Heart problem. • Pancreatitis.	Consult doctor.
• Pain in lower abdomen. • Unexplained vaginal bleeding.	Several disorders.	See Vaginal Bleeding, Unexpected (in Symptoms section).

Abdominal or Pelvic Pain (cont.)

SYMPTOMS & FACTORS	POSSIBLE PROBLEM	WHAT TO DO
• Abdominal cramps. • Intermittent diarrhea. • Gas and abdominal bloating.	Parasitic infection (amebiasis).	Consult doctor.
• Vague discomfort in lower abdomen. • Gastrointestinal upset. • Irregular menstrual periods. • Excessive hair growth.	Cancer.	See Ovarian Cancer.
• Pain in upper abdomen. • Belching.	Heartburn.	See Heartburn during Pregnancy.

Abdominal Swelling

SYMPTOMS & FACTORS	POSSIBLE PROBLEM	WHAT TO DO
• Lower abdominal swelling that is slowly increasing. • No signs of pregnancy. • Persistent constipation.	• Constipation. • Tumor.	• Consult doctor. • See Ovarian Tumor, Benign.
Abdominal swelling 1 to 5 days before or during menstrual period.	Fluid retention caused by hormone changes.	See Premenstrual Syndrome.
• Abdominal swelling; bloated and full feeling. • Gas or belching. • Abdominal pain or discomfort.	• Heartburn. • Gallstones.	Consult doctor.
• Abdominal swelling in last 24 hours. • Severe abdominal pain. • Fever. • Diarrhea or constipation. • Vomiting.	• Serious abdominal disorder. • Intestinal obstruction.	Call doctor now.
• Abdominal swelling. • Swollen ankles. • Breathing difficulty, especially at night.	Fluid in abdomen and other body parts caused by heart condition.	Consult doctor.
• Abdominal swelling. • Puffy ankles that hold a dent when pressed with finger. • Decreased urination.	Glomerulonephritis.	Consult doctor.
• Abdominal swelling. • Yellow skin and eyes.	Cirrhosis of the liver.	Consult doctor.
• Abdominal swelling. • Overweight.	Obesity.	Consult doctor.
• Abdominal swelling in woman of childbearing age. • Tender, enlarged breasts. • Morning nausea. • No menstrual period for 2 months or longer.	Pregnancy.	Consult doctor to confirm pregnancy.

Anxiety and Nervousness

SYMPTOMS & FACTORS	POSSIBLE PROBLEM	WHAT TO DO
• Anxiety, plus any of following: • Inability to listen attentively and remember. • Clinging dependency. • Cold or hot flashes. • Cool, sweaty hands. • Abdominal cramps. • Diarrhea or constipation. • Dizziness. • Dry mouth. • Lack of concentration. • Faintness. • Rapid heartbeat. • Impotence in men. • Low frustration level. • Muscle tension and pain (backache, neck ache, headache). • Painful menstruation. • Painful sexual intercourse. • Pale or flushed skin. • Restlessness. • Tightness in chest. • Frequent urination.	Effect of stress or unrecognized fear.	See Anxiety.
Anxiety about any of following: enclosed spaces; airplanes; crowds; heights; "going crazy"; infection; or death.	Psychological disorder.	See Phobias.
• Anxiety, plus 2 or more of following: • Weight loss. • Bulging eyes. • Excessive sweating. • Fatigue. • Rapid or irregular heartbeat.	Overactive thyroid gland.	See Hyperthyroidism.
Persistent anxiety without other symptoms.	Effect of stress.	See Anxiety.
• Anxiety. • Dizziness or lightheadedness. • Rapid breathing. • Frequent sighing.	Decreased carbon dioxide in blood.	See Panic Disorder.
• Anxiety. • Use of prescription or non-prescription drug.	Adverse reaction or side effect of drug.	• Consult doctor about prescription drug. • Discontinue use of non-prescription drug if symptoms persist.
• Nervousness and irritability. • Menstrual period is due in 7 to 14 days.	Hormone fluctuation.	See Premenstrual Syndrome.

Anxiety and Nervousness (cont.)

SYMPTOMS & FACTORS	POSSIBLE PROBLEM	WHAT TO DO
• Anxiety. • Recent withdrawal from tobacco, alcohol or drug, such as sleeping pills.	Withdrawal symptom.	• Consult doctor about drug withdrawal. • See Substance Abuse & Addiction. • See Alcoholism.
• Anxiety behavior. • Restlessness; inability to be still. • Unable to pay attention to directions.	Attention deficit hyperactivity disorder.	Consult doctor.
• Anxiety involving recurrent, intrusive and distressing recollection of an event. • Reliving of an event.	Post traumatic stress disorder.	Consult doctor.

Appetite Loss

SYMPTOMS & FACTORS	POSSIBLE PROBLEM	WHAT TO DO
• Appetite loss. • Nausea and vomiting. • Fever.	Gastroenteritis.	Consult doctor.
• Appetite loss. • Use of vitamins or prescription or nonprescription drug, especially anticancer drugs; digitalis; aminophylline; narcotics; antihistamines; ephedrine; methylphenidate; diphenyl-hydantoin or amphetamines.	Adverse reaction or side effect of drug.	• Consult doctor about prescription drug. • Discontinue use of non-prescription drugs.
• Appetite loss, plus 2 or more of following: • Fever. • Sore throat. • Headache. • Painful swelling in neck, armpit or groin. • Fatigue. • Jaundice (yellow skin and eyes). • Pain in upper right abdomen.	Infectious mononucleosis.	Consult doctor.
• Appetite loss. • Pain or pressure in stomach. • Excessive consumption of alcohol or food.	Gastritis.	Consult doctor.
• Appetite loss. • Depression or anxiety.	Effect of stress.	• See Depression. • See Anxiety. • See Anorexia Nervosa. • See Postpartum Depression or Blues.
• Decrease in appetite (especially in a child). • Low grade fever. • Runny nose. • Cough.	Respiratory syncytial virus.	Consult doctor.
• Appetite loss. • Emotional upset such as grief.	Temporary emotional situation.	Appetite will return in time. Drink plenty of fluids.
• Appetite loss (sudden). • Headache. • Nausea or vomiting. • Bloody urine. • Decreased urination. • Puffy face.	Kidney disorder (glomerulonephritis).	Consult doctor.
• Appetite loss. • Nausea at sight of food, plus 2 or more of following: • Jaundice (yellow skin and eyes). • Vomiting. • Tenderness over liver area. • Fever. • Weakness and fatigue.	• Viral hepatitis. • Cirrhosis of the liver.	Consult doctor.

Appetite Loss (cont.)

SYMPTOMS & FACTORS	POSSIBLE PROBLEM	WHAT TO DO
• Appetite loss. • Weight loss. • Vague feeling of illness or fatigue.	Early signs of cancer or other disorder.	Consult doctor.
• Appetite loss. • Fatigue. • Weight loss. • Hair loss. • Craving for salt. • Skin that darkens. • Dizziness on standing.	Addison's disease.	Consult doctor.
• Appetite loss with weight gain. • Loss of energy, fatigue. • Puffy face. • Decreased sex drive. • Dry skin and hair. • Constipation. • Low voice.	Underactive thyroid gland.	See Hypothyroidism.
• Appetite loss. • Excessive alcohol consumption.	Vitamin deficiency caused by alcohol.	See Alcoholism.
• Appetite loss. • Weight loss, plus 2 or more of following: • Paleness. • Sore, red, smooth, burning tongue. • Yellowish skin.	Vitamin B-12 and folic-acid deficiency (pernicious anemia).	Consult doctor.
• Gradual appetite loss in woman 45 or older. • Fatigue. • Menstrual changes.	Normal occurrence with the decreasing estrogen level of menopause.	See Menopause.
• Appetite loss. • Fluid retention. • Reduced urine production.	Kidney disease (nephrotic syndrome).	Consult doctor.
• Appetite loss in child. • Irritability. • Paleness.	Disorder of red blood cells.	See Anemia, Iron Deficiency.
• Appetite loss. • Nausea. • Pregnancy or possible pregnancy.	Effect of hormone change during pregnancy.	Eat small, frequent meals.
• Poor appetite. • Sleeping problems. • Lack of energy. • Feelings of hopelessness; self-pity.	Chronic mild depression.	See Low Grade Depression.
• Appetite loss and weight loss. • Tender mass in upper right abdomen. • Pain in upper right abdomen.	Liver cancer.	Consult doctor.

Backache

SYMPTOMS & FACTORS	POSSIBLE PROBLEM	WHAT TO DO
• Sudden backache. • Recent fall or injury to back. • Pain only at injury site.	• Muscle injury or muscle spasm. • Ruptured disk. • Sprain or strain.	Consult doctor.
• Sudden sharp pain down back of leg. • Recent heavy lifting or strenuous exercise.	Pressure on large nerve in leg (sciatica).	Consult doctor.
• Sudden backache in person over age 60. • Sharp pain in one place over the spine. OR • Recent confinement to bed or wheelchair.	Bone damage caused by softening of bones.	• Consult doctor. • See Osteoporosis.
• Backache. • Fever. • Painful urination.	• Kidney infection. • Virus infection (influenza). • Bladder infection.	• Consult doctor. • See Bladder Infection.
• Backache in person older than 60. • Pain in other joints.	Degenerative condition (osteoarthritis).	Consult doctor.
• Backache. • Overweight plus any of following: • Use of chair too high or too low for desk. • Recent heavy lifting or strenuous exercise. • Recent use of jackhammer or other heavy equipment.	Strain of back muscle or ligament.	• See Obesity. • Consult doctor.
• Chronic backache. • Numbness or tingling in extremities that is worsening.	Pressure on spinal cord (spinal cord tumor).	Consult doctor.
• Sudden backache. • Recent fall or injury to back, plus any of following: • Difficulty moving arm or leg. • Loss of bladder or bowel control. • Numbness or tingling in extremities.	Damaged spinal cord.	• Call doctor now. • Don't move injured person.
• Backache. • Wearing high heels.	Poor weight distribution.	Wear lower heels.
• Chronic backache. • Repetitive work such as computer use or typing.	Poor posture, incorrect chair or desk height.	Correct problem with posture or equipment.
Backache that is worse in morning.	• Lack of adequate back support during sleep. • Chronic inflammation. • Ankylosing spondylitis.	• Sleep on back or side. Use mattress that is neither too firm nor too soft. • Consult doctor.

Backache (cont.)

SYMPTOMS & FACTORS	POSSIBLE PROBLEM	WHAT TO DO
• Backache that worsens with lifting. • Lump in back or front of the vagina or projecting outside of it.	Fallen uterus.	See Uterine Prolapse.
• Pain in bones in back. • Weight loss. • Symptoms of anemia.	Cancer (multiple myeloma).	Consult doctor.
• Back pain. • Pain with sexual intercourse. • Blood in the urine.	Disorder of the uterus.	See Endometriosis.
• Back pain. • Visible curving of the upper body.	Curvature of the spine (scoliosis).	Consult doctor.

Behavioral or Emotional Changes

SYMPTOMS & FACTORS	POSSIBLE PROBLEM	WHAT TO DO
• Behavior that involves negative thoughts and thoughts of failure, inadequacy. • Lack of energy. • Sleeping problems. • Poor appetite.	Mild or clinical depression.	• See Low Grade Depression. • See Depression.
• Behavioral changes. • Use of a prescription or non-prescription drug.	Adverse reaction or side effect of drug.	• Consult doctor about prescription drug. • Discontinue non-prescription drug. • See Pregnancy & Drug Dependence.
Obsessions and/or compulsive behaviors that consume more than an hour a day.	Psychological disorder (obsessive compulsive disorder).	Consult doctor.
Anxiety symptoms when exposed to, or thinking of, a particular stimulus.	Psychological disorder.	See Phobias.
• Recurrent, intrusive and distressing recollection of an event. • Reliving of an event.	Psychological disorder (post traumatic stress disorder).	Consult doctor.
• Start of winter season. • Depression. • Irritability. • Tiredness.	Lack of light.	See Seasonal Affective Disorder.
• Fear of going crazy. • Fear of dying. • Sense of terror or doom. • Palpitations. • Rapid heartbeat.	Severe anxiety.	See Panic Disorder.
• Behavioral changes. • Week to 14 days before menstrual period. OR • Beginning of menopause.	Hormone fluctuations.	• See Premenstrual Syndrome. • See Menopause.
• Irritability. • Paleness, fatigue, lethargy. • Abdominal discomfort. • Headache. • Tremor.	Inhalation or ingestion of lead (lead poisoning).	Consult doctor.
Behavioral changes in an elderly person.	• Mental deterioration. • Alzheimer's disease. • Dementia.	Consult doctor.

Behavioral or Emotional Changes (cont.)

SYMPTOMS & FACTORS	POSSIBLE PROBLEM	WHAT TO DO
• Behavioral changes. • Recent withdrawal from tobacco, alcohol or drug, such as sleeping pills.	Withdrawal symptom.	• Consult doctor about drug withdrawal. • See Substance Abuse & Addiction. • See Alcoholism.
• Behavioral or personality changes. • Stiff neck. • General ill feeling. • Headache, vomiting, fever.	• Brain inflammation. • Viral encephalitis.	Consult doctor.
• Confusion. • Restlessness and anxiety. • Weakness. • Muscle cramps.	Electrolyte disorder (sodium imbalance).	Consult doctor.
• Behavioral or personality changes. • Binge eating. • Termination of binge with purging measures.	Psychological eating disorder.	• Consult doctor. • See Bulimia Nervosa.

Breast Pain, Tenderness or Lumps

SYMPTOMS & FACTORS	POSSIBLE PROBLEM	WHAT TO DO
Breast pain or lump that can be felt or seen.	• Cyst. • Tumor.	• Consult doctor. • See Fibrocystic Breast Changes. • See Breast Cancer.
• Pain or tenderness in breasts before menstrual periods. • Irregular periods. • Woman over age 38.	Thickening of gland tissue in breasts caused by hormonal changes.	See Menopause.
• Throbbing pain in breast of new mother. • Hard, tender, red lump on breast, or inflamed nipple. • Fever.	Breast infection.	See Mastitis.
• Breast pain. • Use of estrogen medications.	Adverse reaction or side effect of drug.	Consult doctor.
• Pain or tenderness in breasts. • Possible pregnancy.	Common sensitivity during pregnancy.	Wear a support bra as breasts enlarge.
Swollen, tender, hard breasts within 4 days of delivering baby.	Engorgement of breast tissue with milk.	Consult doctor.
• Sore nipples in woman who is breast-feeding. OR • Sharp pain in nipple of nursing mother when breast-feeding baby. • No fever. • No other symptoms related to breast.	Cracked or sore nipples. Common occurrence during first weeks of breast-feeding.	• Wash nipples and apply lanolin cream after breast-feeding. • Consult doctor if fever develops.
• Pain or tenderness in breasts. • Menstrual period due in a few days.	Discomfort caused by hormone changes.	See Premenstrual Syndrome.
• Pain or tenderness in breasts. • Body aches. • Fever and chills.	Breast infection.	See Breast Abscess.

Depression

SYMPTOMS & FACTORS	POSSIBLE PROBLEM	WHAT TO DO
• Depression. • Chronic illness, especially rheumatoid arthritis, multiple sclerosis or chronic heart disease.	Any illness, severe or mild, can cause significant depression.	• Consult doctor. • See Depression.
• Depression. • Use of prescription or non-prescription drug. OR • Excessive alcohol consumption.	Adverse reaction or side effect of drug or alcohol.	• Consult doctor. • See Alcoholism.
• Depression. • Recent virus infection with fever such as flu, infectious mononucleosis or hepatitis.	Common occurrence following infection.	Consult doctor if depression worsens or lasts longer than 2 weeks.
Depression following traumatic or sad event, such as death in family.	Normal occurrence for 3 to 6 months following such experiences.	Feelings are a normal part of mourning and will gradually improve over time. Seek medical help if depression worsens.
Depression experienced at the start of winter season.	Lack of light.	See Seasonal Affective Disorder.
Chronic depressive mood.	Mild depression.	See Low Grade Depression.
Depression following childbirth.	Common occurrence for several weeks after delivery.	See Postpartum Depression or Blues.
• Depression. • Persistent fatigue over the last 6 months.	Unknown cause.	See Chronic Fatigue Syndrome.
• Depression. • Anger. • Low self-esteem. • Muscle tension. • Headache.	Effect of stress.	See Stress.

Diarrhea

SYMPTOMS & FACTORS	POSSIBLE PROBLEM	WHAT TO DO
• Diarrhea. • Nausea or vomiting.	Viral, bacterial or parasitic infection of digestive tract.	Consult doctor.
• Diarrhea for 24 hours or longer. • Vomiting. • Abdominal pain. • Consumption of spoiled food or contaminated food or water.	Effect of toxins in food.	Consult doctor.
• Recurrent attacks of diarrhea. • Pain in lower abdomen.	• Intestinal parasites. • Several disorders.	Consult doctor.
• Diarrhea. • Use of prescription or non-prescription drug.	Adverse reaction or side effect of drug.	• Consult doctor about prescription drug. • Discontinue use of non-prescription drug.
• Diarrhea. • Blood in stool.	Inflammation of large intestine.	Consult doctor.
Recurrent attacks of diarrhea during periods of stress.	Effect of stress.	See Anxiety.
• Diarrhea. • Use of sorbitol, a common sweetener found in many diet products.	The sugar is not absorbed by the small intestine.	Discontinue use of the product with sorbitol.
• Diarrhea. • Abdominal pain. • Flatulence and bloating.	Reaction to a swallowed substance (food allergy).	Consult doctor.
• Explosive diarrhea. • Weakness and faintness. • Recent stomach surgery.	Intestinal disorder.	Consult doctor.

Fatigue or Tiredness (continued on next page)

SYMPTOMS & FACTORS	POSSIBLE PROBLEM	WHAT TO DO
• Fatigue. • Appetite loss. • Weight loss.	• Cancer. • Disorder of red blood cells.	• Consult doctor. • See Anemia (all charts).
• Fatigue, plus 2 or more of following: • Appetite loss. • Fever. • Headache. • Painful swelling in neck, armpit or groin. • Jaundice (yellow skin and eyes). • Sore throat.	Virus infection (mononucleosis).	Consult doctor.
• Fatigue. • Use of prescription or non-prescription drug.	Adverse reaction or side effect of drug.	• Consult doctor about prescription drug. • Discontinue use of non-prescription drug.
• Fatigue. • Coarse skin and hair. • Low voice. • Loss of sex drive. • Puffy face.	Underactive thyroid gland.	See Hypothyroidism.
• Fatigue. • Fever. • Headache, plus any of following: • Nausea, vomiting or diarrhea. • Drowsiness. • Cough. • Sore throat. • Pain in neck. • Aches in bones or joints. • Skin rash. • Pain in back. • Painful urination.	Bacterial or viral infection.	Consult doctor.
• Fatigue in woman at menopause. • Appetite loss.	Normal occurrence with decreasing estrogen level of menopause.	See Menopause.
• Fatigue. • Pregnancy. • Shortness of breath.	Dietary deficiency during pregnancy, particularly of protein, calcium, vitamins or iron.	• Consult doctor. • Eat extra protein foods. • Drink 2 extra glasses of skim milk daily. • Take iron supplement and prenatal vitamin supplement.
• Fatigue. • Depression or anxiety.	Effect of stress.	• See Depression. • See Anxiety.
• Ongoing fatigue for several months. • Numerous other symptoms.	Unknown infection or problem.	See Chronic Fatigue Syndrome.

Fatigue or Tiredness (cont.)

SYMPTOMS & FACTORS	POSSIBLE PROBLEM	WHAT TO DO
• Fatigue. • Chest discomfort with exertion that is relieved by rest.	Narrowing of coronary arteries.	Consult doctor.
• Tiredness. • Depression. • Increased appetite. • Beginning of winter.	Lack of light.	See Seasonal Affective Disorder.
• Fatigue and weakness. • Intermittent fever, chills, sweating. • Weight loss.	Heart valve or heart lining infection.	Consult doctor.
• Fatigue. • Fever; rash (usually on the cheeks). • Joint pain.	Autoimmune disorder.	Consult doctor.
• Fatigue. • Appetite loss. • Weight loss. • Hair loss. • Craving for salt. • Skin that darkens.	Inadequate cortisone hormone.	Consult doctor.
• Fatigue. • Cough. • Fever. • Weight loss. • Shortness of breath.	• Lung infection. • Tumor.	Consult doctor.
• Fatigue. • Headache and nausea. • Recent travel to foreign country.	Parasite infection.	Consult doctor.
• Fatigue. • Shortness of breath. • Irregular heartbeat.	Heart inflammation.	Consult doctor.
• Fatigue. • Chills, fever, sweating. • Tenderness along spine.	Bacterial infection.	Consult doctor.
• Fatigue. • Excess thirst. • Weight loss. • Frequent urination.	Several disorders.	• Consult doctor. • See Pregnancy & Diabetes Mellitus, Pregestational.

Fatigue or Tiredness (cont.)

SYMPTOMS & FACTORS	POSSIBLE PROBLEM	WHAT TO DO
• Fatigue and lethargy. • Paleness. • Behavioral changes. • Abdominal discomfort.	Inhalation or ingestion of lead (lead poisoning).	Consult doctor.
• Tiredness. • Fever. • Swollen lymph glands.	Protozoan infection.	See Toxoplasmosis.
• Fatigue and weakness. • Tingling sensation in arms, hands, legs and feet. • Urinary frequency.	Endocrine disorder.	Consult doctor.
• Fatigue. • Appetite loss. • Nausea at sight of food, plus 2 or more of following: • Jaundice (yellow skin and eyes). • Vomiting. • Tenderness over liver. • Fever. • Weakness.	Liver disorder.	Consult doctor.
• Fatigue. • Weight loss. • Recurrent skin and respiratory infections. • Fever. • Swollen lymph glands.	Infection.	See HIV & AIDS in Pregnancy.

Fever

SYMPTOMS & FACTORS	POSSIBLE PROBLEM	WHAT TO DO
• Fever. • Cough. • Headache. • Aches in bones or joints. • Stuffy or runny nose.	Virus infection (cold; influenza).	Consult doctor.
• Fever for 24 hours without other symptoms. OR • Recurrent fever with normal temperature between fevers.	Several disorders.	Consult doctor.
• Fever. • Nausea or vomiting. • Diarrhea.	Infection of digestive tract.	Consult doctor.
Any of the following symptoms: • Fever. • Pain in back below last rib. • Painful urination. • Frequent urination.	Urinary tract infection.	Consult doctor.
Fever after several hours in strong sunshine or hot environment.	Excess heat exposure.	• Limit exposure to sun. • Consult doctor.
• Fever. • Cough. • Shortness of breath, even when resting.	Lung infection.	Consult doctor.
• Fever. • Cough with gray-yellow sputum. OR • Wheezing.	Infection of bronchial tubes.	Consult doctor.
• Fever. • Use of prescription or non-prescription drug.	Adverse reaction or side effect of drug.	• Consult doctor about prescription drug. • Discontinue use of non-prescription drug.
• Fever. • Sore throat.	Infection (tonsillitis; pharyngitis; agranulocytosis).	Consult doctor.
• Fever. • Rash.	Several disorders.	Consult doctor.
• Sudden high fever. • Vomiting and watery diarrhea. • Rash resembling sunburn.	Blood poisoning.	See Toxic Shock Syndrome.

Fever (cont.)

SYMPTOMS & FACTORS	POSSIBLE PROBLEM	WHAT TO DO
• Fever. • Other symptoms similar to cold (cough, tiredness, chills).	Fungal infection or tick-caused disorder, depending on location in U.S.	Consult doctor.
• Fever. • Headache, plus any of following: • Pain bending forward. • Lethargy. • Confusion. • Nausea or vomiting.	Infection of membranes around brain.	Call doctor now.
• Intermittent fever and chills. • Fatigue and weakness. • Weight loss. • Vague aches and pains.	Heart valve or lining infection.	Consult doctor.
• Fever and chills. • General ill feeling. • Headache. • Muscle ache.	Bacterial infection.	Consult doctor.
• Low grade fever. • Weight loss. • Recurrent respiratory and skin infections.	Virus infection.	See HIV & AIDS.
• Fever (rapid temperature rise). • Shaking chills. • Pounding heartbeat. • General ill feeling.	Severe bacterial infection.	Consult doctor.
• Intermittent fever. • Chills. • Marked fatigue. • Enlarged lymph glands.	Bacterial infection.	Consult doctor.
• Fever. • Chills, muscle aches, cough. • Listlessness. • Exposure to field mice or other rodents.	Virus infection (hantavirus).	Consult doctor.
• Fever. • Tiredness. • Swollen lymph glands.	Protozoan infection.	See Toxoplasmosis.
• Fever. • Breast pain, tenderness, redness or hardness. • Body aches.	Infection.	See Breast Abscess.

Genital Sores, Blisters, Warts or Boils

SYMPTOMS & FACTORS	POSSIBLE PROBLEM	WHAT TO DO
Painless blister on genitals.	Sexually transmitted disease.	See Granuloma Inguinale.
• Painless red sore on genitals for months or less. • Enlarged lymph glands in neck, armpit or groin. • Headache. • Rash on skin.	Sexually transmitted disease.	See Syphilis.
Small painful lesion surrounded by a red border.	Sexually transmitted disease.	See Chancroid.
• Small flesh-colored bumps or tiny cauliflower-like bumps. • Warts may cause itching, burning, tenderness or pain.	Sexually transmitted disease.	See Warts, Genital.

Hair Growth in Women, Excessive

SYMPTOMS & FACTORS	POSSIBLE PROBLEM	WHAT TO DO
• Excessive hair growth over 4 or 5 months. • Unexplained weight gain. • Menstrual changes or absent periods. • Deep voice.	Disorder or tumor of ovaries or adrenal gland.	• See Ovarian Tumor, Benign. • See Ovarian Cancer. • See Polycystic Ovarian Syndrome.
• Excessive hair growth over 2 months or less. • Use of prescription drug, such as hormones, cortisone drugs or anticonvulsants.	Adverse reaction or side effect of drug.	Consult doctor.
• Excessive hair on face or body that developed before age 20. • Similar hairiness in other female family members.	Genetic causes; no underlying disorder.	Consult cosmetologist for removal of unwanted hair.
Excessive hair growth, especially on face, in woman who has had ovaries removed or is over age 40.	Normal occurrence with decreasing estrogen level of menopause.	• Consult doctor. • Consult cosmetologist for removal of unwanted hair.
Excessive hair growth during pregnancy.	Hormone changes of pregnancy.	Nothing. Hair growth decreases after delivery.
• Hair thickens and grows in a male pattern. • Irregular or no menstruation. • Acne. • Infertility.	Excessive production of androgens (male hormones).	See Hirsutism.

Headache

SYMPTOMS & FACTORS	POSSIBLE PROBLEM	WHAT TO DO
• Headache. • Use of prescription or nonprescription drug.	Adverse reaction or side effect of drug.	• Consult doctor about prescription drug. • Discontinue use of nonprescription drug.
• Severe headache. • Fever.	Common occurrence with infection.	See Fever chart (in Symptoms section).
• Headache. • Recent head injury. • No other symptoms.	Common occurrence after head injury.	Consult doctor.
• Headache. • Vision disturbance before headache. • Nausea or vomiting.	Severe vascular headache.	Consult doctor.
• Headache in forehead or back of head. • Tense, stressed feeling. • Sleeping difficulty.	Effect of stress.	• See Anxiety. • See Depression.
• Sudden onset of headache. • Pain around eyes. • Headache occurs at same time every day.	Chronic headache disorder.	Consult doctor.
• Pain or tenderness around eyes and cheekbones that worsens when bending head forward. • Recent cold or nasal allergies.	Sinus infection (sinusitis).	Consult doctor.
• Headache without pain around eyes and cheekbones. • Runny or stuffy nose.	Virus infection.	Consult doctor.
• Headache. • Decreased consumption of caffeine-containing beverages (coffee, colas, cocoa, tea).	Caffeine withdrawal.	• Reduce consumption of caffeine gradually. • Use a nonprescription pain reliever, such as acetaminophen.
• Headache, plus any of following: • Unusually long time since eating. • Excessive alcohol consumption. • Stuffy, smoky or noisy room. • Exposure to strong sunlight.	Circumstantial headache. No underlying disorder.	Use a nonprescription pain reliever, such as acetaminophen.
• Headache after excessive alcohol consumption. • Nausea or vomiting.	"Hangover."	Use a nonprescription pain reliever, such as acetaminophen.
• Severe headache that worsens when bending head forward. • Eyes sensitive to light. • Lethargy. • Confusion. • No recent head injury.	Bleeding in membrane around brain.	Call doctor now.

Headache (cont.)

SYMPTOMS & FACTORS	POSSIBLE PROBLEM	WHAT TO DO
• Headache that worsens when bending head forward. • Fever. • Eyes sensitive to light.	Infection of membranes around brain (meningitis).	Call doctor now.
• Headache. • Eye pain. • Blurred vision. • Nausea or vomiting. • No injury to eye.	Excess pressure in eye.	Call doctor now.
• Habitual headache on waking; no excessive alcohol consumption. • Double vision. • Nausea or vomiting.	• High blood pressure. • Brain tumor.	Consult doctor.
Headache after reading or straining to see.	Strain on neck muscles (not strain on eyes).	Consult doctor.
• Headache, nausea, vomiting. • Ascent to higher altitude.	Lack of oxygen.	Consult doctor.
• Headache. • Dizziness. • Nausea, vomiting. • Faintness.	Gas inhalation (carbon monoxide poisoning).	Consult doctor.
• Headache. • Stiff neck. • Fever.	Fungal infection (cryptococcosis).	Consult doctor.
• Headache. • General ill feeling. • Chills and fever. • Muscle aches.	Bacterial infection.	Consult doctor.
• Headache. • Fatigue and nausea. • Travel to foreign country.	Parasite infection (malaria).	Consult doctor.

Heartbeat Irregularity

SYMPTOMS & FACTORS	POSSIBLE PROBLEM	WHAT TO DO
• Irregular heartbeat. • General ill feeling. • History of heart disease.	Disorder of heart rate or rhythm.	Call doctor now.
• Irregular heartbeat. • Use of prescription or nonprescription drugs, such as thyroid medication; digitalis preparations; diuretics; diet pills; stimulants; caffeine; decongestants; cold remedies, including nasal sprays; illegal drugs, including marijuana, cocaine, psychedelics, amphetamines.	Adverse reaction or side effect of drug.	• Consult doctor about prescription drug. • Discontinue use of nonprescription or illegal drug.
• Irregular heartbeat. • Unexplained weight loss. • Anxiety. • Excessive sweating. • Fatigue.	Overactive thyroid gland.	See Hyperthyroidism.
• Rapid or irregular heartbeat. • Recent tension or worry.	Effect of stress.	• See Anxiety. • See Panic Disorder. • See Phobias.
• Irregular heartbeat. • Excessive smoking. OR • Excessive consumption of caffeine-containing beverages such as coffee, cola, tea or cocoa.	Effect of nicotine or caffeine.	Decrease nicotine or caffeine use.
• Rapid or irregular heartbeat. • Fever.	Infection.	See Fever chart (in Symptoms section).
• Heartbeat irregularity. • Shortness of breath. • Fatigue.	Heart inflammation.	Consult doctor.
• Rapid heartbeat following exercise, emotional upset or exposure to cold. • Tremors and nervousness. • Feelings of doom.	Adrenal tumor.	Consult doctor.

Itching

SYMPTOMS & FACTORS	POSSIBLE PROBLEM	WHAT TO DO
• Itching hands. • Hands are frequently wet or exposed to chemicals.	Effect of chemicals or moisture (contact dermatitis).	Consult doctor.
• Itching on head or between toes. • Small bald patches on scalp.	Fungus infection (ringworm; athlete's foot).	Consult doctor.
• Itching on head. • Tiny white spots on hair that won't come off.	Parasites (lice).	Consult doctor.
• Itching. • Insect bite or sting.	Reaction.	Consult doctor.
• Itching or bleeding around anus. • Painful bowel movements.	• Varicose veins in anus. • Split in skin around anus (hemorrhoids; anal fissure).	Consult doctor.
Itching around anus following severe diarrhea.	Normal response to irritation.	Apply ointment containing zinc oxide.
• Itching. • Diarrhea. • Abdominal pain. • Flatulence and bloating. • Rash.	Reaction to a swallowed substance (food allergy).	Consult doctor.
• Intense itching and burning. • Bright red skin rash. • Contact with poisonous plant.	Allergic reaction to plant (poison ivy, oak, sumac).	Consult doctor.
• Itching. • Fluid-filled blisters. • Skin disorder elsewhere on body.	Allergic reaction (id reaction).	Consult doctor.
• Itching. • Yellow skin and eyes.	• Liver disorder. • Blood disorder.	Call doctor now.
• Itching. • General ill feeling. • Use of prescription or nonprescription drugs.	• Blood disorder. • Kidney disorder. • Overactive thyroid gland. • Adverse reaction or side effect of drug. • Cancer.	• Consult doctor. • See Hyperthyroidism.
• Itching. • Rash. • No fever.	Several skin disorders.	See Rash without Fever (in Symptoms section).
Itching in genital area.	Irritation or infection.	See Vaginal Itching (in Symptoms section).
Itching around anus, especially at night.	• Parasites. • Several causes.	Consult doctor.
• Itching. • Wheezing, coughing, sneezing. • Swelling around face and hands. • Difficulty breathing.	Allergic reaction (anaphylaxis).	Call doctor now.

Menstrual Periods, Late or Absent

SYMPTOMS & FACTORS	POSSIBLE PROBLEM	WHAT TO DO
• Menstrual periods absent, plus 1 or more of following: • Unexplained weight gain. • Masculine voice. • Abnormal hairiness.	Hormone imbalance.	• Consult doctor. • See Hirsutism.
Menstrual periods absent in woman over age 38.	Normal menstrual irregularities at this age.	See Menopause.
• Menstrual periods absent. • Recent quick weight loss from drastic dieting. OR • Current participation in strenuous exercise program. OR • Recent illness. OR • Tension or worry. OR • Change in lifestyle such as new job or new home. OR • Menstrual periods absent since discontinuing use of oral contraceptives.	• Hormone changes. • Effect of stress. • Hormone changes caused by discontinuing pill.	See Amenorrhea.
• Menstrual periods absent. • Use of prescription drug.	Adverse reaction or side effect of drug.	• Consult doctor. • See Amenorrhea (all charts).
• Menstrual period late by 2 or more weeks. • Sexual intercourse within last month.	Pregnancy.	• Consult doctor to confirm pregnancy. • Take home-pregnancy test.
Menstrual periods absent since delivery of baby.	Normal occurrence caused by hormone changes following childbirth.	• If bottle-feeding, consult doctor if periods do not resume within 8 weeks after delivery. • If breast-feeding, consult doctor if periods do not resume within 4 weeks after weaning.
Menstrual periods have never started.	Hormone changes of puberty have not occurred.	• Consult doctor if older than 16. • See Amenorrhea, Primary.
• Irregular menstrual periods. • Gastrointestinal upsets. • Discomfort or pain in lower abdomen.	• Cyst. • Cancer.	• See Polycystic Ovarian Syndrome. • See Ovarian Cancer.

Menstrual Periods, Painful or Heavy

SYMPTOMS & FACTORS	POSSIBLE PROBLEM	WHAT TO DO
• Excessive menstrual flow. • Menstrual period lasts more than 7 days.	Menstrual irregularity.	See Menorrhagia.
Menstrual period more painful or heavier than usual, especially during last days of period.	Disorder of lining of pelvic organs.	• See Endometriosis. • See Dysmenorrhea.
• Current menstrual period more painful or heavier than usual. • Period arrived 1 week or more late.	• Early pregnancy and miscarriage. • Pregnancy outside uterus.	• Consult doctor. • See Miscarriage. • See Ectopic Pregnancy.
Menstrual periods more painful or heavier since receiving intrauterine contraceptive device (IUD).	Common side effect of using IUD.	Consult doctor.
• Menstrual periods more painful or heavier than usual. • No other pelvic or genital symptoms.	Benign growth in uterus.	See Fibroid Tumor, Uterine.
Menstrual periods painful or heavy since discontinuing use of oral contraceptives.	Hormone changes caused by discontinuing pill.	Consult doctor.
• Menstrual periods painful. • Periods began within last 3 years. • Healthy otherwise.	No disease.	See Dysmenorrhea.
Menstrual period heavy in woman who has recently delivered a baby.	Normal occurrence during first 2 menstrual periods following childbirth.	Consult doctor if heavy periods persist.
Menstrual flow always heavy.	No underlying disorder.	Consult doctor for blood test for anemia.
• Heavy menstrual flow. • Bleeding between normal menstrual periods.	Excessive estrogen.	See Endometrial Hyperplasia.
Painful, prolonged or irregular bleeding through the vagina.	Several causes.	See Uterine Bleeding, Dysfunctional.
• Menstrual periods more painful or heavier than usual. • Bad-smelling vaginal discharge. • Fever.	Infection of reproductive organs.	• Call doctor now. • See Pelvic Inflammatory Disease.
• Menstrual period abnormally heavy. • Spotting or bleeding between periods. • Persistent vaginal discharge. • Pain and bleeding after intercourse. • Pelvic pain which radiates to hips and thighs.	Cervical cancer.	• Call doctor now. • See Cervical Cancer.

Rash with Fever

SYMPTOMS & FACTORS	POSSIBLE PROBLEM	WHAT TO DO
• Raised, red, itching bumps that become blisters on face, trunk and genitals. • Fever.	Virus infection (chickenpox).	Consult doctor.
• Red rash. • Fever. • Swelling on both sides of neck or at base of skull.	Virus infection (rubella).	Consult doctor.
• Red spots or blotches on face or trunk. • Fever, plus 2 or more of following: • Dry cough. • Sore, red eyes. • Runny nose. • Sore throat. • Headache.	• Virus infection. • Rickettsia infection. • Measles. • Rocky Mountain spotted fever.	Consult doctor.
• Painful, red, blister-like rash on body. • Fever. • General ill feeling.	Virus infection.	See Genital Herpes.
• Purple spots, plus 2 or more of following: • Fever. • Headache. • Pain when bending head forward. • Eyes sensitive to light. • Vomiting.	Infection of membranes around brain (meningitis).	Call doctor now.
• Red rash in woman of childbearing age. • Fever of 101F (38.3C) or higher. • Rapid heartbeat. • Fatigue and weakness. • Excessive thirst.	Bacterial infection.	• Call doctor now. • See Toxic Shock Syndrome.
• Purple rash. • Fever.	Allergic disorder.	Call doctor now.
• Red rash. • Paleness around mouth. • Fever of 102F (38.9C) or higher. • Bright red sore throat. • Swollen tonsils. • Enlarged glands in neck.	Complication of preceding streptococcal infection.	Call doctor now.

Rash with Fever (cont.)

SYMPTOMS & FACTORS	POSSIBLE PROBLEM	WHAT TO DO
• Mild skin rash on chest, back and abdomen. • Fever, fatigue and paleness. • Pain caused by joint inflammation.	Complication of preceding streptococcal infection.	Consult doctor.
• Red rash or spots that begin on palms, soles, arms and legs. • Rash develops into blisters. • Fever (sometimes).	Inflammatory disorder (erythema multiforme).	Consult doctor.

Rash without Fever

SYMPTOMS & FACTORS	POSSIBLE PROBLEM	WHAT TO DO
• Light red bumps with raised edges. • Severe itching.	Allergic reaction (hives).	Consult doctor.
• Itching rash. • Use of prescription or non-prescription drug.	Adverse reaction or side effect of drug.	Call doctor now.
Itching, red, scaling or moist rash under cosmetics, jewelry or new clothing.	Allergic reaction.	Consult doctor.
Itching, red, scaling or moist rash, especially on hands.	Skin disorder aggravated by stress.	Consult doctor.
• Itching, red, scaling or moist rash, plus: • Recent contact with plant, such as poison ivy, poison oak, poison sumac, primrose or mango. OR • Recent contact with irritating detergents or other chemicals.	Allergic reaction.	Consult doctor.
• Itching rash around genitals or anus. • No other symptoms or factors.	• Sugar in urine. • Vaginal infection.	Consult doctor.
Red bumps in a small area without other symptoms.	Insect bites.	Consult doctor.
• Red rash. • Rash is located in areas of heavy perspiration.	Obstruction of sweat glands.	Consult doctor.
• Red rash scattered over body. • Severe itching at night. • Gray lines or red, sore spots between fingers or on wrists.	Parasites.	See Scabies.
• Rash that consists of small white blisters with pus inside. • Blisters are located in hair follicles of the skin.	Bacterial or fungal skin infection (folliculitis).	Consult doctor.
Red, scaling patch that spreads into a ring.	Fungus infection (ringworm).	Consult doctor.
• Red rash that begins on palms, soles, arms and legs. • Rash develops into blisters.	Inflammatory disorder (erythema multiforme).	Consult doctor.

Rash without Fever (cont.)

SYMPTOMS & FACTORS	POSSIBLE PROBLEM	WHAT TO DO
• Red, raised rash or skin lesions. • Rash appears on cheeks in a "butterfly" appearance.	Autoimmune disorder.	Consult doctor.
• Rash starting on cheeks then spreading. • Slight tiredness or fatigue.	Virus infection.	Consult doctor.
• Skin rash, progressing to thin, raised lines on the skin. • Contact with soil or sand.	Hookworm infestation (larva migrans).	Consult doctor.
• Skin rash (that may itch) on face, shoulders, arms and over joints. • Weakness in the pelvic or shoulder muscles.	Connective tissue disorder (polymyositis).	Consult doctor.
• Red skin rash, sometimes with small blisters. • A burning reaction similar to those that follow prolonged sun exposure. • Dizziness, nausea, vomiting. • Brief sun exposure.	Sensitivity to sun.	Consult doctor.

Sexual Intercourse, Painful

SYMPTOMS & FACTORS	POSSIBLE PROBLEM	WHAT TO DO
• Painful intercourse only when partner penetrates vagina deeply. • Heavy, painful periods.	Disorder of lining of pelvic organs.	See Endometriosis.
• Painful intercourse. • Abnormal vaginal discharge.	Several disorders.	• See Vaginal Discharge, Abnormal (in Symptoms section). • See Vaginitis (all charts).
• Painful intercourse. • Tenderness over bladder. • Frequent, painful urination.	Bladder inflammation.	See Bladder Infection.
Painful intercourse in woman past menopause or over age 45.	Normal occurrence caused by decreased vaginal secretions.	• See Vaginismus. • See Dyspareunia. • See Menopause.
• Painful intercourse. • Recent childbirth.	Inflammation or scarring caused by a stretched or torn vagina or episiotomy repair.	• Wait at least 3 weeks before resuming sexual relations after childbirth. • Consult doctor if pain lasts longer than 8 weeks.
• Painful intercourse. • Vaginal itching.	Several disorders.	See Vaginal Itching (in Symptoms section).
• Painful intercourse. • Vagina seems too tight.	Muscle spasm.	• See Vaginismus. • See Dyspareunia.
• Painful intercourse. • Recent start or increase in sexual activity.	No underlying disorder.	• Wait 2 to 3 days for symptoms to disappear before resuming sex. • See Vaginismus. • See Dyspareunia.
• Dryness of vagina causing painful intercourse. • Dryness of eyes and mouth.	Autoimmune disorder (Sjögren's syndrome).	Consult doctor.
• Pain with intercourse. • Bad smelling vaginal discharge. • Frequent, painful urination.	Infection.	See Pelvic Inflammatory Disease.
• Pain with intercourse. • Lump in back of the vagina or projecting outside of it. • Vague backache.	Fallen uterus.	See Uterine Prolapse.
• Painful intercourse. • Swelling without pain in lower abdomen or severe abdominal pain. • Stinging or burning with urination.	Cysts.	See Polycystic Ovarian Syndrome.
• Painful intercourse. • No other symptoms or factors.	• Vaginal malformation. • Lack of experience and education.	Consult doctor.
• Painful intercourse. • Formation of a nonpainful lesion. • Vaginal discharge with unpleasant odor.	Sexually transmitted disease.	See Granuloma Inguinale.

Sweating, Excessive

SYMPTOMS & FACTORS	POSSIBLE PROBLEM	WHAT TO DO
• Excessive sweating. • Anxiety or excitement.	Normal occurrence with stress.	See Anxiety.
• Excessive sweating. • Overweight.	Effect of excess weight.	See Obesity.
• Excessive sweating in woman older than 38. • Irregular menstrual periods.	Hormone changes; end of menstrual cycles approaching.	See Menopause.
• Excessive sweating in woman during menstrual period. OR • Excessive sweating due to tension or apprehension. OR • Excessive sweating following coffee consumption.	No underlying disorder.	Nothing.
Excessive sweating in teenager.	Normal occurrence during adolescence.	Nothing.
• Sweating. • Palpitations, tremors, flushing. • Symptoms of anxiety when exposed to, or thinking of, a particular stimulus.	Fears.	See Phobias.
• Excessive sweating. • Unpleasant body odor.	Several disorders.	Consult doctor.
• Skin is cool and moist. • Prolonged exposure to hot temperature.	Excessive fluid loss.	Consult doctor.
• Excessive sweating. • Chest pain.	Heart attack.	Call doctor now.
• Excessive sweating at night. • Weight loss. • Persistent cough with blood in sputum. • Fever. • Fatigue.	• Lung inflammation or infection. • Cancer.	Consult doctor.
• Excessive sweating, plus 2 or more of following: • Weight loss. • Increased appetite. • Anxiety. • Sleeping problems.	Overactive thyroid gland.	See Hyperthyroidism.
• Excessive sweating. • Use of prescription, non-prescription or illegal drug.	Adverse reaction or side effect of drug.	• Consult doctor about prescription drug. • Discontinue use of non-prescription or illegal drug.
• Excessive sweating. • Fever.	Normal occurrence with fever.	See Fever charts (in Symptoms section).

Swelling or Lump

SYMPTOMS & FACTORS	POSSIBLE PROBLEM	WHAT TO DO
Firm swelling in groin that does not disappear when pressed.	• Infection in leg or genitals. • Protruding intestinal tissue (hernia).	Consult doctor.
• Nodule or bump under the skin. • Nodule feels "doughy," smooth and easily movable.	Benign fat-cell tumor (lipomas).	Consult doctor.
• Painful, red lump or swelling. • Recent injury to area.	Bleeding under skin (sprain or strain; tendinitis).	Consult doctor.
Lump in breast.	• Cyst. • Cancer.	• Consult doctor. • See Fibrocystic Breast Changes. • See Breast Cancer.
Soft lump or swelling in groin or near navel that disappears when pressed or enlarges with cough.	Protruding intestinal tissue.	Consult doctor.
Swelling between ear and jaw.	• Virus infection of glands. • Infection around tooth. • Disorder or tumor of salivary gland.	Consult doctor.
• Lump or swelling in neck, armpit or groin. • Fever.	Virus infection.	Consult doctor.
• Swelling on both sides of neck, toward front. • Sore throat.	Bacterial or viral infection (tonsillitis; pharyngitis; mononucleosis).	Consult doctor.
• Swelling at both sides of back of neck. • Pink rash. • Fever.	Virus infection (rubella).	Consult doctor.
• Tender swelling in armpit, groin, elbow or base of neck. • Sore, cut or bite on hand, arm, leg or shoulder on same side as swelling.	Infected bite or wound.	Consult doctor.
• Tender lump on elbow or in armpit. • Fever. • Exposure to cats.	Virus infection.	Consult doctor.
Swelling in front of neck with movement when swallowing.	Thyroid goiter.	Consult doctor.

Swelling or Lump (cont.)

SYMPTOMS & FACTORS	POSSIBLE PROBLEM	WHAT TO DO
• Swelling in neck, armpit or groin. • Recent vaccination, such as tetanus or typhoid.	Swelling caused by vaccination.	Consult doctor.
Painless swelling near joint that is overused.	Ganglion cyst.	Consult doctor.
• Mass in abdomen that can be felt, especially in young child. • Cramping abdominal pain.	Intestinal obstruction (intussusception).	Call doctor now.
Lump or swelling in neck, armpit or groin without other symptoms or factors.	• Infection. • Tumor.	Consult doctor.
• Lump or swelling in neck, armpit or groin. • Use of prescription drug, especially for epilepsy or thyroid disorder.	Adverse reaction or side effect of drug.	Consult doctor.
• Swollen lymph nodes. • Low grade fever. • Weight loss. • Recurrent respiratory and skin infections.	Virus infection.	See HIV & AIDS.
• Hard mass in right, upper abdomen. • Unexplained weight loss and appetite loss. • Bleeding tendency.	Liver tumor (hepatoma; liver cancer).	Consult doctor.

Trembling or Twitching

SYMPTOMS & FACTORS	POSSIBLE PROBLEM	WHAT TO DO
• Trembling or twitching, especially of tongue and face muscles. • Use of prescription or nonprescription drug, especially phenothiazine.	Adverse reaction or side effect of drug.	• Consult doctor about prescription drug. • Discontinue use of nonprescription drug.
Trembling in one part of body, especially when affected part is at rest.	Disorder of central nervous system (Parkinson's disease).	Consult doctor.
• Trembling. • Alcohol withdrawal.	Withdrawal symptom.	See Alcoholism.
• Trembling. • Excessive consumption of coffee or tea. OR • Use of nonprescription drug containing caffeine.	Adverse effect of caffeine.	Decrease use of caffeine.
• Trembling, plus 2 or more of following: • Weight loss. • Fatigue. • Excessive sweating.	Overactive thyroid gland.	See Hyperthyroidism.
• Painful twitching on side of face. • Pain is triggered by stroking or touching the face.	Nerve disorder (trigeminal neuralgia).	Consult doctor.
Twitching in one small part of body, such as eyelid.	Fatigue or tension. Usually no underlying disorder.	• Nothing. • Consult doctor if you feel ill or if muscles seem weak.
Trembling in any part of body without other symptoms or factors.	Inherited tendency to tremble, especially from anxiety or stress.	Consult doctor to confirm diagnosis.
Unexpected body jerks when falling asleep.	Involuntary muscle spasms. No underlying disorder.	Nothing.
• Trembling or twitching. • Loss of conciousness. • Loss of bladder control.	Seizure.	See Pregnancy and Seizure Disorder, Pregestational.

Urination, Frequent (continued on next page)

SYMPTOMS & FACTORS	POSSIBLE PROBLEM	WHAT TO DO
• Frequent urination, especially at night. • Increased urine production. • Excessive consumption of tea, coffee, cola or alcohol.	Effect of caffeine or alcohol.	Decrease consumption of caffeine or alcohol.
• Frequent urination, especially at night. • Increased urine production. • Use of diuretic drug for heart disease or high blood pressure.	Effect of diuretic drug.	Consult doctor if uneasy.
• Frequent urination. • Anxiety or excitement. OR • Cold weather.	Normal occurrence.	Nothing.
• Frequent urination. • Burning and stinging on urination. • Increased urge to urinate.	Bladder infection.	See Bladder Infection.
• Frequent urination. • Painful urination. • Blood in urine.	Stones (urinary calculi).	Consult doctor.
• Frequent urination. • Possible pregnancy.	Normal occurrence during first 3 months and last 3 months of pregnancy.	Consult doctor to confirm pregnancy.
• Frequent urination. • Pain with urination.	Several disorders.	Consult doctor.
• Frequent urination, especially at night. • Increased urine production, plus 2 or more of following: • Increased hunger and thirst. • Itching around genitals or anus. • Fatigue. • Weight loss.	Sugar in urine (diabetes mellitus).	Consult doctor.
• Frequent urination. • Intense urge to urinate followed quickly by uncontrollable urine leak.	Urge incontinence.	See Incontinence, Urge.
• Frequent urination. • Difficulty controlling bladder.	Several disorders.	See Urination, Lack of Control (in Symptoms section).
• Frequent urination. • Vaginal discharge. • Backache. • Lower abdominal pain.	Cervicitis.	See Cervicitis.

Urination, Frequent (cont.)

SYMPTOMS & FACTORS	POSSIBLE PROBLEM	WHAT TO DO
• Frequent urination. • Discharge from urethra.	Inflammatory disease (Reiter's syndrome).	Consult doctor.
• Passage of large amounts of urine. • Colorless urine. • Excessive thirst.	Hormone disorder (diabetes insipidus).	Consult doctor.
• Frequent urination. • Pelvic pain and pressure. • Sensation of incomplete emptying of the bladder. • Pain during intercourse.	Inflammation of the bladder wall.	See Interstitial Cystitis.

Urination, Lack of Control

SYMPTOMS & FACTORS	POSSIBLE PROBLEM	WHAT TO DO
Small urine leak in female when coughing, sneezing, laughing or running.	Stress incontinence.	See Incontinence, Stress.
• Lack of urinary control. • Use of prescription drug.	Adverse reaction or side effect of drug.	Consult doctor.
• Lack of urinary control. • Cloudy, bad-smelling urine.	Infection of urinary tract.	• See Bladder Infection. • See Urethritis.
• Lack of urinary control. • Lack of bowel control.	Decreased blood supply to brain (stroke).	Call doctor now.
• Lack of urinary control. • Constipation for longer than 1 week.	Pressure on bladder from fecal impaction.	Consult doctor.
• Lack of urinary control in person over age 60, plus 2 or more of following: • Inability to remember recent events. • Decline in attention to personal appearance or cleanliness. • Personality change.	• Poor nutrition. • Mental deterioration. • Vitamin B deficiency. • Alzheimer's disease. • Dementia.	Consult doctor.
• Lack of urinary control. • Chronic illness.	Several disorders.	Call doctor now.
• Lack of urinary control. • Incomplete emptying of bladder. • Increased urinary frequency.	Pelvic weakness.	See Vaginal Hernias.

Urination, Painful

SYMPTOMS & FACTORS	POSSIBLE PROBLEM	WHAT TO DO
• Painful urination. • Pain in one side of back, between waist and last rib. • Fever.	Kidney infection.	Consult doctor.
• Painful urination. • Frequent urination.	Bladder inflammation.	See Bladder Infection.
• Painful urination. • Painful blisters on genitals. • Fever.	Sexually transmitted virus infection.	See Genital Herpes.
• Painful urination. • Green-yellow or white discharge from vagina. • Itching around genitals.	Vaginal infection.	• See Vaginitis, Candidal. • See Vaginitis, Trichomonal.
• Painful urination. • Bad-smelling vaginal discharge. • Pain or tenderness in lower abdomen. • Fever.	Sexually transmitted infection.	• See Gonorrhea. • See Urethritis.
• Burning urination. • Blood in urine. • Pain in pelvic area.	Abnormal growth in bladder (bladder tumor).	Consult doctor.
• Painful urination or inability to urinate. • Forceful blow, injury or wound in lower abdomen.	Injury to genital tract.	Consult doctor.
• Discomfort on urinating. • Vaginal discharge.	Infection.	See Chlamydia Infection.
• Burning sensation on urination. • Urge to urinate when bladder is empty. • Pain in lower abdomen.	Infection.	See Urinary Tract Infection in Pregnancy.

Urine, Abnormal Color

SYMPTOMS & FACTORS	POSSIBLE PROBLEM	WHAT TO DO
• Pink, red, smoky-brown or other color change in urine. • Use of new prescription drug in last 24 hours.	Side effect of drug.	Consult doctor if color change not expected.
• Dark yellow or orange urine. • Recent use of laxatives containing senna. OR • Recent consumption of rhubarb.	Effect of chemicals in these substances.	Nothing.
• Pink, red or smoky-brown urine. • Recent consumption of beets, blackberries or other red food.	Effect of natural or artificial color.	Nothing.
Pink, red or smoky-brown urine.	Disorder of urinary tract.	Consult doctor.
• Clear or dark brown urine. • Pale stool. • Yellow skin and eyes.	Liver disorder (viral hepatitis).	Call doctor now.
• Dark yellow or orange urine. • Fever. OR • Very hot weather. OR • Decreased fluid intake.	Concentrated urine (heatstroke; heat exhaustion; dehydration).	• See Fever chart (in Symptoms section). • Increase fluid intake.
• Dark yellow or orange urine. • Vomiting. • Diarrhea.	Concentrated urine.	• See Vomiting, Recurrent Attacks (in Symptoms section). • See Diarrhea (in Symptoms section).
Green or blue urine.	Effect of artificial color in food or drug.	Nothing.
• Colorless urine. • Excessive thirst. • Passage of large amounts of urine.	Hormone disorder (diabetes insipidus).	Consult doctor.

Vaginal Bleeding, Unexpected

SYMPTOMS & FACTORS	POSSIBLE PROBLEM	WHAT TO DO
Vaginal bleeding during first 3 months of pregnancy.	Spontaneous abortion.	• Call doctor now. • See Miscarriage.
Vaginal bleeding during 4th to 9th month of pregnancy.	Abnormal location of placenta.	• Call doctor now. • See Placenta Previa. • See Abruptio Placentae.
• Unexpected vaginal bleeding. • Severe abdominal pain. • Pregnancy possible. OR • Current use of intrauterine contraceptive device (IUD).	Pregnancy developing outside uterus.	• Call doctor now. • See Ectopic Pregnancy.
• Unexpected vaginal bleeding in woman over age 45. • Last menstrual period more than 6 months ago.	• Hormone changes. • Tumor or cancer.	• See Menopause. • See Uterine Bleeding, Postmenopausal. • See Uterine Malignancy. • See Cervical Cancer. • See Ovarian Cancer. • See Vaginal or Vulvar Cancer.
• Unexpected vaginal bleeding in woman over age 45. • Use of prescription drug for hormone replacement therapy.	Breakthrough bleeding.	Consult doctor.
• Unexpected vaginal bleeding. • Vaginal discharge.	• Several disorders. • Cancer. • Cervical erosion.	• See Cervical Polyps. • See Cervical Cancer. • See Uterine Cancer. • See Vaginal or Vulvar Cancer.
• Unexpected vaginal bleeding. • Pain in lower abdomen.	• Uterine fibroids. • Cancer.	• See Cervical Polyps. • See Uterine Bleeding, Dysfunctional. • See Fibroid Tumor, Uterine. • See Ovarian Cancer.
• Unexpected vaginal bleeding. • Recent insertion of intrauterine contraceptive device (IUD).	Complications caused by IUD.	Consult doctor.
• Unexpected vaginal bleeding. • Use of oral contraceptives.	Breakthrough bleeding; common occurrence in women taking pill.	Consult doctor.
• Excessive menstrual flow. • Menstrual period lasts more than 7 days.	Menstrual irregularity.	See Menorrhagia.
• Menstrual disorders. • Coarse skin. • Sleepiness.	Underactive thyroid gland.	See Hypothyroidism.
• Unexpected vaginal bleeding. • Insertion of foreign object into vagina.	Vaginal injury.	Consult doctor.

Vaginal Bleeding, Unexpected (cont.)

SYMPTOMS & FACTORS	POSSIBLE PROBLEM	WHAT TO DO
• Vaginal bleeding after sexual intercourse. • Uterine cramping. • Enlarged uterus.	Cancer.	• Call doctor now. • See Uterine Malignancy.
• Vaginal bleeding. • Morning sickness that is excessive. • Passage of vesicle.	Pregnancy disorder.	See Gestational Trophoblastic Disease.

Vaginal Discharge, Abnormal

SYMPTOMS & FACTORS	POSSIBLE PROBLEM	WHAT TO DO
• Heavy vaginal discharge. • Vaginal pain.	Irritation or infection of cervix.	See Cervicitis.
• Green-yellow, bad-smelling vaginal discharge. • No other symptoms.	Vaginal infection.	See Vaginitis, Trichomonal.
• Heavy vaginal discharge that is normal in color and consistency. • Vaginal itching or soreness.	Irritation or infection.	See Vaginal Itching (in Symptoms section).
White, curd-like vaginal discharge.	Vaginal fungus infection.	See Vaginitis, Candidal.
• Green-yellow, bad-smelling vaginal discharge. • Tampon, diaphragm or cervical cup left in vagina.	Vaginal infection.	• Remove tampon, diaphragm or cup if you can. • If not, consult doctor.
• Heavy vaginal discharge that is normal in color and consistency. • Use of oral contraceptives. OR • Possible pregnancy.	Normal occurrence caused by hormone changes.	Consult doctor to confirm pregnancy.
Heavy vaginal discharge that is normal in color and consistency during ovulation occurring during middle days between periods.	Normal occurrence.	Nothing.
• Vaginal discharge. • Reddening of vagina.	Vaginal infection.	• See Chlamydia Infection. • See Vaginitis, Bacterial. • See Vaginitis, Postmenopausal.
• Vaginal discharge, which may or may not smell bad. • Redness, itching around genital area. • Young girl (before puberty).	Infection.	See Vulvovaginitis before Puberty.
• Red or brown vaginal discharge. • Occasional spotting of blood between menstrual periods.	Several disorders.	• See Cervical Polyps. • See Vaginal Bleeding, Unexpected (in Symptoms section).
• Green-yellow, bad-smelling vaginal discharge. • Pain in lower abdomen. • Frequent or painful urination.	Infection of reproductive organs.	• See Pelvic Inflammatory Disease. • See Gonorrhea.
• Heavy, bad-smelling vaginal discharge 2 or more days after childbirth. • Fever. • Abdominal pain.	Infection of uterus (puerperal infection).	Consult doctor.
• Leakage or gush of blood-tinged amniotic fluid from vagina. • Bad-smelling vaginal discharge.	Tear in amniotic fluid sac.	See Premature Rupture of the Membranes.

Vaginal Itching

SYMPTOMS & FACTORS	POSSIBLE PROBLEM	WHAT TO DO
• Vaginal itching. • Unusual vaginal discharge.	Several disorders.	• See Vulvovaginitis before Puberty (children only). • See Vaginitis, Bacterial. • See Vaginitis, Postmenopausal (women over 45). • See Pruritis Vulvae. • See Vaginal Discharge, Abnormal (in Symptoms section).
• Vaginal itching. • Use of antibiotics.	Vaginal infection.	• Consult doctor. • See Vaginitis, Candidal.
• Vaginal itching. • Use of chemical spray, ointment, cream, douche or contraceptive foam.	Irritation caused by chemical or drug.	• Consult doctor. • Discontinue use of possible irritant.
Vaginal itching in woman over age 38.	Decreasing level of estrogens at menopause.	See Pruritis Vulvae.
• Vaginal itching, plus 2 or more of following: • Unexplained weight loss. • Increased hunger and thirst. • Frequent urination. • Fatigue.	Sugar in urine (diabetes mellitus).	Consult doctor.

Vomiting, Recurrent Attacks

SYMPTOMS & FACTORS	POSSIBLE PROBLEM	WHAT TO DO
• Recurrent vomiting. • Burning sensation in chest or upper abdomen, especially when bending forward or lying down.	Stomach acid in esophagus (gastroesophageal reflux disease).	Consult doctor.
• Recurrent vomiting. • Occasional pain or tenderness in upper right abdomen. • No fever.	Gallbladder disorder.	Consult doctor.
• Recurrent vomiting. • Occasional pain or tenderness in upper right abdomen. • Fever.	Gallbladder inflammation (cholecystitis; cholangitis).	Consult doctor.
• Recurrent vomiting. • Poor appetite. • Jaundice (yellow skin and eyes).	Gallbladder or liver disorder.	Consult doctor.
• Recurrent vomiting. • Use of prescription or non-prescription drug.	Adverse reaction or side effect of drug.	• Consult doctor. • Discontinue use of nonprescription drug.
• Recurrent vomiting. • Pain or tenderness in center of upper abdomen. • Discomfort relieved by vomiting.	Peptic-ulcer disease.	Consult doctor.
Vomiting within hours after drinking alcohol.	Stomach inflammation (gastritis).	Consult doctor.
• Recurrent vomiting. • Pregnancy.	• Vomiting of early pregnancy. • Other pregnancy disorder.	• See Morning Sickness during Pregnancy. • See Hyperemesis Gravidarum.
Recurrent, self-induced vomiting.	Psychological disorder.	See Bulimia Nervosa.
• Vomiting. • Extreme dizziness. • Loss of balance.	Inner ear disorder (labyrinthitis).	Consult doctor.
• Recurrent vomiting. • Poor appetite. • Constant pain in upper abdomen.	Tumor.	Consult doctor.
• Recurrent vomiting without nausea. • Recurrent headaches, especially in morning.	• Bleeding inside skull. • Tumor.	Consult doctor.
• Bloody vomit. • Bleeding from several body parts.	Blood-clotting problem.	Consult doctor.
• Vomiting. • Extreme abdominal pain, swelling and gas.	Disorder of the pancreas (pancreatitis).	Consult doctor.

Vomiting, Sudden Attack (continued on next page)

SYMPTOMS & FACTORS	POSSIBLE PROBLEM	WHAT TO DO
• Vomiting. • Diarrhea. • Fever.	Infection of digestive tract (gastroenteritis).	Consult doctor.
• Vomiting. • Feelings of nervousness and apprehension (such as before going on stage).	Emotional upset.	• Vomiting should stop when emotions calm down. • See Anxiety. • See Panic Disorder.
• Vomiting. • Headache.	Headache disorder (migraine).	Consult doctor.
• Vomiting. • Use of prescription or nonprescription drug.	Adverse reaction or side effect of drug.	• Consult doctor about prescription drug. • Discontinue use of nonprescription drug.
• Vomiting. • Jaundice (yellow skin or eyes).	Gallbladder or liver disorder (hepatitis; gallstones).	Consult doctor.
Recent, recurrent vomiting attacks.	Several disorders.	See Vomiting, Recurrent Attacks (in Symptoms section).
• Vomiting. • Consumption of spoiled, contaminated or improperly prepared food.	Effect of toxins in food.	Consult doctor.
• Vomiting. • Dizziness.	Infection or disorder of inner ear (labyrinthitis; Meniere's disease).	Consult doctor.
• Vomiting. • Excessive consumption of alcohol or rich food.	Stomach inflammation (gastritis).	Consult doctor.
Vomiting of blood or dark "coffee ground" material.	Bleeding in stomach (ulcer; gastric erosion).	Call doctor now.
• Vomiting. • Severe abdominal pain. • No pain relief from vomiting.	Several disorders.	Call doctor now.
• Vomiting. • Dizziness, headache, faintness.	Gas inhalation (carbon monoxide poison).	Consult doctor.
• Vomiting. • Headache, plus any of following: • Eyes sensitive to light. • Drowsiness or confusion. • Pain when bending head forward.	Infection or bleeding in membranes around brain (meningitis).	Call doctor now.
• Vomiting. • Headache. • Head injury in last 24 hours.	Brain injury.	Call doctor now.

Vomiting, Sudden Attack (cont.)

SYMPTOMS & FACTORS	POSSIBLE PROBLEM	WHAT TO DO
• Vomiting. • Abdominal pain or swelling. • Inability to have bowel movement.	Blockage in intestines.	Call doctor now.
• Vomiting. • Eye pain. • Blurred vision.	Excess pressure inside eye (glaucoma).	Call doctor now.
• Vomiting and watery diarrhea. • Sudden high fever. • Rash that resembles sunburn.	Blood poisoning.	See Toxic Shock Syndrome.

Weight Gain

SYMPTOMS & FACTORS	POSSIBLE PROBLEM	WHAT TO DO
• Weight gain. • Change from active to sedentary lifestyle.	Calorie intake too high for current activity level.	Decrease food consumption and increase physical activity.
• Weight gain. • No other symptoms.	More calories consumed than burned.	See Obesity.
• Weight gain. • Depression.	Compensatory overeating.	See Depression.
• Weight gain. • Feeling of depression and tiredness. • Start of, or during, winter season.	Lack of light.	See Seasonal Affective Disorder.
• Weight gain. • Use of prescription or non-prescription drug that causes fluid retention, such as steroids, cortisone drugs, oral contraceptives or nonsteroid anti-inflammatory drugs.	Adverse reaction or side effect of drug.	Consult doctor.
• Weight gain. • Decreased tolerance for cold. • Dry skin or hair. • Fatigue. • Constipation.	Underactive thyroid gland.	See Hypothyroidism.
• Weight gain. • Recently discontinued smoking.	Normal occurrence.	Weight gain will soon stop. But be careful about what you eat. Get plenty of exercise.
Rapid weight gain during pregnancy.	Complication of pregnancy.	See Preeclampsia & Eclampsia.
• Weight gain. • High blood pressure or history of heart, kidney or liver disease.	Fluid retention caused by disorder of blood vessels, heart, liver or kidney.	Consult doctor.
• Weight gain with accumulation of fat over upper back and trunk. • Round face and puffy eyes.	Endocrine disorder (Cushing's syndrome).	Consult doctor.
Weight gain due to fluid retention.	Several disorders.	Consult doctor.

Weight Loss

SYMPTOMS & FACTORS	POSSIBLE PROBLEM	WHAT TO DO
• Weight loss, plus 2 or more of following: • Increased hunger. • Increased thirst. • Fatigue. • Family history of diabetes. • Frequent urination. • Itching rash in genital area.	Sugar in urine (diabetes mellitus).	Consult doctor.
• Weight loss, plus 2 or more of following: • Bulging eyes. • Excessive sweating. • Fatigue. • Anxiety. • Rapid heartbeat.	Overactive thyroid gland.	See Hyperthyroidism.
• Weight loss of 10 or more pounds. • Anxiety or depression.	• Effect of stress. • Psychological disorder.	• See Anxiety. • See Depression. • See Anorexia Nervosa. • See Bulimia Nervosa.
• Weight loss. • Current use of prescription drug.	Adverse reaction or side effect of drug.	Consult doctor.
• Weight loss. • Recurrent diarrhea or constipation. • Recurrent pain in lower abdomen. • Black stool.	• Inflammation of intestine. • Tumor.	Consult doctor.
• Weight loss. • Recurrent pain in upper abdomen.	• Peptic-ulcer disease. • Tumor. • Stress or emotional conflicts. • Intestinal inflammatory disorder.	Consult doctor.
• Weight loss, plus 2 or more of following: • Excessive sweating at night. • Fever. • Fatigue. • Persistent cough with blood in sputum.	Lung inflammation or infection (tuberculosis; bronchitis; bronchiectasis).	Consult doctor.
• Weight loss. • Recurrent diarrhea. • Pale, bulky, bad-smelling stool.	Poor digestion (malabsorption).	Consult doctor.
• Weight loss. • Increased physical activity.	Normal occurrence.	Consult doctor if weight loss is not expected and continues longer than 2 weeks.
• Weight loss. • Recurrent respiratory and skin infections.	Virus infection.	See HIV & AIDS.

Weight Loss (cont.)

SYMPTOMS & FACTORS	POSSIBLE PROBLEM	WHAT TO DO
• Unexplained weight and appetite loss. • Abdominal discomfort. • Hard mass in upper right abdomen.	Liver tumor (hepatoma).	Consult doctor.

Breasts

Breast Abscess

GENERAL INFORMATION

DEFINITION—An infected area of breast tissue that becomes filled with pus when the body fights the infection. It involves breast tissue, nipple, milk glands and milk ducts.

SIGNS & SYMPTOMS
- Breast pain, tenderness, redness or hardness.
- Body aches.
- Fever and chills.
- A general ill feeling.
- Drainage (pus) from the affected breast.
- Tender lymph glands in the underarm area.

CAUSES—Bacteria that enter the breast through the nipple (usually a cracked nipple during the early days of breast-feeding).

RISK INCREASES WITH
- Postpartum mastitis.
- Diabetes mellitus.
- Rheumatoid arthritis.
- Use of steroid medications.
- Heavy cigarette smoking.
- Lumpectomy with radiation.
- Silicone implants.

HOW TO PREVENT
- Clean the nipples and breasts thoroughly before and after nursing.
- Lubricate the nipples after nursing with vitamin A & D ointment, or other topical medication if recommended, to keep the nipple from drying out and the tissue from cracking and fissuring.
- Avoid clothing that irritates the breasts.

PROBABLE OUTCOME—Usually curable in 8 to 10 days with treatment. Draining the abscess is occasionally necessary to hasten healing.

POSSIBLE COMPLICATIONS
- It is usually recommended that breast-feeding from the infected breast be discontinued until the abscess has healed. However, it is rarely necessary to discontinue nursing from the unaffected breast. Antibiotics may be necessary, particularly if mastitis is also present. Most antibiotics and painkillers can be continued along with breast-feeding. Specific questions in regard to the newborn should be directed to your pediatrician.
- Rarely, a fistula (abnormal passage between two organs or between the body and the outside) may develop.

HOW TO TREAT

GENERAL MEASURES
- Use warm water (or cold water if it is more soothing) soaks to relieve pain and hasten healing.
- Discontinue nursing the baby from the infected breast until it heals. Use a breast pump to express milk regularly from the infected breast until you can resume nursing on that side.
- Surgery to drain the abscess.

MEDICATION
- Antibiotics, if needed to fight infection. Antibiotics may reduce the effectiveness of some oral contraceptives. If you are using oral contraceptives for birth control, discuss this with your doctor.
- Prescription pain medication should generally be required for only 2 to 7 days following the procedure.

ACTIVITY—After treatment, resume normal activity as soon as symptoms improve.

DIET—No special diet.

CALL YOUR DOCTOR IF

- You or a family member has symptoms of a breast abscess.
- Any of the following occur during treatment:
  Fever.
  Pain becomes unbearable.
  Infection seems to be spreading, despite treatment.
  Symptoms don't improve in 72 hours.
- New, unexplained symptoms develop. Drugs used in treatment may produce side effects.

Breast Abscess

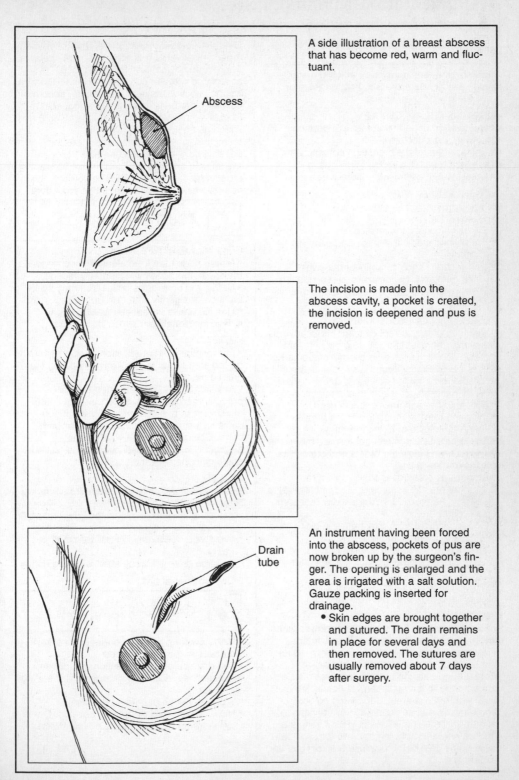

A side illustration of a breast abscess that has become red, warm and fluctuant.

Abscess

The incision is made into the abscess cavity, a pocket is created, the incision is deepened and pus is removed.

Drain tube

An instrument having been forced into the abscess, pockets of pus are now broken up by the surgeon's finger. The opening is enlarged and the area is irrigated with a salt solution. Gauze packing is inserted for drainage.
- Skin edges are brought together and sutured. The drain remains in place for several days and then removed. The sutures are usually removed about 7 days after surgery.

Breast Augmentation
(Augmentation Mammoplasty)

 ## GENERAL INFORMATION

DEFINITION—Implantation of artificial material inside the female breasts to enlarge them or give them a different shape.

REASONS FOR PROCEDURE
• Restoration of normal breast appearance following a mastectomy.
• Enlargement of the breasts in patients who have less breast tissue than they desire.
• Correction of asymmetry of the breasts.

RISK INCREASES WITH
• Smoking.
• Obesity.
• Excess alcohol consumption.
• Preexisting medical illness (e.g., diabetes, hypertension).
• Use of drugs such as antihypertensives, muscle relaxants, tranquilizers, sleep inducers, insulin, sedatives, beta-adrenergic blockers or cortisone.

DESCRIPTION OF PROCEDURE
• Because of the current concern about adverse reactions to breast implants, the only implant type presently available for cosmetic augmentation is saline-filled; silicone gel implants are still available, on a limited basis and under clinical trial, to some breast reconstruction patients.
• A local or general anesthesia is used.
• Incisions may be made under the breast, through the nipple or in the armpit.
• The breast tissue is brought forward by raising muscles from below the breast or the muscles next to the chest wall.
• A pocket is created, and the implant (a mammary prosthesis usually filled with saline) is inserted. The procedures are usually repeated on the other breast.
• Occasionally, a drain may be left in place for a few days to promote healing.
• The skin is closed with sutures or clips, which usually can be removed about 1 week after surgery. A light bandage is applied.
• A bra or elastic bandage is fitted to give support and to reduce possible bleeding.

PROBABLE OUTCOME
• Expect complete healing without complications. Allow about 2 weeks recovery from surgery.
• You should have realistic expectations about the results this type of surgery can deliver. Breast augmentation usually improves physical appearance, but results can vary considerably from woman to woman, depending on your anatomy, as well as your surgeon's technique and ability. You should ask to view a variety of "before and after" photographs so that you can have some idea of the possible results you may experience.

POSSIBLE COMPLICATIONS
Over the past few years, there have been many reports of adverse reactions to breast implants. There are known risks including those associated with the surgical procedure (surgical-wound infection, risks of anesthesia, abnormal bleeding, etc.); implant risks (leaking, scar formation, infection, calcium deposits, etc.) and concerns about interference with mammography. In addition, there are the possible risks of autoimmune (such as rheumatoid arthritis) and connective tissue disorders (such as lupus). Be sure you are aware of all the risks and benefits of this procedure.

 ## FOLLOW-UP CARE

GENERAL MEASURES
• A hard ridge may form along the incisions. As they heal, the ridges will gradually recede.
• Bathe and shower as usual. You may wash the incisions gently with mild unscented soap.
• Use ice packs to reduce swelling and to relieve incisional pain.

MEDICATION
• Prescription pain medication should generally be required for only 2 to 7 days following the procedure.
• Antibiotics may be prescribed to fight or prevent infection. Antibiotics may reduce the effectiveness of oral contraceptives. If you are currently using oral contraceptives for birth control, discuss this with your doctor.
• You may use nonprescription drugs, such as acetaminophen, for minor pain.

ACTIVITY
• Have someone drive you home from surgery. Resume normal activities slowly. You will be provided with specific instructions depending on individual requirements.
• Avoid vigorous exercise for 6 weeks after surgery.
• Resume driving 1 week after returning home.

DIET—No special diet.

 ## CALL YOUR DOCTOR IF

• Pain, swelling, redness, drainage or bleeding increases in the surgical area.
• You develop signs of infection: headache, muscle aches, dizziness or a general ill feeling and fever.
• You experience nausea or vomiting.
• New, unexplained symptoms develop. Drugs used in treatment may produce side effects.

Breast Augmentation
(Augmentation Mammoplasty)

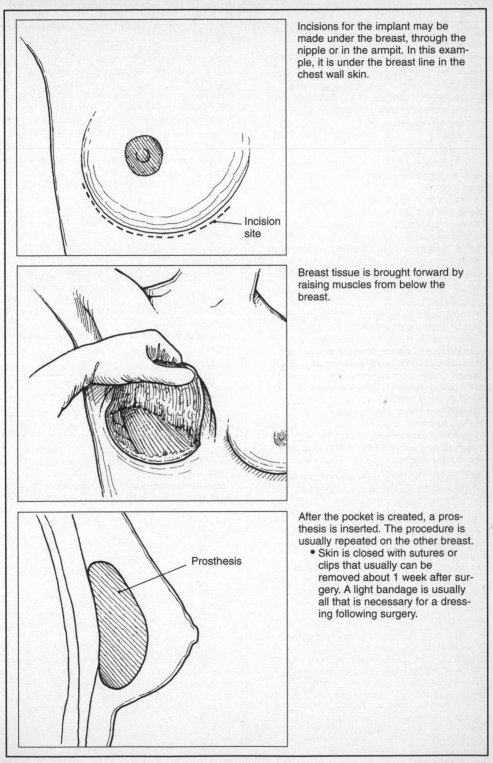

Incisions for the implant may be made under the breast, through the nipple or in the armpit. In this example, it is under the breast line in the chest wall skin.

Incision site

Breast tissue is brought forward by raising muscles from below the breast.

After the pocket is created, a prosthesis is inserted. The procedure is usually repeated on the other breast.

• Skin is closed with sutures or clips that usually can be removed about 1 week after surgery. A light bandage is usually all that is necessary for a dressing following surgery.

Prosthesis

Breast Biopsy by Incision

GENERAL INFORMATION

DEFINITION—Removal of a lump or cyst from one of the breasts.

REASONS FOR PROCEDURE—Signs or symptoms that may indicate breast cancer or the results of mammography suggestive of breast cancer. Pathologic examination of the removed tissue aids in diagnosis.

RISK INCREASES WITH
• Obesity.
• Smoking.
• Poor nutrition.
• Preexisting medical illness (e.g., diabetes, hypertension).
• Poor nutrition, especially inadequate iron intake that has led to anemia.
• Use of drugs such as antihypertensives, muscle relaxants, tranquilizers, sleep inducers, insulin, sedatives, beta-adrenergic blockers or cortisone.

DESCRIPTION OF PROCEDURE
• Biopsy is performed under local or general anesthesia.
• Needles may be inserted into the breast to localize the lump or cyst.
• An incision is made over the cyst or lump to be removed. It is often possible to make a cosmetic incision by cutting at the edge of the areola.
• The cyst or lump is cut free of surrounding tissue and removed.
• Bleeding is controlled with sutures or electrocautery.
• The skin is closed with sutures or surgical clips, which usually can be removed about 1 week after surgery.

PROBABLE OUTCOME—Expect complete healing without complications. Allow about 2 weeks for recovery from surgery.

POSSIBLE COMPLICATIONS
• Excessive bleeding.
• Surgical-wound infection.
• Unsightly scar on breast (rare).
• In cases of a large biopsy, or if the tissue removed is close to the skin, there can be some minor changes in the contour of the breast.

FOLLOW-UP CARE

GENERAL MEASURES
• A hard ridge should form along the incision. As it heals, the ridge will recede gradually.
• Use an electric heating pad, a heat lamp or a warm compress to relieve incisional pain.
• Bathe and shower as usual. You may wash the incision gently with mild unscented soap.
• Wear a supportive bra. Apply bandages to the surgical wound, and change them as directed.

MEDICATION
• Your doctor may prescribe pain relievers. Don't take prescription pain medication for longer than 4 to 7 days. Use only as much as you need.
• You may use nonprescription drugs, such as acetaminophen, for minor pain.

ACTIVITY
• Have someone drive you home following the procedure.
• To help recovery and aid your well-being, resume daily activities, including work, as soon as possible.
• Avoid vigorous exercise for 2 weeks after surgery.
• Resume driving 3 to 5 days after returning home.

DIET—No special diet.

CALL YOUR DOCTOR IF

• Pain, swelling, redness, drainage or bleeding increases in the surgical area.
• You develop signs of infection: headache, muscle aches, dizziness or a general ill feeling and fever.
• New, unexplained symptoms develop. Drugs used in treatment may produce side effects.

Breast Biopsy by Incision

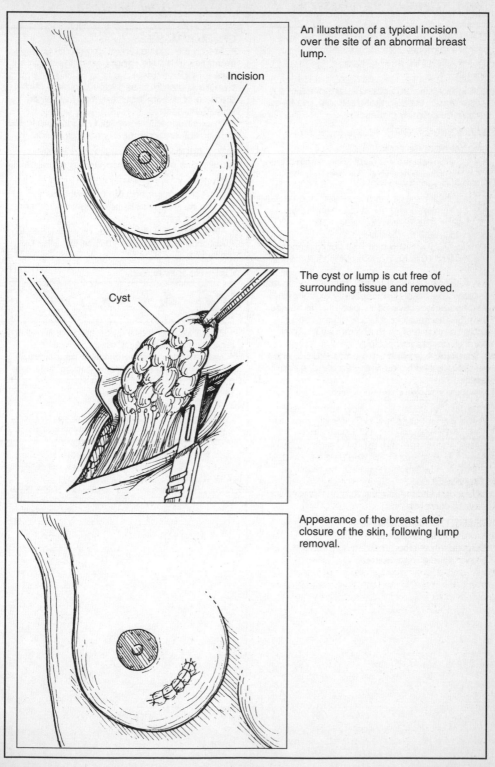

An illustration of a typical incision over the site of an abnormal breast lump.

Incision

The cyst or lump is cut free of surrounding tissue and removed.

Cyst

Appearance of the breast after closure of the skin, following lump removal.

Breast Biopsy by Needle Aspiration

 GENERAL INFORMATION

DEFINITION—Removal of fluid or tissue from one of the breasts. Needle aspirations are often the best first step for diagnosis of a lump in the breast.

REASONS FOR PROCEDURE—Diagnosis of a thickening or lump so that treatment and follow-up can be properly planned.

RISK INCREASES WITH—None expected.

DESCRIPTION OF PROCEDURE
• A local anesthetic will usually be administered.
• A small hollow needle is inserted into the thickening or lump.
• If the thickening or lump is a cyst, fluid usually can be removed and the cyst will shrink or disappear. This is often considered both diagnostic and therapeutic.
• In some cases, the removed fluid is sent to the laboratory to be examined for abnormal cells.
• If a solid tumor is detected, tissue is removed through the needle for laboratory examination. The tissue is recovered by passing the needle through the suspicious tissue several times, while using a syringe to aspirate as big a sample of cells as possible.
• The needle is withdrawn; pressure is exerted on the site of the biopsy, then a bandage is applied.

PROBABLE OUTCOME
• Usually, the results will show normal breast tissue without abnormal cells. Most lumps are benign (noncancerous), fluid-filled cysts.
• Abnormal tissue may exhibit a wide range of benign or malignant cells and follow-up tests will be conducted to determine the exact diagnosis.
• Expect complete healing from the procedure without complications.

POSSIBLE COMPLICATIONS
• Infection in surgical area (rare).
• Collection of blood (hematoma) under the skin where needle was inserted.

 FOLLOW-UP CARE

GENERAL MEASURES
• Use an electric heating pad or a warm compress to relieve minor pain in the surgical area.
• Bathe and shower as usual. You may wash the area of needle insertion gently with mild unscented soap.
• Wear a supportive bra. Apply bandages to the biopsy site, and change them as directed.

MEDICATION—You may use nonprescription drugs, such as acetaminophen, for minor pain.

ACTIVITY
• To help recovery and aid your well-being, resume daily activities, including work, as soon as you are able.
• Allow about 1 week for recovery from surgery. Avoid vigorous exercise for 2 weeks after the procedure.

DIET—No special diet.

 CALL YOUR DOCTOR IF

• Pain, swelling, redness, drainage or bleeding increases in the surgical area.
• You develop signs of infection: headache, muscle aches, dizziness or a general ill feeling and fever.

Breast Biopsy by Needle Aspiration

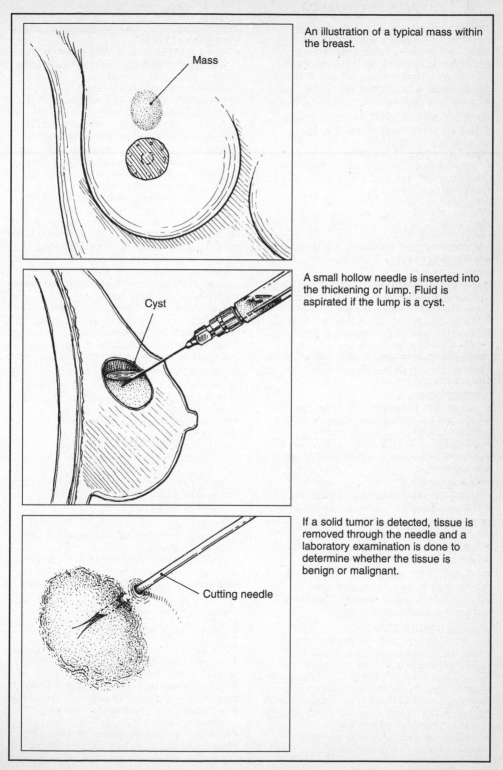

An illustration of a typical mass within the breast.

Mass

A small hollow needle is inserted into the thickening or lump. Fluid is aspirated if the lump is a cyst.

Cyst

If a solid tumor is detected, tissue is removed through the needle and a laboratory examination is done to determine whether the tissue is benign or malignant.

Cutting needle

Breast Cancer

GENERAL INFORMATION

DEFINITION—A malignant growth of breast tissue. Breast cancer can spread to nearby lymph glands, lungs, pleura, bone (especially the skull and spinal column), pelvis and liver. Breast cancer is rare before age 30; the peak ages are from 45 to 65.

SIGNS & SYMPTOMS—No symptoms in early stages, but presymptom stages may be detected by mammogram.
- Swelling or lump in the breast.
- Vague discomfort in the breast without pain.
- Retraction of the nipple.
- Distorted breast contour.
- Dimpled or pitted skin in the breast.
- Enlarged nodes under the arm (late stages).
- Bloody discharge from the nipple (rare).

CAUSES—Unknown.

RISK INCREASES WITH
- Women over 50.
- Women who have not had children or who conceived in the late fertile years.
- Family history of breast cancer.
- Genetic factors or markers (BRCA1; BRCA2).
- Previous breast biopsy showing atypical cells.
- Early menstruation (before age 12); late menopause; first pregnancy after age 30.
- Previous breast cancer in one breast.
- Obesity or a high-fat diet.
- Radiation exposure.
- Patients with endometrial or ovarian cancer.
- Additional risk factors may include prolonged estrogen intake and excessive alcohol consumption. Studies are still being conducted to determine the risks associated with these and other factors.

HOW TO PREVENT
- Eat a well-balanced diet that is low in fat.
- If you are pregnant, consider breast-feeding your baby. Women who have breast-fed have a lower incidence of breast cancer.
- A drug, such as tamoxifen, may be prescribed for women at high risk for breast cancer.

PROBABLE OUTCOME—Breast cancer is often curable if diagnosed and treated early. The 10-year survival rate is related to the clinical stage of the disease at diagnosis.

POSSIBLE COMPLICATIONS
- Spread to vital organs if not treated early.
- Adverse reactions to drugs and radiation.
- Lymphedema (a painful swelling of soft tissues) can develop in the arm or hand on the affected side. The radiation or removal of lymph nodes can interfere with the normal flow of fluid through the lymphatic vessels, causing swelling, decreased mobility and infection.
- Postsurgical complications (e.g., wound infection, limited shoulder motion).

HOW TO TREAT

GENERAL MEASURES
- The following measures will not prevent breast cancer but will help by allowing early diagnosis should breast cancer develop:
  Monthly breast self-examinations.
  Regular professional examinations.
  A baseline mammogram between ages 35 to 40. Have mammograms every 1 to 2 years to age 49, and annually after age 50.
- Diagnostic tests will include a physical exam, biopsy and mammogram. Following the initial diagnosis, ultrasound, bone scan, chest x-ray and liver scans are often performed.
- The decision for treatment is very complex, and often confusing. Be sure all options are explained and that the risks and benefits of each are thoroughly understood. It is important for you to be an informed and participating member of your health-care team.
- Surgery (mastectomy) to remove the lump, or breast, lymph glands, and lymphatic channels and muscles under the breast.
- Other treatment options include radiation therapy, hormonal or chemotherapy, and bone marrow transplant (still experimental).
- See the Resource section of this book for additional information.

MEDICATION
- For minor discomfort during treatment, you may use nonprescription drugs such as acetaminophen, ibuprofen or aspirin.
- Other drugs that may be prescribed:
  Pain relievers.
  Anticancer drugs, such as fluorouracil, cyclophosphamide, methotrexate, chlorambucil, vincristine, doxorubicin or melphalan.
  Hormones (male and female).
  Cortisone drugs.

ACTIVITY
- If surgery is performed, resume your normal activities gradually.
- Exercise for rehabilitation following surgery will depend on how much tissue has been removed and your general physical condition.

DIET—No special diet. Maintain good nutrition.

CALL YOUR DOCTOR IF

- You or a family member discovers a lump or other change in the breast.
- Following surgery or radiation, you experience nausea, vomiting, fever or swelling in the arm.
- You have pain that is not controlled by medication.
- New, unexplained symptoms develop. Drugs used in treatment may produce side effects.

Breast Implant Safety

 GENERAL INFORMATION

DEFINITION—Breast implants have been marketed since the early 1960s, long before the first medical device law was enacted in 1976 that gives regulation authority to the FDA (Food and Drug Administration). Over a million American women have had implant surgery for augmentation (to enlarge or reshape their breasts) or for reconstruction following mastectomy (removal of the breast) to treat breast cancer. Prior to 1992, most of the implants consisted of rubber silicone envelopes filled with silicone gel; about 10% were filled with saline (saltwater). A growing number of reports of adverse reactions raised safety concerns about the breast implants. The FDA ordered the silicone-filled implants off the market in April 1992. They are currently available only in clinical studies, to women seeking breast reconstruction after breast cancer surgery. The saline-filled implants were allowed to stay on the market for both reconstruction and augmentation. (Information adapted in part from the *FDA Consumer* magazine.)

MEDICAL STUDIES ON IMPLANTS
• Numerous medical studies have been conducted and more are ongoing to assess the risks of breast implants.
• Some recent studies comparing the rate of immune-related diseases in women with implants do provide some reassurance to women with implants that they are not at a greatly increased risk of these disorders.
• Several studies have indicated there is no increased risk of breast cancer in women with implants. However, many of the women are not yet in the age group that is more prone to cancer so future effects are unknown. Long-term studies to look at this are under way.
• Other ongoing studies are intended to assess short-term safety data; rates of capsular contracture (hardening of the breast due to excessive contracting of scar tissue); rupture; complications such as infection and hematoma (collection of blood that may cause swelling, pain and bruising); quality-of-life benefits; extent of interference with mammography as well as other safety concerns.
• Though saline-filled implants are still available, studies are being conducted on them as well.

KNOWN RISKS OF BREAST IMPLANTS
Surgical risks:
• Possible complications of general anesthesia.
• Infection (which can sometimes necessitate temporary removal of the implant).
• Hematoma.
• Hemorrhage (abnormal bleeding).
• Thrombosis (abnormal clotting).
• Skin necrosis (skin tissue death).
• Excessive scarring.

Implant risks:
• Capsular contracture (hardening of the breast due to scar tissue).
• Leak or rupture (silicone implants may leak or rupture slowly, releasing silicone into surrounding tissue); saline implants may rupture suddenly and deflate (usually requires immediate removal or replacement).
• Temporary or permanent change or loss of sensation in the nipple or breast tissue.
• Formation of calcium deposits in surrounding tissue, possibly causing pain and hardening.
• Shifting from the original placement, giving the breast an unnatural look.
• Interference with mammography readings, possibly delaying breast cancer detection by "hiding" a suspicious lesion. Also, it may be difficult to distinguish calcium deposits formed in the scar tissue from a tumor when interpreting a mammogram. Advise any mammogram technician that you have implants.

POSSIBLE RISKS OF BREAST IMPLANTS
• Autoimmune or connective tissue disorders. Signs include joint pain and swelling; skin tightening, redness or swelling; swelling of hands or feet; rash; swollen glands or lymph nodes; unusual fatigue; general aching; greater chance of getting colds, viruses and flu; unusual hair loss; memory problems; headaches; muscle weakness or burning; nausea or vomiting; and irritable bowel syndrome. Recent studies have shown there is not a large increased risk.
• Fibrositis/fibromyalgia-like disorders (pain, tenderness and stiffness of muscles, tendons and ligaments).

CONSIDERATIONS
• For cosmetic breast enlargement, saline-filled implants are the only type currently available. Prior to any surgery, information will be provided that details risks and benefits and a consent form will need to be signed.
• For breast reconstruction following mastectomy, both silicone-filled and saline-filled implants are currently available. Prior to any surgery, information will be provided that details risks and benefits of each and a consent form will need to be signed.
• Women with existing implants should see their doctor if any symptoms listed as known risks or possible risks develop. Recognize that many of these symptoms can be caused by a number of disorders that have no association with breast implants.
• See the Resource section of this book for additional information.

CALL YOUR DOCTOR IF

You have questions or concerns about breast implants.

Breast Reconstruction

GENERAL INFORMATION

DEFINITION—Reconstruction of the female breast during mastectomy or at a later date. You and your surgeon should have a clear understanding of what is to be done during surgery, but the surgeon will need some leeway in case unexpected problems occur.

REASONS FOR PROCEDURE—Reconstruction of the breast following a mastectomy for breast cancer is usually done for psychological and cosmetic reasons. It is becoming the standard procedure and is normally covered by medical insurance.

RISK INCREASES WITH
- Obesity.
- Smoking.
- Excess alcohol consumption.
- Preexisting medical illness (e.g., diabetes, hypertension).
- Poor nutrition, especially inadequate iron intake that has led to anemia.

DESCRIPTION OF PROCEDURE—Several options are available and additional methods are undergoing development:
- During mastectomy: If there is sufficient muscle and skin to cover the implant, a simple silicone gel bag implant may be all that is required. If additional muscle and skin is needed, it is brought in (usually from a nearby location on the body) to cover the implant.
- Temporary expander: During the mastectomy or later, a silicone bag with an attached valve is implanted under the skin and muscle. The bag is inflated at scheduled intervals over a period of time (usually several months) by the addition of a saltwater solution. This inflation (or expansion) is done in the doctor's office and should not produce any pain. In a subsequent operation, the surgeon will remove the tissue expander and place a new, permanent silicone- or saline-filled implant in the newly enlarged space.
- Tissue to form a "new breast" is obtained from the abdominal wall or back. An implant is not necessary. This procedure produces the most normal and natural breast in appearance and feel, but usually requires more surgery than with the other methods described.
- In some patients, the other (noncancerous) breast may be altered to better match the reconstructed breast.
- The nipple-areola area can also be reconstructed. This is generally done after breast reconstruction healing so that the positioning is correct. Skin may be grafted from the inner thigh near the groin. Color may be added by tattooing. For some patients, the nipple area may be preserved during mastectomy and used in reconstruction.

PROBABLE OUTCOME
- Expect complete healing without complications. Allow about 6 weeks for recovery from surgery.
- There is no evidence that breast reconstruction might increase the risk of the cancer recurring.

POSSIBLE COMPLICATIONS—Over the past few years, there have been many reports of adverse reactions to breast implants. There are known risks including those associated with the surgical procedure; implant risks (leaking, scar formation, calcium deposits, etc.) and concerns about interference with mammography. In addition, there are the possible risks of autoimmune (such as rheumatoid arthritis) and connective tissue disorders (such as lupus). Be sure you are aware of all the risks and benefits of this procedure if implants are used. A consent form will need to be signed before the surgery is scheduled.

FOLLOW-UP CARE

GENERAL MEASURES
- Bathe and shower as usual. You may wash the incision gently with mild unscented soap.
- Use warm compress to relieve incisional pain.
- See the Resource section of this book for additional information.

MEDICATION
- Your doctor may prescribe pain relievers. Don't take prescription pain medication for longer than 4 to 7 days. Take only as much as you need.
- Antibiotics to prevent or fight infection. Antibiotics may interfere with the effectiveness of oral contraceptives. If you are currently using oral contraceptives for birth control, discuss this with your doctor.
- You may use nonprescription drugs, such as acetaminophen, for minor pain. Avoid aspirin.

ACTIVITY
- Return to work and normal activity as soon as possible.
- Perform implant exercises to help reduce the risk of capsular contracture.
- Special exercises to aid in recovery of arm mobility may be recommended.

DIET—No special diet.

CALL YOUR DOCTOR IF

- Pain, swelling, redness, drainage or bleeding increases in the surgical area.
- You develop signs of infection: headache, muscle aches, dizziness or a general ill feeling and fever.
- New, unexplained symptoms develop. Drugs used in treatment may produce side effects.

Breast Reconstruction

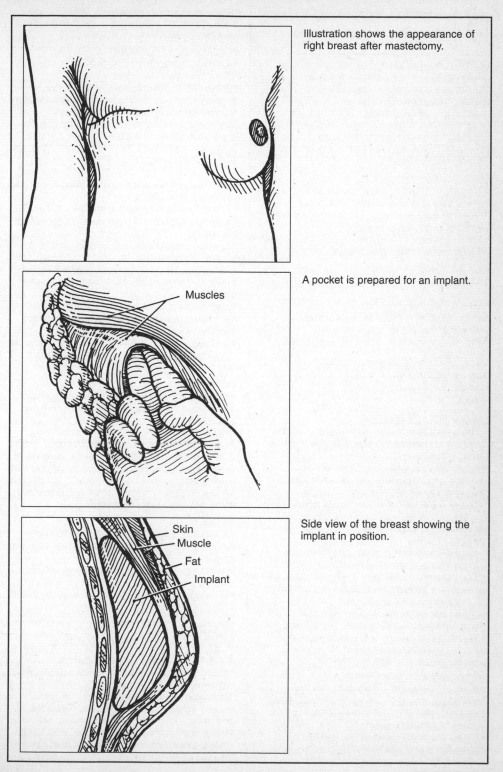

Illustration shows the appearance of right breast after mastectomy.

A pocket is prepared for an implant.

Muscles

Side view of the breast showing the implant in position.

Skin
Muscle
Fat
Implant

Breast Reduction
(Reduction Mammoplasty)

 GENERAL INFORMATION

DEFINITION—Removal of excess tissue and overlying skin from the female breasts. Usually, this surgery also includes reconstruction of breast shape. Often, this surgery is covered by medical insurance, particularly if minimum requirements are met for the amount of tissue removed from each breast. Many insurance companies require a minimum removal of 10 to 16 ounces per breast.

REASONS FOR PROCEDURE
• Reduction of overly large breasts to improve appearance and/or emotional well-being.
• Relief of back and neck pain caused by the weight of overly large breasts.
• Reconstruction of a breast to match a surgical change made in the other breast.

RISK INCREASES WITH
• Obesity.
• Smoking.
• Excess alcohol consumption.
• Poor nutrition, especially inadequate iron intake that has led to anemia.
• Preexisting medical illness (e.g., diabetes, hypertension).
• Use of drugs such as antihypertensives, muscle relaxants, tranquilizers, sleep inducers, insulin, sedatives, beta-adrenergic blockers or cortisone.

DESCRIPTION OF PROCEDURE
• The breast is marked where the skin will be removed and where the nipple will be after tissue is removed.
• A general anesthetic is administered by injection and inhalation, with an airway tube placed in the windpipe.
• The skin between the new nipple location and the natural nipple location is incised and removed. The nipple stays attached to underlying tissue.
• Another incision is made below the nipple. Excess tissue is removed through this incision.
• The tissue removed from the breasts should be sent to a pathology laboratory and analyzed for any early sign of breast cancer.
• Drains are left in place to prevent fluid or blood from accumulating under the sutures.
• The skin is closed with fine sutures, which usually can be removed about 10 to 14 days after surgery.

PROBABLE OUTCOME
• Expect complete healing without complications. Allow about 4 weeks for recovery from surgery.
• The breasts may take 3 to 12 weeks to assume their final shape.
• Some women experience heightened or decreased nipple sensitivity following surgery.

• The ability to breast-feed in the future cannot be guaranteed.

POSSIBLE COMPLICATIONS
• Excessive bleeding.
• Surgical-wound infection.
• Abnormal scarring (called keloids) may necessitate a second surgery for a scar revision.
• Development of small, tumor-like cysts (seromas) or collections of blood and serum in the breast tissue as it heals.

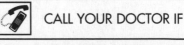 FOLLOW-UP CARE

GENERAL MEASURES
• A small ridge may form along the incision. The ridge should heal and gradually recede without treatment.
• Use ice packs to reduce swelling and to relieve incisional pain.
• Move and elevate your legs often while resting in bed to decrease the likelihood of deep-vein clots.
• Bathe and shower as usual. You may wash the incision gently with mild unscented soap.
• Women over age 30 should have a mammogram both before and six months following surgery. The postoperative mammogram will serve as a baseline for future mammograms.

MEDICATION
• Prescription pain medication should generally be required for only 2 to 7 days following the procedure.
• Antibiotics to fight infection, if necessary. Antibiotics may reduce the effectiveness of oral contraceptives. If you are currently using oral contraceptives for birth control, discuss this with your doctor.
• You may use nonprescription drugs, such as acetaminophen, for minor pain.

ACTIVITY
• To help recovery and aid your well-being, resume daily activities, including work, as soon as you are able.
• Avoid vigorous exercise for 6 weeks after surgery.
• Resume driving 1 month after returning home.

DIET—No special diet.

CALL YOUR DOCTOR IF

• Pain, swelling, redness, drainage or bleeding increases in the surgical area.
• You develop signs of infection: headache, muscle aches, dizziness or a general ill feeling and fever.
• New, unexplained symptoms develop. Drugs used in treatment may produce side effects.

Breast Reduction (Reduction Mammoplasty)

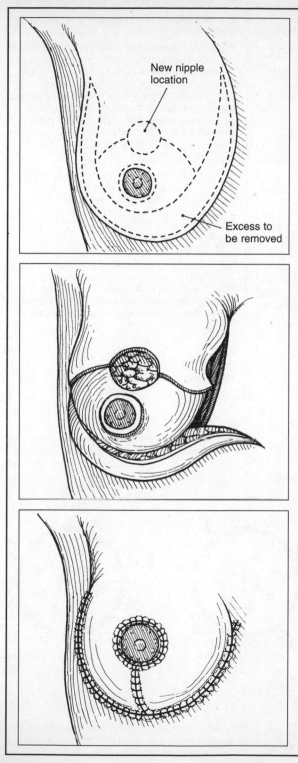

An illustration showing markings on the breast where skin will be removed and the nipple will be placed after the reduction procedure.

New nipple location

Excess to be removed

Skin between the new nipple location and the natural nipple location is incised and removed. The nipple stays attached to the underlying tissue.

Another incision is made below the nipple. Excess tissue is removed, drains are left in place to prevent collection of fluid, and skin is closed with fine sutures. Sutures are usually removed about 10 to 14 days after surgery.

Breast Self-Examination

WHEN TO DO BSE

The best time is about a week after your period ends when your breasts are not tender or swollen. If you are not having regular periods, do BSE on the same day every month.

HOW TO DO BSE

1. Lie down with a pillow under your right shoulder. Place your right arm behind your head.

2. Use the finger pads of the three middle fingers on your left hand to feel for lumps in the right breast. The finger pads are the top third of each finger.

3. Press firmly enough to know how your breast feels. A firm ridge in the lower curve of each breast is normal. If you're not sure how hard to press, talk with your health-care provider, or try to copy the way the doctor or nurse does it.

4. Move around the breast in a set way. You can choose either the up and down line, the circle or the wedge, but be sure to do it the same way every time. Go over the entire breast area, and remember how your breast feels from month to month.

5. Repeat the exam on your left breast, using the finger pads of the right hand.

6. If you find any changes, see your doctor right away.

7. Repeat the examination of both breasts while standing, with your one arm behind your head. The upright position makes it easier to check the upper, outer part of the breasts (toward your armpit). This is where about half of breast cancers are found. You may want to do the upright part of the BSE while you are in the shower. Your soapy hands will make it easy to check how your breasts feel as they glide over the wet skin.

8. For added safety, you might want to check your breasts by standing in front of a mirror right after your BSE each month. See if there are any changes in the way your breasts look, such as dimpling of the skin, changes in the nipple, redness or swelling.

Note: Reprinted from the American Cancer Society web page (www.cancer.org) by the permission of the American Cancer Society Inc.

BREAST SELF EXAMINATION (BSE) PATTERNS

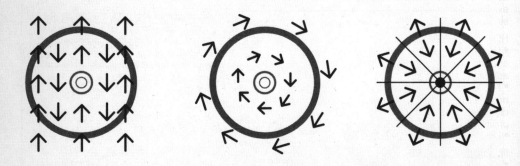

Fibrocystic Breast Changes (Breast Lump)

GENERAL INFORMATION

DEFINITION—A common condition of the female breast characterized usually by nonmalignant lumps and pain. It can affect females from puberty to around age 50 (about 20% of premenopausal women have the disorder). It often disappears after menopause (unless estrogen-replacement therapy is used). Since it is so common, it is no longer considered a disease and is usually not a cause for concern.

SIGNS & SYMPTOMS
• Lumps are usually in both breasts. Solitary lumps may occur, but multiple lumps are common.
• Lumps offer resistance when pressed with fingertips; they may be tender.
• Generalized breast pain, especially just before menstrual periods.
• Lumps often enlarge before menstrual periods and shrink afterward.
• Lumps come in different sizes. When the lumps are relatively large and near the surface, they can be moved freely within the breast.
• Lumps deep within the breast may be indistinguishable from breast cancer.
• Nipple discharge.

CAUSES—Unknown but probably related to estrogen and other hormones produced by the ovaries and possibly to dietary fat intake.

RISK
• Unknown.
• Often, there is a family history of benign breast lumps or cysts.
• Some studies indicate that drinking caffeinated beverages, having a high dietary fat intake, and smoking cigarettes are all associated with a higher incidence and greater extent of fibrocystic breast changes. Other studies have failed to show them as risk factors.

HOW TO PREVENT
• Until research is conclusive, do not smoke and avoid drinking caffeinated beverages. Also adhere to a low-fat diet.
• Monthly breast self-examination to check breasts for lumps and changes in lumps after diagnosis. Report any changes to your physician.
• Routine mammogram studies.

PROBABLE OUTCOME
• Women with fibrocystic breast changes continue to have breast lumps that appear and dissolve; some remain permanently. They do not jeopardize your health.
• Some cysts can be aspirated (removal of the fluid with a hollow needle) in a doctor's office, causing the lump to disappear. If the lump does not disappear completely after aspiration, it may be cancerous and should be diagnosed by biopsy and microscopic analysis.

POSSIBLE COMPLICATIONS—Rarely, some lumps appear benign but are cancerous. Diagnostic studies, including biopsy, are often necessary to rule out malignancy.

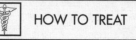

HOW TO TREAT

GENERAL MEASURES
• Diagnostic tests include mammogram, ultrasound (useful for distinguishing cystic from solid lesions) and surgical diagnostic procedures such as biopsy or cyst aspiration.
• Examine your breasts carefully each month. The best time to do the exam is 7 to 10 days after the start of your menstrual cycle, when breasts are usually least lumpy or tender.
• Visit the doctor at least every year for a breast exam or other studies. If you have a family history of cancer, more frequent examinations may be recommended.
• Cold compresses may help relieve discomfort or pain.
• Wear a well-fitting, supportive bra.
• Sometimes excision of benign tumors or fat necrosis lesions is recommended.

MEDICATION
• For pain, spironolactone and vitamin B-6 or iodine (kelp tablets) may be recommended.
• A mild diuretic for 7 to 10 days before menstruation may help some patients.
• For more severe symptoms, danazol or bromocriptine may be prescribed.
• There is some evidence that vitamin E may be beneficial.

ACTIVITY—No restrictions.

DIET
• Avoid beverages that contain caffeine (coffee, tea, some soft drinks).
• Avoid fatty and fried foods; reduce salt in the diet.

CALL YOUR DOCTOR IF

• You have undiagnosed lumps in the breast.
• You detect a change in a lump, or new lumps appear.
• You experience breast swelling, pain, redness, skin dimpling, nipple inversion (nipple turns "inside out") or discharge from the nipple.
• You have not had a breast exam in 2 years.
• New, unexplained symptoms develop. Drugs used in treatment may produce side effects.

Mammography

GENERAL INFORMATION

DEFINITION—Mammography is a procedure that involves taking x-rays of the breasts to detect breast cysts or tumors, especially those that cannot be felt (palpable) by the fingers during a physical examination. A mammogram is the photographic result. The procedure does not prevent breast cancer; it is used to detect cancer early when it is more likely to be successfully treated. However, there are some breast cancers that are not visible even on mammograms.

REASONS FOR PROCEDURE
• Evaluate breast symptoms such as lumps, persistent pain, or nipple discharge.
• Screen for breast cancer.
• Help differentiate between noncancerous breast disease and breast cancer.

RISK INCREASES WITH—None expected.

DESCRIPTION OF PROCEDURE
• All clothing above the waist is removed and a gown provided that opens in the front.
• You will stand in front of the x-ray equipment.
• Each breast in turn will be compressed between 2 plastic plates in 2 or more positions for the x-rays. Compressing the breasts can be uncomfortable, but it minimizes the amount of radiation required to get a clear image and allows for a more accurate reading of the mammogram.
• After the films are taken, they are checked to make sure they are readable. If not, the procedure will be repeated.

PROBABLE OUTCOME
• There are normally no physical side effects from the test itself.
• As a screening test, results usually reveal normal breast tissue with no abnormal masses or calcification.
• Any findings that suggest cancer require further tests (such as biopsy) for confirmation.

POSSIBLE COMPLICATIONS—Misdiagnosis: missing cancers that are there or mistaking benign lumps for cancerous ones.

FOLLOW-UP CARE

GENERAL MEASURES
• Many facilities have been approved and accredited by the American College of Radiology (ACR) and meet minimum standards that assure consistency and quality in the techniques used for mammography. Facilities which have ACR accreditation usually use only equipment that has been designed specifically for breast x-rays. Many of these facilities limit their services to providing breast x-rays only and, therefore, tend to do a higher number of mammograms per day. Because these facilities specialize in mammography, many people feel that the results of their mammogram at an ACR accredited facility will be more accurate and reliable. You may want to ask your doctor whether the facility you will use has ACR accreditation.
• If you menstruate, you may want to schedule your mammogram for 7 to 10 days after the start of your menstrual cycle, when your breasts are less likely to be swollen and tender.
• Do not use any deodorant, antiperspirant, talcum powder or lotion on your upper body on the day of your mammogram, as these can interfere with the results of the x-rays.
• There are no special self-care measures to take following the test.
• Test results that are suggestive often require a needle aspiration, biopsy and/or ultrasound testing.
• Further testing may be recommended even if the mammogram results are negative, such as when there is an undiagnosed abnormality on physical examination or when unexplained symptoms occur.
• Follow-up treatment steps will depend on the specific diagnosis.
• Routine mammograms are recommended for the following age groups:
  Around the age of 40, all women should have their first mammogram.
  Between ages 40 and 50, women should have a mammogram every 1 to 2 years.
  After age 50, all women should have a mammogram every year.
  Women who have had breast cancer should have a mammogram at least once a year, regardless of their age.
  Women at high risk for breast cancer (anyone with a close relative who has had breast cancer) should have a mammogram every 1 to 2 years, beginning at age 35.
• See the Resource section of this book for additional information.

MEDICATION—Medicine is not necessary for the procedure itself.

ACTIVITY—No restrictions.

DIET—No special diet.

CALL YOUR DOCTOR IF

• You have not had a mammogram as recommended for your age group.
• You detect any changes in your breasts, including lumps, pain, swelling, redness, skin dimpling, nipple inversion (nipple turns "inside out"), or discharge from the nipple.

Mastitis

 GENERAL INFORMATION

DEFINITION—An inflammatory and infectious condition of the breast which occurs in about 1% of new mothers and is more likely in women who are breast-feeding.

SIGNS & SYMPTOMS—Symptoms may occur anytime while nursing but usually begin 1 week or more after delivery. Common symptoms include:
• Fever.
• Body aches or a general feeling of illness.
• Tender, swollen, hard, hot breast(s).
• Purulent drainage (pus) from the breast(s).
• Redness and red streaking of the breast(s).

CAUSES—Infection from bacteria that enter the mother's breast from the nursing baby's nose or throat. The most common bacteria are Staphylococcus aureus and beta-hemolytic streptococci. Infection with the mumps virus is another cause.

RISK INCREASES WITH
• Abrasion of the nipple.
• Blocked milk ducts from wearing too-tight bras, sleeping on your stomach or waiting too long between feedings.
• Use of an electric or manual breast pump.
• Silicone breast implants.
• Diabetes mellitus.
• Steroid use.
• Smoking.

HOW TO PREVENT
• Wash nipples before nursing. Wash hands before touching breasts. Nipple and areola care is essential to prevent the skin from drying and cracking, which significantly increases a woman's risk of infection.
• If a nipple cracks or fissures, apply lanolin cream or other topical medication (e.g., vitamin A & D ointment) to promote healing.
• Wear a comfortable bra that is not too tight.
• Don't sleep on your stomach.

PROBABLE OUTCOME—Usually curable in 10 days with antibiotic treatment.

POSSIBLE COMPLICATIONS—Without treatment, may lead to breast abscess.

 HOW TO TREAT

GENERAL MEASURES
• Diagnostic tests may include laboratory blood studies, culture of pus or fluid and, occasionally, ultrasound, mammography and breast biopsy if something other than infection may be causing symptoms.
• Apply an ice pack (ice in a plastic bag, covered with a thin towel) to the engorged breast 3 to 6 times a day. Use for 15 to 20 minutes at a time. Don't use ice packs within 1 hour of nursing; use warm compresses instead.
• Wear an uplift bra during treatment.
• Continue to breast-feed, even though breasts are infected. Offer the affected breast first to promote complete emptying.
• Massage nipples with cocoa butter or a cream recommended by the doctor.
• If an abscess develops, stop breast-feeding on the affected side. Use a breast pump to empty the infected breast regularly and continue breast-feeding on the unaffected side.

MEDICATION
• Antibiotics to fight infection. Finish the prescription, even if symptoms subside quickly.
• Pain relievers. For minor discomfort, you may use nonprescription drugs such as acetaminophen.

ACTIVITY—Rest in bed until fever and pain diminish.

DIET—No special diet. Drink extra fluids while you have fever.

CALL YOUR DOCTOR IF

• You or a family member has symptoms of mastitis.
• During treatment, temperature rises to over 101°F (38.3°C).
• You have signs of a developing abscess (a localized area with increasing redness, pain, tenderness and fluctuance that feels like pushing on an inflated inner tube).
• New, unexplained symptoms develop. Drugs used in treatment may produce side effects.

Partial Mastectomy (Lumpectomy)

GENERAL INFORMATION

DEFINITION—Removal of a lump from the female breast that is known or suspected to be cancerous. It is the least invasive procedure for breast cancer surgery and is the most likely to leave the breast looking normal. Be sure you understand the rationale for any recommended procedure, the risks and benefits involved as well as any possible alternative treatments. Surgeries to treat breast cancer are controversial and vary considerably.

REASONS FOR PROCEDURE—Cancer or suspected cancer of the breast.

RISK INCREASES WITH
• Obesity.
• Smoking.
• Stress.
• Poor nutrition, especially inadequate iron intake that has led to anemia.
• Recent or chronic illness (e.g., diabetes, hypertension).
• Use of drugs such as antihypertensives, muscle relaxants, tranquilizers, sleep inducers, insulin, sedatives, beta-adrenergic blockers or cortisone.

DESCRIPTION OF PROCEDURE
• A general anesthetic is administered by injection and inhalation with an airway tube placed in the windpipe.
• An incision is made over the lump to be removed.
• The lump and a small surrounding area of normal tissue are cut free and removed. Bleeding is controlled with ties and electrocauterization.
• It is frequently necessary to make a separate incision in the axilla (under the armpit) to sample or significantly remove the axillary lymph nodes.
• The skin is closed with sutures or clips, which usually can be removed about 1 week after surgery.

PROBABLE OUTCOME
• Expect complete healing of the surgical wound. Allow about 2 weeks for recovery from surgery.
• If the lump removed was a large one, you may see some difference in the size or contours of the affected breast.

POSSIBLE COMPLICATIONS
• Excessive bleeding.
• Surgical-wound infection.
• Need for additional surgery or radiation (sometimes).

• Lymphedema (swelling of the soft tissues in the arm or hand on the side of the body where the surgery was performed). The removal of lymph nodes during mastectomy can interfere with the normal flow of lymphatic fluid through the lymphatic vessels. Painful swelling, decreased mobility, and infection can occur when lymphedema is present.

FOLLOW-UP CARE

GENERAL MEASURES
• A hard ridge should form along the incision. As it heals, the ridge will gradually recede.
• Use an electric heating pad, a heat lamp or a warm compress to relieve incisional pain.
• Bathe and shower as usual. You may wash the incision gently with mild unscented soap.
• See the Resource section of this book for additional information.

MEDICATION
• Prescription pain medication should generally be required for only 2 to 7 days following the procedure.
• You may use nonprescription drugs, such as acetaminophen, for minor pain.
• Stool softener laxative to prevent constipation.
• Antibiotics to fight infection. Antibiotics may reduce the effectiveness of some oral contraceptives. If you are currently using oral contraceptives for birth control, discuss this with your doctor.

ACTIVITY
• To help recovery and aid your well-being, resume daily activities, including work, as soon as you are able. Most regular activities can be resumed within 2 weeks.
• Avoid vigorous exercise for 4 weeks after surgery.
• Resume driving 1 week after returning home.

DIET—Clear liquid diet until the gastrointestinal tract functions again. Then eat a well-balanced diet to promote healing.

CALL YOUR DOCTOR IF

• Pain, swelling, redness, drainage or bleeding increases in the surgical area.
• You develop signs of infection: headache, muscle aches, dizziness or a general ill feeling and fever.
• You experience nausea or vomiting.
• New, unexplained symptoms develop. Drugs used in treatment may produce side effects.

Partial Mastectomy
(Lumpectomy)

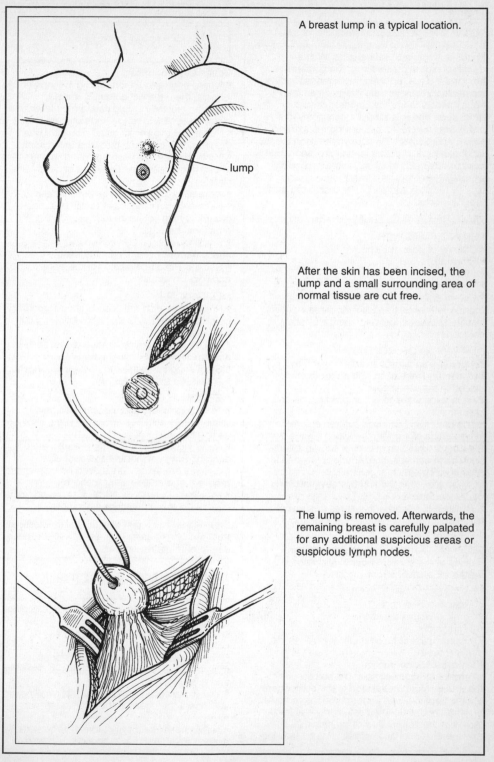

A breast lump in a typical location.

After the skin has been incised, the lump and a small surrounding area of normal tissue are cut free.

The lump is removed. Afterwards, the remaining breast is carefully palpated for any additional suspicious areas or suspicious lymph nodes.

Total Mastectomy (Modified Radical Mastectomy)

 GENERAL INFORMATION

DEFINITION—A radical mastectomy removes the breast, all the axillary (under the arm) lymph nodes and the pectoral muscles. With a modified radical mastectomy, the pectoral muscles are not removed. An extended radical mastectomy removes the internal mammary nodes in addition to the standard radical procedure; and in a simple mastectomy, the entire breast is removed, leaving the axillary lymph nodes intact. Be sure you understand the rationale for any recommended procedure, the risks and benefits involved, and any possible alternative treatments. Breast reconstruction is usually feasible and should be discussed prior to a mastectomy.

REASONS FOR PROCEDURE—Breast cancer.

RISK INCREASES WITH
• Obesity or poor nutrition.
• Smoking.
• Stress.
• Recent or chronic illness.
• Use of drugs such as antihypertensives, muscle relaxants, tranquilizers, sleep inducers, insulin, sedatives, beta-adrenergic blockers or cortisone.

DESCRIPTION OF PROCEDURE
• A general anesthetic is administered by injection and inhalation with an airway tube placed in the windpipe.
• An incision is made encompassing the entire breast.
• The underlying tissue is cut free and removed in one piece along with the lymph glands from the armpit. Bleeding is controlled with sutures and electrocauterization. A tube is inserted for drainage. The drain is generally removed by your doctor within the first few days following the procedure.
• The skin is closed with sutures or surgical clips, which usually can be removed about 1 week after surgery.

PROBABLE OUTCOME—Expect complete healing of the surgical wound. Allow about 6 weeks for recovery from surgery.

POSSIBLE COMPLICATIONS
• Excessive bleeding.
• Surgical-wound infection.
• Depression.
• Accumulation of blood under the skin in the surgical area.
• Limited shoulder motion.
• Lymphedema (swelling of the soft tissues in the arm or hand on the side of the body where the mastectomy was performed). The removal of lymph nodes during mastectomy can interfere with the normal flow of lymphatic fluid through the lymphatic vessels. Painful swelling, decreased mobility, and infection can occur when lymphedema is present.
• Nerve damage.

 FOLLOW-UP CARE

GENERAL MEASURES
• A hard ridge should form along the incision. As it heals, the ridge will gradually recede.
• Use an electric heating pad, a heat lamp or a warm compress to relieve incisional pain.
• Bathe and shower as usual. You may wash the incision gently with mild unscented soap.
• Move and elevate your legs often while resting in bed to decrease the likelihood of deep-vein clots.
• A breast prosthesis can be used if desired.
• Seek help from friends or family or support groups to help you learn to cope with the emotional feelings.
• Swelling (edema) can be reduced in the affected arm by elevating it frequently.
• See the Resource section of this book for additional information.

MEDICATION
• Prescription pain medication should generally be required for only 2 to 7 days following the procedure.
• You may use nonprescription drugs, such as acetaminophen, for minor pain.
• Stool softener laxative to prevent constipation.
• Antibiotics to fight infection.

ACTIVITY
• To help recovery and aid your well-being, resume daily activities, including work, as soon as you are able.
• Avoid vigorous exercise for 6 weeks after surgery. Physical therapy and/or special exercises are usually prescribed (to help speed recovery and reduce complications).
• Resume driving 2 weeks after returning home.
• Resume sexual relations when able.

DIET—Clear liquid diet until the gastrointestinal tract functions again. Then eat a well-balanced diet to promote healing.

 CALL YOUR DOCTOR IF

• Pain, swelling, redness, drainage or bleeding increases in the surgical area.
• You experience nausea, vomiting or constipation.
• You develop signs of infection: headache, muscle aches, dizziness, or a general ill feeling and fever.
• You experience redness, warmth, swelling, stiffness or hardness in the affected arm or hand.
• New, unexplained symptoms develop. Drugs used in treatment may produce side effects.

Total Mastectomy (Modified Radical Mastectomy)

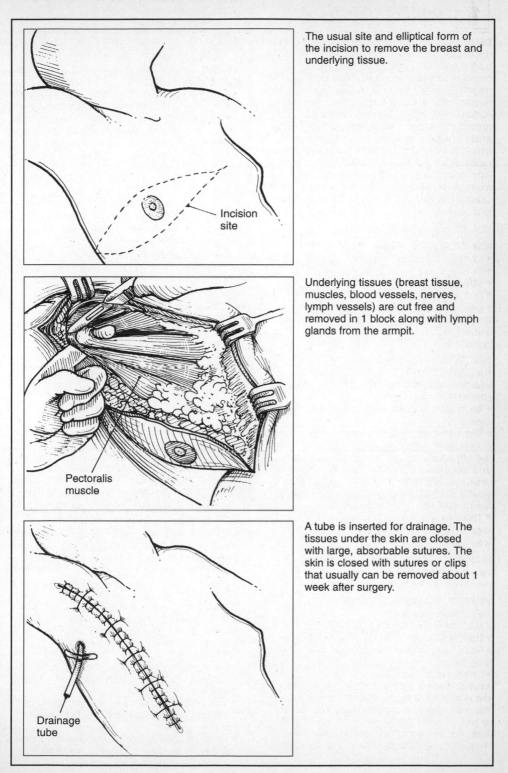

The usual site and elliptical form of the incision to remove the breast and underlying tissue.

Incision site

Underlying tissues (breast tissue, muscles, blood vessels, nerves, lymph vessels) are cut free and removed in 1 block along with lymph glands from the armpit.

Pectoralis muscle

A tube is inserted for drainage. The tissues under the skin are closed with large, absorbable sutures. The skin is closed with sutures or clips that usually can be removed about 1 week after surgery.

Drainage tube

Gynecology

Amenorrhea, Primary

GENERAL INFORMATION

DEFINITION—Complete absence of menstruation in a young woman who is at least 16 years old, or at age 14 with a lack of normal growth or absence of normal sexual development. It is a rare disorder as over 95% of girls have their first menstrual period by age 15.

SIGNS & SYMPTOMS—Lack of menstrual periods after puberty. Most girls begin menstruating by age 14; average age is 12 years and 8 months.

CAUSES
Usually unknown. Possible causes include:
• Delayed puberty.
• Congenital abnormalities, such as the absence or abnormal formation of female organs (vagina, uterus, ovaries).
• Intact hymen (membrane covering the vaginal opening) that has no opening to allow passage of menstrual flow.
• Pregnancy.
• Polycystic ovarian disease (Stein-Leventhal syndrome).
• Disorders (tumors, infections or other problems) of the endocrine system, including the pituitary, hypothalamus, thyroid, parathyroid, adrenal and ovarian glands.
• Chromosome disorders.
• Systemic disease.
• Severe nutritional or physical stressor such as anorexia or competitive sports.
• Rarely, prior gynecological surgery.

RISK INCREASES WITH
• Stress.
• Use of drugs, including oral contraceptives, anticancer drugs, barbiturates, narcotics, cortisone drugs, chlordiazepoxide and reserpine.
• Excessive exercise.
• Family tendency to start menstruation late.
• Excessive dieting or weight loss.

HOW TO PREVENT
• Don't use drugs unless prescribed by doctor.
• Reduce athletic activities if they are too strenuous.
• Obtain medical treatment for any underlying disorder.
• Maintain proper nutrition and body weight.

PROBABLE OUTCOME
• The absence of menstruation is not a health risk in itself, but the cause should be identified. If an ovarian cyst or tumor is the cause, it requires removal.
• Amenorrhea is usually curable with hormone treatment directed at the underlying cause. Treatment may be delayed to age 18 unless the cause can be identified and treated safely.

• Causes which sometimes cannot be corrected include chromosome disorders and abnormalities of the reproductive system.

POSSIBLE COMPLICATIONS
• Psychological distress about sexual development.
• Some of the causes may result in infertility (inability to conceive).
• Rare endocrinological condition may require surgical treatment in addition to hormone replacement.

HOW TO TREAT

GENERAL MEASURES
• Diagnostic tests may include a thorough physical examination, a medical and personal history, laboratory studies of blood samples to check for hormone levels, plus thyroid and adrenal function studies. In addition, your doctor may order ultrasound studies, as well as x-rays or laparoscopy.
• Treatment usually involves hormone replacement therapy. Treatment for amenorrhea not related to hormone deficiency depends on the cause.
• Psychotherapy or counseling, if amenorrhea is related to stress or results from eating disorders.
• Surgery (minor) to create an opening in the hymen, if necessary.
• Surgery to correct abnormalities of the reproductive system (sometimes).

MEDICATION—You may be prescribed progesterone (hormone) treatment to induce bleeding. If bleeding begins when progesterone is withdrawn, the reproductive system is functioning. This also indicates that pituitary disease is unlikely. If progesterone withdrawal does not induce bleeding, gonad stimulants such as clomiphene or gonadotrophins may be used for the same purpose.

ACTIVITY
• No restrictions. Exercise regularly, but not to excess.
• Sleep at least 8 hours every night.

DIET
• Eat 3 well-balanced meals a day.
• If you are overweight or underweight, get medical advice about diets. Don't try to lose weight by crash-dieting.

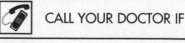

CALL YOUR DOCTOR IF

• You are 16 years old and have never had a period.
• Periods don't begin in 6 months, despite treatment.
• New, unexplained symptoms develop. Drugs used in treatment may produce side effects.

Amenorrhea, Secondary

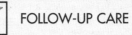

GENERAL INFORMATION

DEFINITION—Cessation of menstruation for at least 3 months in a woman who has previously menstruated.

SIGNS & SYMPTOMS—Absence of menstrual periods for 3 or more months in a woman who has menstruated at least once.

CAUSES
- Pregnancy (if a woman has had sexual intercourse).
- Breast-feeding an infant.
- Discontinuing use of birth control pills.
- Menopause (if a woman is over 35 and not pregnant).
- Emotional stress or psychological disorder.
- Surgical removal of the ovaries or uterus.
- Polycystic ovarian disease (Stein-Leventhal syndrome).
- Disorder of the endocrine system, including the pituitary, hypothalamus, thyroid, parathyroid, adrenal and ovarian glands.
- Diabetes mellitus.
- Tuberculosis.
- Obesity, anorexia nervosa or bulimia.
- Strenuous program of physical exercise, such as long-distance running.

RISK INCREASES WITH
- Stress.
- Poor nutrition.
- Use of certain drugs, such as narcotics, phenothiazines, reserpine or hormones.
- Excessive exercise.

HOW TO PREVENT
- If your amenorrhea is caused by an underlying disease, such as tuberculosis, diabetes or anorexia nervosa, obtain treatment for the primary disorder.
- Don't use drugs unless prescribed by your doctor.
- If the cause of your amenorrhea is unknown, there are no specific preventive measures.
- Maintain proper nutrition and body weight.

PROBABLE OUTCOME—Amenorrhea is not a threat to health. Whether it can be corrected varies with the underlying cause:
- If from pregnancy or breast-feeding, menstruation will resume when these conditions cease.
- If from discontinuing use of oral contraceptives, periods should begin in 2 months to 2 years (rarely does it take this long).
- If from menopause, periods will become less frequent or may never resume. Hysterectomy also ends menstruation permanently.
- If from endocrine disorders, hormone replacement usually causes periods to resume.
- If from eating disorders, successful treatment of that disorder is necessary for menstruation to resume.
- If from diabetes or tuberculosis, menstruation may never resume.
- If from strenuous exercise, periods usually resume when exercise decreases.

POSSIBLE COMPLICATIONS
- None expected if no serious underlying cause can be discovered.
- May experience estrogen deficiency symptoms, such as hot flushes or vaginal dryness.
- May affect fertility.

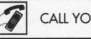

FOLLOW-UP CARE

GENERAL MEASURES
- To aid in diagnosis, laboratory studies, such as a pregnancy test, blood studies of hormone levels and Pap smear are usually necessary. Surgical diagnostic procedures, such as laparoscopy or hysteroscopy may be recommended.
- Dilatation and curettage, often referred to as D & C (dilation of the cervix and a scraping out of the uterus with a curette) may be performed.
- Treatment of underlying disorder if one is diagnosed.
- Psychotherapy or counseling, if amenorrhea is related to stress.
- Keep a record of menstrual cycles to aid in early detection of recurrent amenorrhea.

MEDICATION
- Therapeutic trial of progesterone and/or estrogen. If bleeding occurs after progesterone is withdrawn, the reproductive system is functional.
- Oral contraceptives may be prescribed to assure contraception and to establish regular menstrual periods.
- Hormone replacement therapy may be prescribed for women who are postmenopausal.
- Your doctor may prescribe a calcium supplement to prevent bone density loss.
- Other drugs to treat underlying disorder may be prescribed.

ACTIVITY–No restrictions. Exercise regularly, but not to excess. Sleep at least 8 hours every night.

DIET
- Usually no special diet is required.
- If overweight or underweight, a change in diet to correct the problem is recommended.

CALL YOUR DOCTOR IF

- You or a family member has symptoms of amenorrhea.
- Periods don't resume in 6 months, despite treatment.
- New, unexplained symptoms develop. Drugs used in treatment may produce side effects.

Bladder Infection (Cystitis) ✓

 GENERAL INFORMATION

DEFINITION—Inflammation or infection of the urinary bladder.

SIGNS & SYMPTOMS
- Painful, burning sensation during urination.
- Frequent urination, although the urine amount may be small.
- Increased urge to urinate.
- Sensation of incomplete bladder emptying.
- Pain in the abdomen over the bladder.
- Low back pain.
- Blood in the urine; bad-smelling urine.
- Low fever.
- Painful sexual intercourse.
- Lack of urinary control (sometimes).

CAUSES
- Bacteria that reach the bladder from another part of the body through the bloodstream.
- Bacteria that enter the urinary tract from skin around the genital and anal area.
- Injury to the urethra.
- Use of a urinary catheter to empty the bladder, such as during childbirth or surgery.

RISK INCREASES WITH
- Frequent or vigorous sexual activity.
- Infection in other parts of the genitourinary system.
- Pregnancy.
- Poor hygiene.
- Diabetes mellitus.
- Certain types of birth control, e.g., diaphragm with a too-tight fit, contraceptive foams or vaginal suppositories that can irritate the urethra, or a nonlubricated condom.
- Underlying abnormalities of the urinary tract, such as tumors, calculi or strictures.
- Incomplete bladder emptying.

HOW TO PREVENT
- Drink a glass of water before sexual intercourse and urinate within 15 minutes after intercourse.
- Use a water-soluble lubricant such as K-Y Lubricating Jelly during intercourse.
- Use female-superior or lateral positions in sexual intercourse to protect your urethra from injury.
- Drink 8 glasses of water every day. Avoid caffeine, which irritates the bladder.
- Seek prompt medical care for symptoms of urinary tract infections.
- Do not douche or use feminine hygiene sprays or deodorants.
- Clean the anal area thoroughly after bowel movements. Wipe from the front to the rear rather than rear to front to avoid spreading fecal bacteria to the genital area.
- Wear underwear and stockings that have a cotton crotch.

- Avoid bubble baths, chlorinated pools and spas.
- Avoid postponing urination.
- If you use a diaphragm, ask your doctor about having it refitted to the smallest effective size, or consider switching to one with a softer, more flexible rim.
- For women with frequent recurrence of infection, antibiotics may be prescribed for use prior to sexual intercourse.

PROBABLE OUTCOME
- Curable in a few days to 2 weeks with prompt medical treatment.
- Recurrence is common.

POSSIBLE COMPLICATIONS—Inadequate treatment can cause chronic urinary tract infections, leading to kidney infection and, in rare cases, kidney failure.

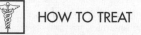 **HOW TO TREAT**

GENERAL MEASURES
- Diagnostic tests usually are limited to urinalysis. On rare occasions when urinary tract infections are recurrent, cystoscopy (see Glossary), ultrasound or intravenous pyelogram (see Glossary) may be performed.
- Treatment is usually with antibiotics.
- Warm baths may help relieve discomfort.
- Pour a cup of warm water over genital area while urinating. It will help to relieve burning and stinging.

MEDICATION
- Antibiotics to fight any bacterial infection. Antibiotics may reduce the effectiveness of oral contraceptives. Discuss this with your doctor.
- Occasionally, urinary analgesics are prescribed for pain. If phenazopyridine (Pyridium) is prescribed, it will turn the urine color to bright orange.

ACTIVITY—Avoid sexual intercourse until you have been free of symptoms for 2 weeks.

DIET
- Drink 6 to 8 glasses of water daily.
- Avoid caffeine and alcohol during treatment.
- Drink cranberry juice to acidify urine. Some antibiotic drugs have increased effectiveness when the urine is more acidic.

 CALL YOUR DOCTOR IF

- You or a family member has symptoms of cystitis.
- Fever occurs or blood appears in the urine.
- Symptoms don't improve in 1 week.
- Symptoms recur after treatment.
- New, unexplained symptoms develop. Drugs used in treatment may produce side effects.

Cervical Cancer

GENERAL INFORMATION

DEFINITION—Cancer of the cervix, the lower third of the uterus which opens into the vagina. Cervical cancer is the third most common malignancy of the female genital tract but, with early diagnosis and treatment, cervical cancer can usually be cured. While the average age of women at diagnosis is about 45, this cancer can affect women of all ages.

SIGNS & SYMPTOMS
In the early, easily treatable stages:
• No symptoms.
In later stages:
• Abnormally heavy menstrual periods.
• Spotting or bleeding between menstrual periods.
• Persistent vaginal discharge.
• Pain and bleeding after intercourse.
• Pelvic pain, which sometimes radiates to the hip and thigh.
In final stages:
• Abdominal pain.
• Leaking of feces and urine through the vagina.
• Appetite and weight loss.
• Weakness.
• Anemia.

CAUSES—Unknown. Probably related to viral infections, specifically human papillomavirus (genital warts).

RISK INCREASES WITH
• Early age of first intercourse.
• Multiple sex partners.
• Multiple pregnancies.
• History of cervical dysplasia.
• Human papillomavirus infection (genital warts).
• HIV infection.
• Recurrent vaginal infections (bacterial or viral, including genital herpes).
• Daughters of women who took DES during pregnancy.
• Smoking.

HOW TO PREVENT
• Avoid the risks listed above as much as possible.
• Obtain regular medical pelvic examinations.
• Obtain regular Pap smears (test done to detect cancer of the cervix in an early and treatable stage).
• Regular pelvic examinations and the Pap smear are very effective in detecting precancerous changes or cervical cancer in its early, symptom-free stage.

PROBABLE OUTCOME
• Usually curable if diagnosed before the tumor has spread.
• After surgery for cervical cancer, you may experience some cramping, tenderness, bleeding or vaginal discharge.

POSSIBLE COMPLICATIONS—If cervical cancer is not treated early, it spreads beyond the uterus to other body parts and leads to death.

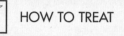

HOW TO TREAT

GENERAL MEASURES
• Diagnostic tests may include a pelvic examination and a Pap test, followed by a biopsy if a suspicious lesion is seen.
• Surgery to remove the cancerous area. During early stages, this may involve only a small area of the cervix, which preserves child-bearing abilities. This surgery is usually performed, on an outpatient basis, through such techniques as loop excision electrosurgical procedure (LEEP). In LEEP, the physician uses a hand-held wire loop, activated by an electrosurgical generator, which makes a very precise and uniform cut across the cervix. Another technique that may be used is cervical conization, where a cone of tissue is removed from the cervix with a surgical knife.
• More advanced stages of cervical cancer may require removal of the reproductive organs and other affected tissue (radical hysterectomy).
• Chemotherapy and radiation therapy (internal, external or both) are possible treatments for advanced cancer.
• See the Resource section of this book for additional information.

MEDICATION—Medicine is usually not necessary for this disorder, if it is diagnosed and treated early. If radical surgery and additional treatment are required, anticancer drugs may be prescribed.

ACTIVITY
• Usually, no restrictions.
• Avoid tampons following surgery.
• Resume sexual activity once you have medical clearance.

DIET—No special diet.

CALL YOUR DOCTOR IF

• You or a family member has persistent vaginal bleeding or other symptoms of cervical cancer.
• You have not had a pelvic examination or Pap smear in at least 1 year.
• New, unexplained symptoms develop. Drugs used in treatment may produce side effects.

Cervical Conization
(Cone Biopsy; LEEP)

 GENERAL INFORMATION

DEFINITION—A minor surgical procedure that involves removal of a cone-shaped piece of tissue of the cervix (the lower third of the uterus). In a cone biopsy, a larger sample of tissue is taken than in a simple biopsy of the cervix.

REASONS FOR PROCEDURE
• Usually follows a Pap smear, visual examination (colposcopy) and a simple biopsy of the cervix that revealed a possible abnormality.
• Investigation of precancerous or cancerous cells of the cervix. Laboratory examination of the removed tissue aids in diagnosis.
• In some cases, the cone biopsy can be a treatment as well as a diagnostic tool by removing all the abnormal tissue.

RISK INCREASES WITH
• History of bleeding disorders.
• Use of drugs such as anticoagulants or aspirin.

DESCRIPTION OF PROCEDURE
• Can be performed in an outpatient surgical facility or hospital; an overnight stay in the hospital may be needed.
• A local, regional or general anesthetic may be used.
• Though several options are available for a cone biopsy, the LEEP (or loop electrosurgical excision procedure) is often the procedure recommended. It involves the use of a specially designed wire loop instrument and a low level of electricity.
• You will lie on the exam table the same way as for a Pap smear.
• With LEEP, the instrument is inserted into the cervix and a cone-shaped tissue specimen is removed from the cervix. The wire loop cuts and cauterizes the tissue.
• Because this specimen is more extensive than a regular biopsy, it can aid in determining the extent and severity of any problem.
• The instrument is removed and the tissue is then sent to the laboratory for microscopic analysis.
• See "Cervix, Biopsy of" in this section of this book for additional information.

PROBABLE OUTCOME
• Tissue obtained successfully without complications in virtually all cases.
• With the removal of all abnormal tissue, many patients are cured of their problem following this procedure.
• You may experience mild cramping or pain during and for a short time after the procedure.

• A brownish-black discharge for the first week is normal. In addition, a thinner discharge may last for up to 6 weeks.

POSSIBLE COMPLICATIONS
• Excessive bleeding or infection.
• A weakening of the cervix that could increase the risk of miscarriage in a future pregnancy.
• Further treatment or a repeat of the procedure may be necessary if all abnormal cells are not removed.

 FOLLOW-UP CARE

GENERAL MEASURES
• Wear cotton panties or pantyhose with a cotton crotch. Avoid panties made from nylon, polyester, silk or other nonventilating materials.
• Use a sanitary pad to protect your clothing. Avoid tampons—they may lead to infection.
• Bathe or shower as usual.
• Don't douche unless it is prescribed for you.
• It is important to go to your doctor's office for follow-up visits and Pap smears.
• If you are diagnosed with cancer, seek emotional help and support of family and friends. See the Resource section of this book for additional information.

MEDICATION
• Vaginal creams to relieve discomfort may be prescribed.
• You may use nonprescription drugs, such as acetaminophen, for minor pain.

ACTIVITY
• Resume driving 24 hours after recovering from surgery.
• Avoid heavy lifting. Do not resume a normal exercise program until your follow-up appointment.
• Abstain from sexual intercourse until your doctor has advised that healing is complete.

DIET—No special diet.

CALL YOUR DOCTOR IF

• You develop signs of infection: headache, muscle aches, dizziness or a general ill feeling and fever.
• Vaginal discharge increases or begins to have an unpleasant odor.
• You experience discomfort that simple pain medication does not relieve quickly.
• Unusual vaginal swelling or bleeding develops.

Cervical Dysplasia
(Cervical Intraepithelial Neoplasia [CIN]; Squamous Intraepithelial Lesions [SIL])

 GENERAL INFORMATION

DEFINITION—Cervical dysplasia is the presence of abnormal cells on the lining of the cervix. It can range from mild to severe, depending on the spread of the abnormal cells. Depending on the severity, dysplasia can be considered a precancerous condition but does not represent cancer of the cervix. Dysplasia occurs in sexually active females of all ages but is most common in those age 25 to 35.

SIGNS & SYMPTOMS—Usually no signs or symptoms occur. The suspected diagnosis results from a routine Pap smear evaluation.

CAUSES—There is an association with human papillomaviruses (genital warts) or similar viruses. The human papillomavirus (HPV) is usually acquired from sexual intercourse but can, in rare instances, be acquired from other skin-to-skin contact.

RISK INCREASES WITH
• Repeated infections.
• Smoking.
• Immunosuppression.
• Pregnancy and the immunologic changes associated with pregnancy.
• Multiple sexual partners.
• Early age of first sexual intercourse.
• Daughters of women who took DES during pregnancy.
• History of infection with the human papilloma-virus (HPV), which causes genital warts.
• Long-term oral contraceptive use.

HOW TO PREVENT
• Sexual monogamy of both partners.
• Yearly Pap smears for all women who are, or have been, sexually active or who have reached the age of 18. Pap smears will not prevent dysplasia but will aid in early diagnosis.
• Don't smoke.
• Use of a diaphragm by the female or a condom by the male for sexual intercourse.

PROBABLE OUTCOME
• With early diagnosis and treatment, the outlook is excellent.
• Spontaneous regression (reversal) occurs in a significant number of patients.

POSSIBLE COMPLICATIONS
• Some severe dysplasia may progress to cancer of the cervix.
• Recurrence is possible, especially in the first two years following treatment. If a woman has completed childbearing, recurrent dysplasia can be treated with a hysterectomy.
• Rarely, complications can result from the treatment, such as excessive bleeding or infection.

HOW TO TREAT

GENERAL MEASURES
• To confirm the diagnosis, a colposcopy (examination of the cervix with a colposcope, a slender optical instrument with a lighted tip) is usually performed and combined with a biopsy.
• Treatment measures will vary depending on the degree and extent of the cervical dysplasia. Possibilities include cryotherapy (freezing), laser surgery, conization of the cervix and cone biopsy. A recently developed treatment for cervical dysplasia is the loop excision electrosurgical procedure (LEEP). In LEEP, the physician uses a hand-held wire loop, activated by an electrosurgical generator, which makes a very precise and uniform cut across the cervix, in much the same way as a laser beam would. LEEP is preferred by many physicians because it allows for a larger tissue sampling in addition to treating the dysplasia, and it is less expensive and faster than either laser surgery or a hospital cone biopsy.
• Follow-up care will depend on the treatment method used.
• Follow-up Pap smears every 3 to 6 months for 1 to 2 years may be recommended to verify the success of treatment and to detect any recurrence. Thereafter, be sure to receive annual Pap smears.
• For patients with recurrent or severe dysplasia, hysterectomy may be an option.

MEDICATION
• Prescription pain medication should generally be required for only 2 to 7 days following the procedure.
• You may use nonprescription drugs, such as acetaminophen, for minor pain.

ACTIVITY
• To help recovery and aid your well-being, resume daily activities, including work, as soon as you are able.
• Delay sexual relations until a follow-up medical examination determines that healing is complete.

DIET—No special diet.

 CALL YOUR DOCTOR IF

• Pain, swelling, redness, drainage or bleeding increases in the surgical area.
• You develop signs of infection: headache, muscle aches, dizziness or a general ill feeling and fever.
• Vaginal discharge increases or begins to have an unpleasant odor.

Cervical Polyps

 GENERAL INFORMATION

DEFINITION—Small, fragile, bulbous growths on stalks protruding through the cervix (lower third of the uterus) from the lining inside the uterus (endometrium). The polyps may be single or numerous. They are relatively common, especially in women over age 20 who have had multiple pregnancies.

SIGNS & SYMPTOMS
• Usually painless.
• Unexpected spotting of blood between monthly menstrual periods.
• Spotting of blood after sexual intercourse or bowel movements.
• Vaginal discharge.

CAUSES—Cervical polyps are caused by cervix inflammation from infection, erosion or ulceration. They frequently accompany chronic infections in the vagina or cervix, although they are not contagious. The small growths are usually benign, but in very rare cases, they represent early cancer of the cervix.

RISK INCREASES WITH
• Diabetes mellitus.
• Recurrent vaginitis or cervicitis (inflammation or infection of the cervix).

HOW TO PREVENT—To prevent vaginal or cervical infections that can precede cervical polyps:
• Wear cotton underpants or pantyhose with a cotton crotch to prevent accumulation of excess heat and moisture, which can make you susceptible to vaginal and cervical infections.
• Avoid contracting sexually transmitted diseases by having your sexual partner wear a condom during sexual activity.

PROBABLE OUTCOME—Usually curable with minor surgery. You may feel brief, mild pain during the procedure and have mild to moderate cramps for several hours. Spotting of blood from the vagina may occur for several days.

POSSIBLE COMPLICATIONS
• Bleeding and some mild pain with removal of the polyps.
• Infection can occasionally develop following surgery to identify or remove polyps.
• In very rare instances, cervical polyps may become malignant.

 HOW TO TREAT

GENERAL MEASURES
• Surgery to remove cervical polyps with a wire snare, electrocautery or liquid nitrogen. This can often be done in a simple office procedure. The cervix may be cauterized after removing the polyp to prevent regrowth of the same or another polyp. If the polyp is large, it may be necessary for the doctor to perform a D & C (dilatation and curettage), either in the office or in a hospital. All tissue removed, by any of these methods, should be sent to a pathology laboratory to be examined for any evidence of cancer.
• Don't douche unless it is recommended.
• Use small sanitary pads to protect your clothing from creams or suppositories.
• A polyp that accompanies cervicitis (inflammation or infection of the cervix) may require more extensive surgery.

MEDICATION—Usually no medications are necessary for this disorder. However, antibiotics may be prescribed if signs of an infection develop. Antibiotics can reduce the effectiveness of oral contraceptives. If you are currently using oral contraceptives for birth control, discuss this with your doctor.

ACTIVITY—No restrictions. Delay sexual relations until a follow-up pelvic examination determines that healing is complete.

DIET—No special diet.

CALL YOUR DOCTOR IF

• You have symptoms of cervical polyps.
• The following occur after treatment:
  Discomfort persists longer than 1 week.
  Symptoms recur.
  Unexplained vaginal bleeding or swelling develops.
• New, unexplained symptoms develop. Drugs used in treatment may produce side effects.

Cervicitis

GENERAL INFORMATION

DEFINITION—Inflammation or infection of the cervix. There are two types and either may be contagious: acute cervicitis, which is usually a bacterial or viral infection with specific symptoms, and chronic cervicitis, which is a long-term infection that may not have symptoms.

SIGNS & SYMPTOMS
Acute cervicitis:
• Vaginal discharge which may be thick and creamy, foamy and greenish-white, white and curdlike, or thin and gray, depending on the type of bacteria present.
Chronic cervicitis:
• Slight, sometimes unnoticeable, vaginal discharge.
• Backache.
• Lower abdominal pain.
• Discomfort with urination.
• Frequent need to urinate.
• Discomfort with sexual intercourse.
Extensive chronic cervicitis:
• Profuse vaginal discharge.
• Vaginal itching or burning.
• Bleeding between menstrual periods.
• Spotting or bleeding after sexual intercourse.

CAUSES
• Acute cervicitis is usually caused by the organisms Neisseria gonorrhoeae or Chlamydia trachomatis. The herpes simplex virus can also be a cause.
• Chronic cervicitis is caused by repeated episodes of acute cervicitis, or one episode that is not treated long enough to heal completely.

RISK INCREASES WITH
• Multiple sexual partners.
• Recent childbirth.
• Diabetes mellitus.
• Acute or recurrent vaginitis.

HOW TO PREVENT
• Have an annual pelvic examination and Pap smear.
• Wear cotton underpants or pantyhose with a cotton crotch. Avoid underpants made from nonventilating materials. Synthetic materials hold in vaginal wetness and warmth, which may trigger vaginal or cervical infections.
• Avoid contracting sexually transmitted diseases by having your sexual partner wear a condom for sexual activity.
• If cervicitis is caused by a sexually transmitted infection, your sexual partner also needs treatment.

PROBABLE OUTCOME
• Mild chronic cervicitis can usually be healed, with treatment, in 4 to 8 weeks.
• Severe chronic cervicitis may require 2 to 3 months of treatment.

• Acute cervicitis caused by venereal disease is contagious through sexual intercourse and is curable with medication.
• Most other cases of cervicitis can be cured with treatment. All women with cervicitis need regular checkups until the condition heals.

POSSIBLE COMPLICATIONS
• Cervical polyps.
• Chronic infection of the upper and lower urinary tract.
• Pelvic inflammatory disease.
• Infertility.
• Cervical hemorrhage following surgical treatment for cervicitis.
• Malignant change in cervix cells (rare).

HOW TO TREAT

GENERAL MEASURES
• Diagnostic tests may include a culture of the vaginal discharge and laboratory blood studies.
• Use sanitary pads instead of tampons during treatment.
• Don't douche unless it is recommended.
• Treatment may involve destruction of abnormal cells with silver nitrate (chemical used for cautery); cryosurgery (destruction of abnormal tissue by applying freezing temperatures, usually with liquid nitrogen); laser therapy or electrocautery (destruction of tissue by heat applied with a controlled electric current).
• If you have chronic cervicitis, your doctor may perform a colposcopy (examination of the cervix with a colposcope, a slender optical instrument with a lighted tip) combined with a biopsy of suspicious areas, in order to rule out cancer of the cervix.

MEDICATION
• Oral antibiotics if infectious cervicitis is suspected.
• Antiviral or antibiotic vaginal creams or suppositories to fight infection.

ACTIVITY—No restrictions, except to avoid sexual relations until determination that the infection has healed.

DIET—No special diet.

CALL YOUR DOCTOR IF

• You or a family member has symptoms of cervicitis.
• During treatment, discomfort persists longer than 1 week or symptoms worsen.
• Unexplained vaginal bleeding or swelling develops during or after treatment.
• New, unexplained symptoms develop. Drugs used in treatment may produce side effects.

Cervix, Biopsy of

GENERAL INFORMATION

DEFINITION—Removal of tissue from the cervix (the lower third of the uterus).

REASONS FOR PROCEDURE
• Usually follows a visual examination or a Pap smear of the cervix that revealed a possible abnormality (e.g., dysplasia).
• Investigation of diseases of the cervix. Laboratory examination of the removed tissue aids in diagnosis.
• May be done for exploratory purposes for conditions such as infertility.
• Sometimes done as a follow-up in women who have previously been treated for early cervical cancer or dysplasia (atypical cells) of the cervix.

RISK INCREASES WITH
• Previous bleeding disorders.
• Use of drugs such as anticoagulants or aspirin.

DESCRIPTION OF PROCEDURE
• Cervical biopsies are usually performed under local anesthesia in the doctor's office.
• A speculum is inserted into the vagina to hold it open and to bring the cervix into view.
• Your physician may perform a colposcopic biopsy, in which a slender optical instrument with a lighted tip is used to pinpoint the areas of the cervix to be biopsied.
• Another instrument is used to gather the tissue. The instrument used will vary, depending on the type of biopsy being performed. In a punch biopsy, the clinician will use an instrument resembling a paper punch to punch out a small sample of cervical tissue; several punches may be necessary. Another common form of biopsy uses a curette, which is a thin metal instrument with a spoon shaped tip, to scrape tissue from the cervix; this is called an endocervical curettage. Still another technique that may be used is called LEEP (loop excision electrosurgical procedure); in this procedure a thin, hand-held wire loop, activated by an electrosurgical generator, is used to make a very precise and uniform cut across the cervix. LEEP can also be used as a treatment for cervical cancer.
• The instruments are removed and the tissue is then sent to the laboratory for microscopic analysis.
• Usually, the procedure is concluded by applying silver nitrate, or a similar agent, to the biopsy sites to prevent bleeding by chemically cauterizing the wounds.

PROBABLE OUTCOME
• Tissue obtained successfully without complications in virtually all cases.
• You may experience mild cramping or pain during the biopsy.
• There may be some spotting of blood for several days, followed by a vaginal discharge, as the biopsy sites heal.

POSSIBLE COMPLICATIONS—Excessive bleeding or surgical-wound infection.

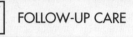

FOLLOW-UP CARE

GENERAL MEASURES
• Wear cotton panties or pantyhose with a cotton crotch. Avoid panties made from nylon, polyester, silk or other nonventilating materials.
• Use a sanitary pad to protect your clothing. Avoid tampons—they may lead to infection.
• Bathe or shower as usual.
• Don't douche unless it is prescribed for you.

MEDICATION
• You may use nonprescription drugs, such as acetaminophen, for minor pain or cramps. If the cramps are severe, your doctor may prescribe additional medication to relieve the pain.

ACTIVITY
• Resume driving 24 hours after recovering from surgery.
• Resume sexual relations 1 to 2 weeks after surgery, unless otherwise specified by your doctor.

DIET—No special diet.

CALL YOUR DOCTOR IF

• You develop signs of infection: headache, muscle aches, dizziness or a general ill feeling and fever.
• Vaginal discharge increases or begins to have an unpleasant odor.
• You experience discomfort that simple pain medication does not relieve quickly.
• Unusual vaginal swelling or bleeding develops.

Cervix, Biopsy of

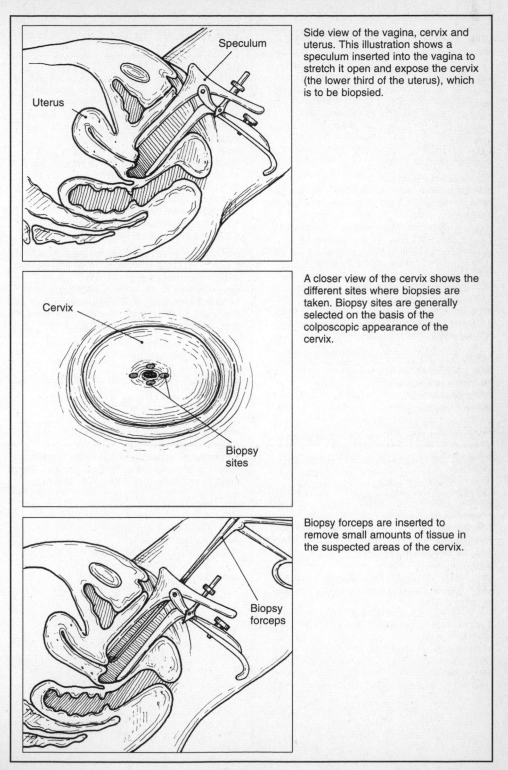

Side view of the vagina, cervix and uterus. This illustration shows a speculum inserted into the vagina to stretch it open and expose the cervix (the lower third of the uterus), which is to be biopsied.

A closer view of the cervix shows the different sites where biopsies are taken. Biopsy sites are generally selected on the basis of the colposcopic appearance of the cervix.

Biopsy forceps are inserted to remove small amounts of tissue in the suspected areas of the cervix.

Chancroid (Soft Chancre)

GENERAL INFORMATION

DEFINITION—A sexually transmitted disease characterized by painful, genital ulcerations, although some women may have no noticeable symptoms of infection. Exposure is usually through sexual intercourse, but accidentally acquired lesions have occurred on the hands. The incubation period is from 3 to 5 days. Chancroid can be transmitted from someone who has no symptoms.

SIGNS & SYMPTOMS
• Small painful lesion (sore or boil), surrounded by a reddish border, that is usually found on the external genitalia. It can become an open, running ulceration. More lesions often develop.
• On women, the lesions most commonly appear on the labia but may appear on the perineum, thigh or cervix. Some women may have no external signs of infection. On men, they appear on the shaft of the penis, the foreskin or the urinary opening.
• The inguinal lymph nodes can become tender, enlarged and matted together, forming an abscess (bubo) in the groin.

CAUSES—Haemophilus ducreyi, a bacterium.

RISK INCREASES WITH
• Multiple sexual partners.
• HIV infection.

HOW TO PREVENT
• Practice safe sex.
• Have a male partner use a condom for sexual activity.
• Liberal use of soap and water on the hands and genitals before and after sexual contact may be somewhat effective in preventing transmission of the disease.

PROBABLE OUTCOME
• Complete healing with appropriate treatment.
• In some patients, the sores heal spontaneously.

POSSIBLE COMPLICATIONS
• Scarring.
• Untreated or inadequately treated cases of chancroid may persist and secondary infection develop.

HOW TO TREAT

GENERAL MEASURES
• Diagnostic tests may include a culture of fluid from the lesions and laboratory blood studies.
• Sexual partners should be examined also.
• Treatment is with medications. The buboes (abscesses) in the lymph nodes may require needle aspiration.
• Warm sitz baths may help ease any pain or discomfort. Sit in a bathtub with warm water 8 to 10 inches deep for 15 to 20 minutes. Do this 2 to 3 times a day.
• Other sexually transmitted diseases are often present and will need to be treated.
• See the Resource section of this book for additional information.

MEDICATION—An antibiotic medication will be prescribed. The treatment regimen may consist of a single dose or treatment for a week depending on the drug used. Antibiotics may reduce the effectiveness of oral contraceptives. If you are currently using oral contraceptives for birth control, discuss this with your doctor.

ACTIVITY—Avoid any sexual activity until healing is complete.

DIET—No special diet.

CALL YOUR DOCTOR IF

• You or your sexual partner has signs and symptoms of chancroid.
• Symptoms worsen after treatment is started.
• New or unexplained symptoms develop. Drugs used in treatment may cause side effects.

Chlamydia Infection

 GENERAL INFORMATION

DEFINITION—Chlamydia are intracellular parasites that have many of the same physical characteristics of viruses. They cause inflammation of the urethra (the tube that allows urine from the bladder to pass outside the body), vagina, cervix, uterus, fallopian tubes, anus and ovaries. This is the most common sexually transmitted disease in the United States. Chlamydia infection may also be transmitted to the eyes or lungs of a newborn infant. If chlamydia are found by microscopic exam and culture of discharge in any person who is sexually active, all sexual partners must be treated.

SIGNS & SYMPTOMS
- Sometimes no symptoms during early stages.
- Vaginal discharge.
- Urethral discharge (males).
- Anal swelling, pain or discharge.
- Reddening of the vagina or tip of the penis.
- Abdominal pain.
- Fever.
- Discomfort on urinating.
- Genital discomfort or pain.

CAUSES—Chlamydia trachomatis bacteria spread by:
- Vaginal sexual intercourse.
- Rectal sexual intercourse.
- Oral-genital contact.
- Vaginal infection during delivery of a newborn, which may infect the baby.

RISK INCREASES WITH
- Unprotected sexual activity, particularly in young females.
- Multiple sex partners.
- Diabetes mellitus.
- General poor health.
- History of other sexually transmitted diseases.

HOW TO PREVENT
- Use of condoms during sexual activity.
- Treatment of all sexual partners of any infected person (usually 2 weeks of an oral antibiotic such as tetracycline).

PROBABLE OUTCOME—Complete cure with adequate antibiotic treatment.

POSSIBLE COMPLICATIONS
- Infertility and/or sterility in females.
- Infecting one's sexual partner.
- Secondary bacterial infections in pelvic organs, genitals or rectum.
- Ectopic pregnancy.
- Abdominal adhesions (scarring).
- Liver infection (perihepatitis).
- Reiter's syndrome.

 HOW TO TREAT

GENERAL MEASURES
- Diagnostic tests may include vaginal smear, rectal smear and urethral smear for laboratory analysis.
- Keep the genital area clean. Use plain unscented soap.
- Take showers rather than tub baths.
- Wear cotton underpants or pantyhose with a cotton crotch. Avoid those made from nonventilating materials, such as nylon.
- After urination or bowel movements, cleanse by wiping or washing from front to back (vagina to anus).
- Lose weight if you are obese.
- Avoid douches.
- If you have diabetes, adhere strictly to your treatment program.
- If urinating causes burning, urinate through a tubular device, such as a toilet-paper roll or plastic cup with the bottom cut out, or pour a cup of warm water over the genital area while urinating.
- A follow-up medical examination, to confirm the absence of chlamydia, is useful after completing the prescribed treatment.
- Testing for other sexually transmitted diseases is usually recommended.

MEDICATION—Oral antibiotics, such as tetracycline or azithromycin (Zithromax), may be prescribed. Antibiotics may reduce the effectiveness of oral contraceptives. If you are currently using oral contraceptives for birth control, discuss this with your doctor.

ACTIVITY
- Delay sexual relations until treatment is completed and symptoms are gone.
- Allow about 3 weeks for recovery.

DIET—No special diet.

 CALL YOUR DOCTOR IF

- You or a family member has symptoms of chlamydia infection.
- Symptoms persist longer than 1 week or worsen despite treatment.
- Unusual vaginal bleeding or swelling develops.
- New, unexplained symptoms develop. Drugs used in treatment may produce side effects.

Colposcopy

GENERAL INFORMATION

DEFINITION—A microscopic examination of the cervix used to diagnose potential abnormalities of the cervix and vagina. Because the colposcope magnifies the tissue by up to 30 times, as well as illuminates the areas to be examined, cervical biopsies performed with a colposcopic examination are more accurate than those done without the use of a colposcope.

REASONS FOR PROCEDURE—It is usually recommended following an abnormal Pap smear test and to select the best area for a biopsy, if needed.

RISK INCREASES WITH—None expected.

DESCRIPTION OF PROCEDURE
• The colposcope is a binocular microscope used to visualize the cervix.
• You will recline on an examining table (as if for a pelvic examination). A speculum is inserted into the vagina to expose the cervix.
• A stain or other chemical agent may be used to help improve the visualization.
• The wheeled colposcope is positioned in front of the vaginal opening and the doctor can locate the abnormalities, determine their extent and possibly identify the cause. Results of the visual examination are available immediately.

PROBABLE OUTCOME—The procedure should take about 15 minutes and in itself cause no discomfort. The instrument never enters the body. If a biopsy is done or endocervical curettage is performed, these procedures may cause some cramping or bleeding.

POSSIBLE COMPLICATIONS—A biopsy done in conjunction with a colposcopy may cause some bleeding and, rarely, an infection.

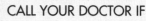

FOLLOW-UP CARE

GENERAL MEASURES—You may bathe or shower as usual.

MEDICATION—Medication is usually not necessary following this procedure.

ACTIVITY—No restrictions.

DIET—No special diet.

CALL YOUR DOCTOR IF

Following the procedure:
• You develop unexplained vaginal bleeding or swelling.
• Vaginal discharge increases or begins to have an unpleasant odor.
• You develop signs of infection: headache, muscle aches, dizziness or a general ill feeling and fever.

Colposcopy

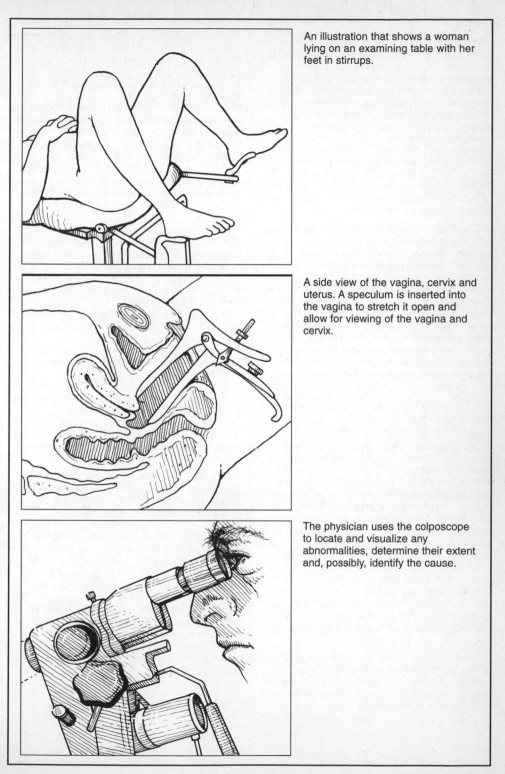

An illustration that shows a woman lying on an examining table with her feet in stirrups.

A side view of the vagina, cervix and uterus. A speculum is inserted into the vagina to stretch it open and allow for viewing of the vagina and cervix.

The physician uses the colposcope to locate and visualize any abnormalities, determine their extent and, possibly, identify the cause.

Condom Usage to Prevent STDs

 GENERAL INFORMATION

WHO SHOULD USE A CONDOM?

• Because male condoms are used for both birth control and reducing the risk of disease, some people think that other forms of birth control will also protect them against disease. This is not true. Even if you use another form of birth control, you need a male condom to reduce the risk of getting STDs (sexually transmitted diseases).

• Condoms do not make sex 100 percent safe, but, if properly used, they can reduce the chance of contracting STDs, including AIDS. This can mean protection not only for you and your partner, but also for any children you may have in the future.

CHOOSING A CONDOM—Read the label and look for the following:

• The condoms should be made of latex (rubber) or polyurethane (a new condom product).

• It should say that the condoms are to prevent disease, and if used properly, latex condoms help reduce risk of HIV transmission and many other STDs. If the package doesn't say anything about preventing disease, the condoms may not provide the protection you want. Novelty condoms, for example, will not be labeled for either disease protection or pregnancy prevention. Condoms that don't cover the entire penis are not labeled for disease prevention and should not be used for this purpose. For proper protection, a condom must unroll to cover the entire penis.

• Check the expiration date (EXP followed by date). The condom should not be purchased or used after that date.

• Condoms are available in many stores and from vending machines. If purchasing condoms from vending machines, check for proper labeling. Do not purchase condoms from a vending machine located where it may be subject to extreme temperatures or direct sunlight.

• Condoms should be stored in a cool, dry place out of direct sunlight. Closets or drawers usually make good storage places. Condoms should not be kept in a pocket, wallet or purse for more than a few hours at a time because they may be exposed to extreme temperatures.

HOW TO USE A CONDOM

• When opening a condom, handle the package gently. Don't use teeth, sharp fingernails, scissors or other sharp instruments as these may damage the condom. And make sure you can see what you're doing!

• After you open the package, inspect the condom. If the material sticks to itself or is gummy, the condom is no good. Check the condom top for other obvious damage such as brittleness, tears and holes, but don't unroll the condom to check it because this could damage it.

• Use a new condom for every act of intercourse and oral sex.

• Put the condom on after the penis is erect and before any contact is made between the penis and any part of the partner's body.

• If using a spermicide (see Spermicides below), put some inside the condom tip.

• If the condom does not have a reservoir tip, pinch the tip enough to leave a half-inch space for semen to collect. Make sure to eliminate any air in the tip to help keep the condom from breaking.

• Holding the condom by the rim (and pinching the half-inch tip, if necessary), place the condom on top of the penis. Then, continuing to hold it by the rim, unroll it all the way to the base of the penis. If you are using a water-based lubricant, you can put more on the outside of the condom.

• If you feel the condom break during sexual activity, stop immediately, withdraw and put on a new condom.

• After ejaculation and before the penis gets soft, grip the rim of the condom and carefully withdraw.

• To remove the condom, gently pull it off the penis, being careful the semen doesn't spill out.

• Wrap the used condom in a tissue and throw it in the trash. Because condoms may cause problems in sewers, don't flush them down the toilet. Afterwards, wash your hands with soap and water.

PRECAUTION—Although condoms afford good protection for vaginal and oral sex (where the penis is in contact with the mouth), the protection they give for anal sex is questionable. The Surgeon General of the Public Health Service has said, "condoms provide some protection, but anal intercourse is simply too dangerous a practice." Condoms may be more likely to break during anal intercourse than during other types of sex because of the greater amount of friction and other stresses involved. Even if the condom doesn't break, anal intercourse is very risky because it can cause rectal tissue to tear and bleed, allowing disease germs to pass more easily from one partner to another.

Condom Usage to Prevent STDs (cont.)

SPERMICIDES
- Spermicides, which kill sperm, are used for birth control either alone or with barrier contraceptives such as the diaphragm or cervical cap. Scientists have observed that, in test tubes, a spermicide called nonoxynol-9 kills organisms that cause STDs. Although it has not been scientifically proven, it is possible that nonoxynol-9 may also reduce the risk of transmission of the AIDS virus during intercourse. Using a spermicide along with a latex condom is therefore advisable and is an added precaution in case the condom breaks. Some condoms come with nonoxynol-9 already added. Their packages are required to be labeled with the expiration date of the spermicide, and they should not be used after that date.
- Some experts think that even if a condom with spermicide is used, additional spermicide in the form of a jelly, cream or foam should be added. These are sold over the counter in pharmacies and some supermarkets. (Although swallowing small amounts of spermicide has not proven harmful in animal tests, it is not known if this is true for humans. For that reason, and because spermicides have a bitter taste, for oral sex only, it may be best to use a condom without spermicide.)

LUBRICANTS—Lubricants may help prevent condoms from breaking during use and may prevent irritation that might increase the chance of infection. Some condoms come lubricated with dry silicone, jelly or cream, or you can add water-based lubricants specifically made for this purpose (for example, K-Y Lubricating Jelly). If you use a separate lubricant, never use a product that contains oils, fats or greases such as a petroleum-based jelly (for example, Vaseline), baby oil or lotion, hand or body lotion, cooking shortenings, or oily cosmetics such as cold creams. These can seriously weaken latex, causing a condom to tear easily. If you use a spermicide, you do not need to use a lubricant because spermicide acts as a lubricant.

ADDITIONAL RESOURCES FOR INFORMATION: See the Resource section of this book for additional information.

 CALL YOUR DOCTOR IF

You have questions about use of a condom.

Cryosurgery
(Cryotherapy)

 GENERAL INFORMATION

DEFINITION—Thermal destruction of abnormal tissue by freezing, usually with liquid nitrogen.

REASONS FOR PROCEDURE
• Primary treatment of mild to moderate cervical dysplasia (abnormal cell growth).
• Sometimes used to treat severe dysplasia.
• Removal of skin lesions such as actinic keratoses (precancerous conditions caused by the sun) and warts.
• Treatment of benign (noncancerous) growths on the cervix (such as polyps) or genital warts.
• Treatment of cervicitis (inflammation of the cervix).

RISK INCREASES WITH—None expected.

DESCRIPTION OF PROCEDURE
• For small skin lesions, liquid nitrogen is applied to a cotton-tipped applicator. The applicator is held to the skin lesions until they are frozen and destroyed.
• Sometimes, a spray can with pressurized liquid nitrogen is used to freeze skin lesions.
• For cryosurgery on the cervix, a special probe instrument is used. Liquid nitrogen circulates in the tip of this instrument causing it to become almost as cold as the liquid nitrogen itself. The instrument tip is held on the affected areas until the abnormal tissue is frozen.

PROBABLE OUTCOME
• For skin lesions: Initial swelling and redness become a blister in 2 or 3 days. The blister will rupture by itself about 2 weeks after surgery. It will leave a scab, but little or no scar after complete healing.
• For cryosurgery of the cervix: Expect complete healing without complications. There may be mild uterine cramping and facial flushing. Vaginal discharge is common; discharge may be profuse, foul-smelling and last for 7-10 days or longer. Allow about 3 weeks for recovery from surgery.

POSSIBLE COMPLICATIONS
• Surgical-wound infection (rare).
• Cervical stenosis (narrowing).
• Failure of the procedure to destroy all of the cervical dysplasia, particularly with severe dysplasia.

 FOLLOW-UP CARE

GENERAL MEASURES
• For cervical therapy, discuss with your doctor when you should be seen for a follow-up examination to be sure healing is complete and to assure that the treatment was effective.
• Bathe and shower as usual. If appropriate, keep any skin wounds dry with bandages for the first 2 or 3 days after surgery. If a bandage gets wet, change it promptly.

MEDICATION—You may use nonprescription drugs, such as acetaminophen, to relieve minor pain.

ACTIVITY—If cryosurgery was for cervical therapy, avoid any sexual activity until healing is complete.

DIET—No special diet.

 CALL YOUR DOCTOR IF

• Pain, swelling, redness, drainage or bleeding increases in the surgical area.
• You develop signs of infection: headache, muscle aches, dizziness or a general ill feeling and fever.
• Vaginal discharge increases or changes.

Cryosurgery
(Cryotherapy)

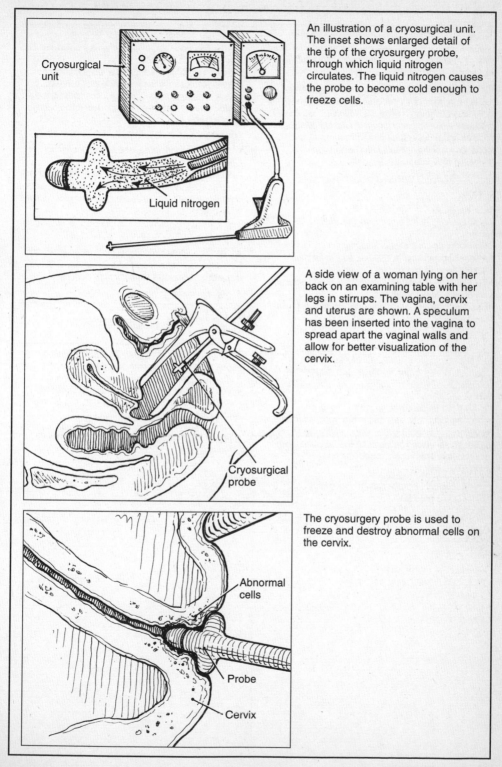

Cryosurgical unit

Liquid nitrogen

An illustration of a cryosurgical unit. The inset shows enlarged detail of the tip of the cryosurgery probe, through which liquid nitrogen circulates. The liquid nitrogen causes the probe to become cold enough to freeze cells.

Cryosurgical probe

A side view of a woman lying on her back on an examining table with her legs in stirrups. The vagina, cervix and uterus are shown. A speculum has been inserted into the vagina to spread apart the vaginal walls and allow for better visualization of the cervix.

Abnormal cells

Probe

Cervix

The cryosurgery probe is used to freeze and destroy abnormal cells on the cervix.

Culdocentesis

 GENERAL INFORMATION

DEFINITION—Piercing the "cul-de-sac," the space deep in the vagina behind and under the cervix, in order to obtain a fluid sample for laboratory examination.

REASONS FOR PROCEDURE—Investigation of possible ailments in the abdomen and pelvis, including bleeding inside the lower pelvic cavity; ruptured ectopic pregnancy; ruptured ovarian cyst; ovarian cancer or pelvic inflammatory disease. Laboratory examination of the removed fluid aids in diagnosis.

RISK INCREASES WITH—Recent or chronic illness.

DESCRIPTION OF PROCEDURE
• A speculum is inserted into the vagina to hold it open.
• The rear lip of the cervix is raised.
• A local anesthetic is applied to the farthest back portion of the vagina (cul-de-sac).
• The posterior wall of the vagina is penetrated with a needle and syringe.
• Fluid, if present, is aspirated. No sutures are necessary.

PROBABLE OUTCOME
• A fluid sample is obtained successfully without complications in virtually all cases. If fluid or blood confirms other findings that suggest a serious disease or condition, you may need further surgery.
• If no fluid is obtained and there are no complications, but you still have your original symptoms, expect further observation or tests to diagnose your condition. Allow about 1 week for recovery from the procedure.

POSSIBLE COMPLICATIONS
• Perforation of bladder or bowel (rare).
• Excessive bleeding.
• Surgical-wound infection.

 FOLLOW-UP CARE

GENERAL MEASURES
• Resume your usual activities as soon as possible.
• Continue to use your usual birth control methods. Your periods should not be disturbed.
• Use sanitary pads for your next menstrual period. Avoid tampons temporarily; they may lead to infection.

MEDICATION
• Will vary, depending upon diagnosis.
• Antibiotics to fight or prevent infection. Antibiotics may reduce the effectiveness of oral contraceptives. If you are currently using oral contraceptives for birth control, discuss this with your doctor.
• You may use nonprescription drugs, such as acetaminophen, to relieve minor pain.

ACTIVITY—Resume normal activities gradually. Resume sexual relations when able. This will depend on various underlying causes.

DIET—No special diet.

CALL YOUR DOCTOR IF

• You experience vaginal bleeding that soaks more than 1 pad or tampon each hour.
• Symptoms recur or worsen.
• You develop signs of infection: headache, muscle aches, dizziness or a general ill feeling and fever.
• New, unexplained symptoms develop. Drugs used in treatment may produce side effects.

Culdocentesis

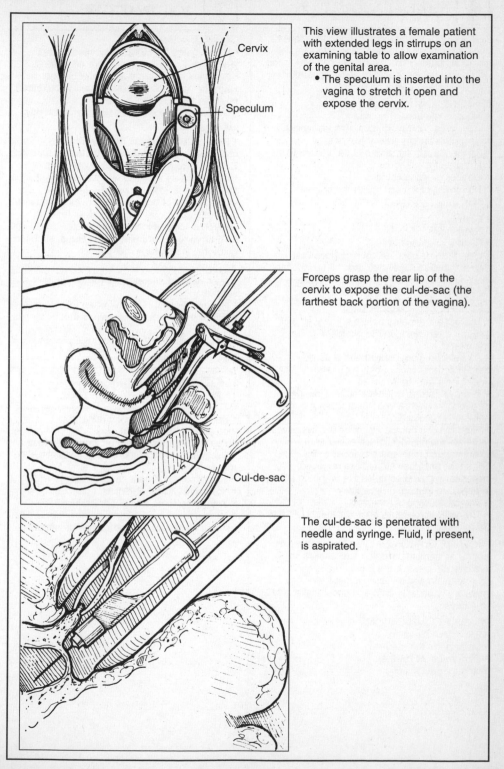

Cervix

Speculum

This view illustrates a female patient with extended legs in stirrups on an examining table to allow examination of the genital area.
- The speculum is inserted into the vagina to stretch it open and expose the cervix.

Forceps grasp the rear lip of the cervix to expose the cul-de-sac (the farthest back portion of the vagina).

Cul-de-sac

The cul-de-sac is penetrated with needle and syringe. Fluid, if present, is aspirated.

Cystoscopy

GENERAL INFORMATION

DEFINITION—Visual examination of the lower urinary tract and collection of a urine sample from the bladder. The examination is performed with a cystoscope, a thin fiber-optic instrument with lenses and a light on its tip.

REASONS FOR PROCEDURE
- Blood in the urine (hematuria).
- Inability to control urination (incontinence).
- Recurrent urinary tract infections.
- Congenital abnormalities of the urinary tract.
- Tumors of the bladder.
- Bladder or kidney stones.
- Tightening of the urethra or the ureters.

RISK INCREASES WITH
- Obesity.
- Smoking.
- Recent or chronic illness.
- Use of drugs such as antihypertensives, muscle relaxants, tranquilizers, sleep inducers, insulin, sedatives, beta-adrenergic blockers or cortisone.

DESCRIPTION OF PROCEDURE
- The patient urinates before surgery so that any urine remaining in the bladder can be measured.
- A local or regional anesthetic is usually administered; occasionally, a general anesthesia may be required.
- The cystoscope is lubricated and inserted through the urethra into the bladder. A urine sample is collected.
- Fluid may be pumped through the cystoscope to inflate the bladder, which allows visual examination of the entire bladder wall.
- Bladder or kidney stones are removed, if necessary. Tissue samples are gathered and lesions are treated, if necessary.
- The cystoscope is removed.
- The entire procedure should take about 20 to 30 minutes.

PROBABLE OUTCOME—Examination completed and urine sample collected successfully in virtually all cases. If the procedure is confined to inspection and minimal manipulation, recovery is usually rapid and should take only 2 to 4 days.

POSSIBLE COMPLICATIONS
- Excessive bleeding.
- Damage to the urethra.
- Perforation of bladder.
- Urinary tract infection.

FOLLOW-UP CARE

GENERAL MEASURES
- Warm baths for 10 to 15 minutes several times a day may help to relieve discomfort.
- You may notice a small amount of blood in your urine following the exam; this should last no more than 24 hours.
- Drink eight 8-ounce glasses of water a day.

MEDICATION
- Pain medication may be prescribed; don't take prescription pain medication for longer than 4 to 7 days. Take only as much as you need.
- Antibiotics as required to fight or prevent infection. Antibiotics may reduce the effectiveness of oral contraceptives. If you are currently using oral contraceptives for birth control, discuss this with your doctor.
- You may use nonprescription drugs, such as acetaminophen, for minor pain.

ACTIVITY
- Avoid vigorous exercise for 2 weeks after surgery.
- Resume sexual relations when follow-up medical examination determines that healing is complete.
- Resume driving 2 days after the procedure.

DIET—No special diet.

CALL YOUR DOCTOR IF

- Pain, swelling, redness, drainage or bleeding increases in the surgical area.
- You develop signs of infection: headache, muscle aches, dizziness or a general ill feeling and fever.
- You experience nausea or vomiting.
- You have painful or difficult urination.
- Your urine turns a bright or dark red color.
- New, unexplained symptoms develop. Drugs used in treatment may produce side effects.

Cystoscopy

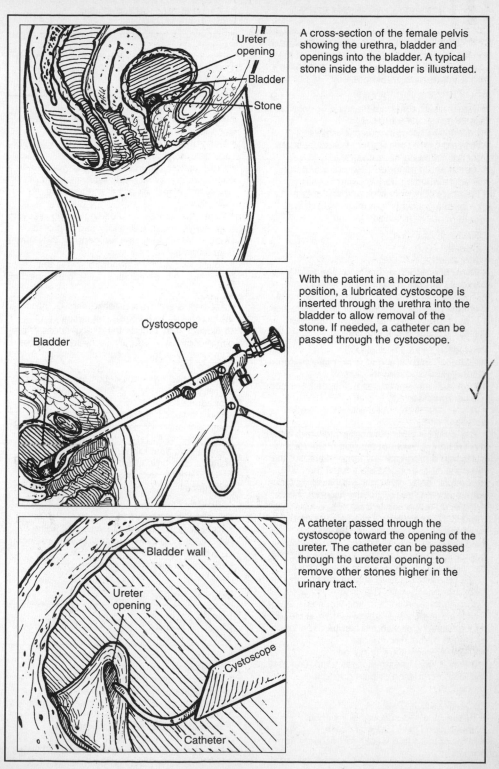

A cross-section of the female pelvis showing the urethra, bladder and openings into the bladder. A typical stone inside the bladder is illustrated.

Ureter opening

Bladder

Stone

With the patient in a horizontal position, a lubricated cystoscope is inserted through the urethra into the bladder to allow removal of the stone. If needed, a catheter can be passed through the cystoscope.

Cystoscope

Bladder

A catheter passed through the cystoscope toward the opening of the ureter. The catheter can be passed through the ureteral opening to remove other stones higher in the urinary tract.

Bladder wall

Ureter opening

Cystoscope

Catheter

Dilatation & Curettage (D & C)

GENERAL INFORMATION

DEFINITION—Opening the cervix and scraping the lining (endometrium) and contents of the uterus. The D & C is often both a diagnostic and a therapeutic procedure.

REASONS FOR PROCEDURE
• Diagnosis of abnormal bleeding or possible cancer inside the uterus.
• Incomplete spontaneous miscarriage.
• Prevent or stop hemorrhage or subsequent infection following miscarriage.
• Treatment of minor diseases of the uterus.
• Elective abortion during early pregnancy.
• Removal of membranes and placenta after childbirth in cases where they fail to deliver spontaneously (retained placenta).

RISK INCREASES WITH
• Obesity.
• Smoking.
• Cervical infection or ongoing uterine infection.
• Excess alcohol consumption.
• Recent or chronic illness, including anemia, diabetes mellitus, and heart or lung disease.
• Use of drugs, such as antihypertensives, cortisone, diuretics or insulin.

DESCRIPTION OF PROCEDURE
• Dilatation and curettage is normally performed in a hospital or a surgery center.
• A general anesthetic, local anesthetic or both will be administered.
• The vagina is cleansed with an antiseptic solution.
• The cervix is carefully opened (dilated) either by inserting a series of tapered metal rods, each with a progressively larger diameter, into the cervical opening at the time of the procedure, or by dilating the cervix in advance with laminaria (freeze-dried seaweed), which are placed in the cervix 8 to 12 hours prior to the D & C, where they will swell and gradually open the cervix to 1 to 2 centimeters.
• Following sufficient opening of the cervix, a curette is inserted into the uterus. The curette can be a suction device or a looped knife.
• The curette is used to scrape the endometrium from the uterine wall. The tissue may be removed for examination and diagnosis, or for treatment of heavy or irregular uterine bleeding.
• Occasionally, ultrasound can be used for guidance of the instruments.
• The instruments are removed.
• If only a local anesthetic was used, you may feel some cramping or pain during the procedure.

PROBABLE OUTCOME
• Tissue obtained successfully without complications in virtually all cases.
• Allow about 4 to 6 weeks for recovery from surgery.

POSSIBLE COMPLICATIONS
• Uterine infection (endometritis).
• Excessive bleeding.
• Inadvertent injury to the uterus, bladder or bowel.

FOLLOW-UP CARE

GENERAL MEASURES
• You may experience mild cramping or back-ache for 2 to 3 days following surgery.
• Don't douche unless your physician recommends it.
• Wear cotton underpants and pantyhose with a cotton crotch. Avoid underpants made from nylon, polyester, silk or other nonventilating materials.
• Expect slight vaginal bleeding during recovery from surgery. Use a sanitary pad to protect clothing. Avoid tampons temporarily; they may lead to infection.
• Your first menstrual period following the procedure may be earlier or later than expected.

MEDICATION
• Antibiotics are often given during, or following, the procedure to help prevent infection. Antibiotics may reduce the effectiveness of oral contraceptives. If you are currently taking oral contraceptives for birth control, discuss this with your doctor.
• Prescription pain medication should generally be required for only 2 to 7 days following the procedure.
• You may use nonprescription drugs, such as acetaminophen, or nonsteroidal anti-inflammatory drugs (NSAIDs) such as ibuprofen or naproxen sodium for minor pain. Follow your dcotor's recommendations.
• Hormones, if necessary to correct an imbalance.

ACTIVITY
• Resume driving in 1 to 2 days.
• To help recovery and aid your well-being, resume daily activities, including work, as soon as you are able.
• Resume sexual relations when spotting ceases.

DIET—No special diet.

CALL YOUR DOCTOR IF

• Vaginal discharge increases or smells unpleasant.
• You experience pain that simple pain medication does not relieve quickly.
• Unusual vaginal swelling or bleeding develops.
• You develop signs of infection: fever, general ill feeling, headache, muscle aches or dizziness.
• New, unexplained symptoms develop. Drugs used in treatment may produce side effects.

Dilatation & Curettage (D & C)

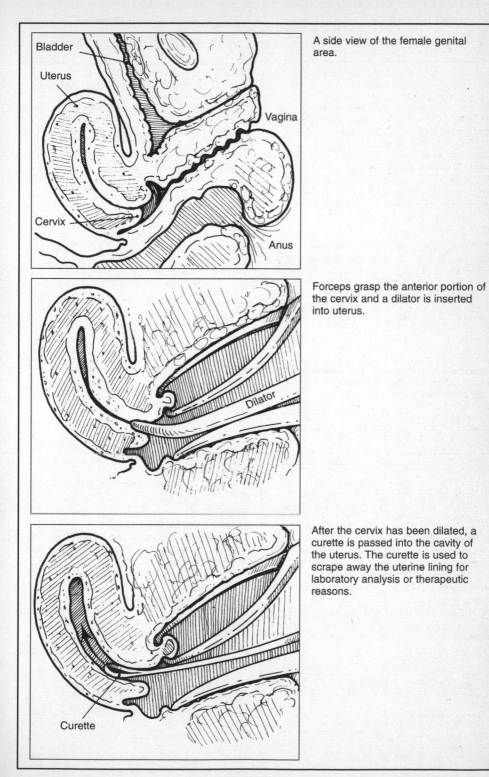

A side view of the female genital area.

Bladder

Uterus

Vagina

Cervix

Anus

Forceps grasp the anterior portion of the cervix and a dilator is inserted into uterus.

Dilator

After the cervix has been dilated, a curette is passed into the cavity of the uterus. The curette is used to scrape away the uterine lining for laboratory analysis or therapeutic reasons.

Curette

Dysmenorrhea
(Menstrual Cramps)

 GENERAL INFORMATION

DEFINITION—Severe, painful cramps during menstruation. Primary dysmenorrhea usually occurs in women who have just begun menstruating; it usually subsides almost completely by the time a woman reaches her late twenties. Secondary dysmenorrhea is menstrual pain that develops in a woman who previously had little or no menstrual pain. The severity of symptoms in both types of dysmenorrhea varies greatly from woman to woman, and from one month to the next in the same woman. Dysmenorrhea usually is less severe after a woman has had a baby.

SIGNS & SYMPTOMS
- Cramping, spasmodic pain in the lower abdomen, lower back and thighs. The pain starts at onset of menses and lasts for hours to days.
- Nausea and vomiting (sometimes).
- Diarrhea (occasionally).
- Irritability, nervousness, depression.

CAUSES
- Strong or prolonged contractions of the muscular wall of the uterus. These may be caused by concentration of prostaglandins (hormones found in the cervix and uterus). Research shows that women with dysmenorrhea produce and excrete more prostaglandins than those who don't have as much discomfort.
- Dilation (stretching) of the cervix to allow passage of blood clots through the cervix.
- Pelvic infections.
- Endometriosis, especially if dysmenorrhea begins after age 20.
- Adenomyosis (endometrial tissue that has become displaced into the wall of the uterus).
- Fibroids or other benign tumors of the uterus.
- Use of intrauterine device (IUD).

RISK INCREASES WITH
- Use of caffeine or nicotine.
- Stress.
- Family history of dysmenorrhea.
- Lack of exercise; poor diet.

HOW TO PREVENT
- Take female hormones that prevent ovulation, such as oral contraceptives.
- Treatment of the underlying cause.

PROBABLE OUTCOME
- Symptoms can be controlled with treatment.
- Symptoms improve with age and with childbirth. Symptoms are rare in postmenopausal women.

POSSIBLE COMPLICATIONS
- Severe pain that regularly interferes with normal activity.
- Infertility from underlying cause.

 HOW TO TREAT

GENERAL MEASURES
- Pelvic exam and a patient history may help suggest the cause of dysmenorrhea.
- Initial treatment aims are to relieve pain. Long-term goals of treatment involve treating any underlying cause with medication, counseling or possibly surgery.
- Heat helps relieve pain. Use a heating pad or hot-water bottle on the abdomen or back, or take hot baths. Sit in a tub of hot water for 10 to 15 minutes as often as necessary.
- Psychotherapy or counseling, if dysmenorrhea is stress-related.
- Hypnosis therapy may help.
- Treatment, as required, for the cause of the secondary dysmenorrhea.
- Surgery may be recommended for women whose pain cannot be controlled by medications.

MEDICATION
- For minor discomfort, use nonsteroidal anti-inflammatory drugs (NSAIDs) such as aspirin, ibuprofen or naproxen, in accordance with your physician's recommendations.
- Oral contraceptives may be prescribed to prevent ovulation.
- In severe cases, hormones (e.g., Lupron or Danazol) can stop ovary function and relieve pain.

ACTIVITY
- No restrictions. When resting in bed, elevate your feet or bend your knees and lie on your side.
- Regular, vigorous exercise reduces discomfort of future periods.

DIET
- Reduce your caffeine intake.
- Vitamin B supplements and herbal teas both help reduce symptoms in some women.

 CALL YOUR DOCTOR IF

- You or a family member has symptoms of dysmenorrhea that cannot be controlled.
- Bleeding becomes excessive (you saturate a pad or tampon more frequently than once each hour).
- Signs of infection develop: fever, a general ill feeling, headache, dizziness or muscle aches.
- New, unexplained symptoms develop. Drugs used in treatment may produce side effects.

Dyspareunia

GENERAL INFORMATION

DEFINITION—Recurrent and persistent genital pain associated with sexual intercourse. Dyspareunia and vaginismus (spasm of the pubic muscles of the lower vagina which prevents penetration) are often linked.

SIGNS & SYMPTOMS—Pain in the genital area during sexual activity, including foreplay, intercourse or attempted intercourse. Pain may be mild or severe, and it may vary with different intercourse positions.

CAUSES
Physical causes:
• Infection of the genitals, including herpes and others involving the vagina, cervix, fallopian tubes or ovaries.
• Scarring from operations or radiation therapy.
• Tight episiotomy scar from vaginal repair after childbirth.
• A fibroid or other uterine tumor.
• Endometriosis.
• A hymen that is imperforate (not opened), torn or thicker than normal.
• A bruised opening to the urethra.
• Inadequate vaginal or condom lubrication.
• Allergic reactions to diaphragms, condoms or contraceptive foams and jellies.
• Dryness and thinness of the vaginal wall after menopause due to estrogen deficiency.
• Pelvic inflammatory disease.
Psychological and emotional causes:
• Fear of pregnancy.
• Fear of injury to the unborn child during pregnancy.
• Lack of sexual arousal and vaginal lubrication caused by inadequate or insufficient sexual foreplay, aversion to a sexual partner, fatigue or anxiety.
• Lack of sexual experience or information.
• Past sexual injury or psychological trauma such as assault.

RISK INCREASES WITH
• Pregnancy and the postpartum period.
• Stress.
• Recent illness.
• Fatigue or overwork.
• Alcohol consumption.
• Menopause.

HOW TO PREVENT
• Obtain prompt medical treatment if you have symptoms of infection of the reproductive organs.
• Discontinue use of contraceptive foams or jellies that produce allergic reactions.
• Discuss the lack of sexual arousal with your partner, including ways to improve foreplay. Enlist your partner's support and patience to overcome the problem. Use a water-based nonallergenic lubricant, if necessary.

• Obtain professional counseling to resolve feelings about past sexual trauma.

PROBABLE OUTCOME—Depends on the cause. Medical disorders are usually curable with treatment. Psychological problems can often be cured with therapy, and interpersonal problems can improve with communication and patience.

POSSIBLE COMPLICATIONS—Damage to personal relationships, permanent inability to enjoy sexual experiences and loss of self-esteem.

HOW TO TREAT

GENERAL MEASURES
• Laboratory studies, such as a Pap smear, blood tests or laparoscopy to diagnose any medical problem that can be treated.
• Appropriate treatment will be directed to physical causes or psychological causes.
• Sitz baths frequently relieve tenderness. Sit in a tub of lukewarm water for 10 to 15 minutes. Repeat baths as often as 3 or 4 times a day.
• Use a nonprescription water-based lubricant, such as K-Y Lubricating Jelly, during sexual intercourse.
• Instructions for exercises or techniques to dilate the vagina. They may involve use of fingers or dilators to condition the body and mind to the sensation of something being inserted into the vagina.
• Try different positions for sexual intercourse to discover new ones that might be pain-free.
• Treatment for psychological causes will vary depending on the needs of the patient. It can involve education about contraception, counseling to uncover hidden conflicts, sensate focus exercises and teaching of appropriate foreplay techniques.
• Surgery to correct an underlying problem may relieve symptoms.

MEDICATION
• Antibiotic, antiviral or antifungal medications may be prescribed for an underlying infection.
• Estrogen therapy may be prescribed for women who are postmenopausal.

ACTIVITY—No restrictions. A regular exercise program, while not a treatment for dyspareunia, is helpful in promoting general well-being.

DIET—No special diet.

CALL YOUR DOCTOR IF

• You or a family member has symptoms of dyspareunia.
• Pain worsens, or symptoms fail to disappear after 3 months of treatment.
• New, unexplained symptoms develop. Drugs used in treatment may produce side effects.

Endometrial Biopsy
(Uterine Biopsy)

 GENERAL INFORMATION

DEFINITION—A diagnostic procedure that involves removal of tissue from the endometrium, the inner lining of the uterus.

REASONS FOR PROCEDURE—Investigation of bleeding between menstrual periods or post-menopausal bleeding. Laboratory examination of the removed tissue aids in diagnosis. If appropriate, the procedure is performed during the last few days of the patient's menstrual cycle. This is the best time to identify possible hormonal problems and to determine if ovulation is occurring for patients undergoing fertility evaluation.

RISK INCREASES WITH—None expected.

DESCRIPTION OF PROCEDURE
• Usually performed in the doctor's office with little or no anesthesia necessary.
• A speculum is inserted into the vagina to bring the cervix into view. In some cases, it is necessary to use a tenaculum (a hooklike instrument that holds and helps stabilize the cervix).
• A small, straw-shaped instrument (or other biopsy instrument) is inserted through the cervix into the uterus. It is gently scraped against the inner lining of the uterus to gather tissue. An alternate method involves obtaining the tissue sample with a suction instrument; this procedure is sometimes referred to as a vacuum aspiration.
• The instruments are removed. The surgery may cause some moderate cramping during the time the tissue is being removed; occasionally, cramping may be more severe.

PROBABLE OUTCOME
• Tissue obtained successfully without complications in virtually all cases.
• Allow about 1 week for recovery from surgery. During this time, you should expect vaginal discharge.
• Laboratory testing on the tissue can confirm ovulation has occurred and may identify other causes of infertility, such as infection.
• Laboratory examination will generally determine if there are any abnormal cells found in the uterine lining.

POSSIBLE COMPLICATIONS
• Excessive bleeding.
• Infection of the uterine lining (endometritis).
• Inadvertent injury to the uterus (rare).

FOLLOW-UP CARE

GENERAL MEASURES
• Bathe or shower as usual. Use nonperfumed soap.
• Wear sanitary pads for the rest of this menstrual period. Avoid tampons temporarily; they may lead to infection. Your menstrual flow may be heavier than usual.
• Wear cotton underpants and pantyhose with a cotton crotch. Avoid underwear made from nylon, polyester, silk or other nonventilating materials.
• Don't douche unless it is prescribed for you.

MEDICATION
• Hormones, if a hormonal imbalance is confirmed.
• If infection is found, your doctor may prescribe oral antibiotics. Antibiotics may reduce the effectiveness of oral contraceptives. If you are currently taking oral contraceptives for birth control, discuss this with your doctor.
• You may use nonprescription drugs, such as acetaminophen or nonsteroidal anti-inflammatory drugs (NSAIDs) such as ibuprofen, for minor pain.

ACTIVITY
• Resume daily activities and work as soon as possible.
• You may resume sexual relations once all bleeding has stopped and medical clearance is given.

DIET—No special diet.

 CALL YOUR DOCTOR IF

• Vaginal discharge increases or begins to have an unpleasant odor.
• You experience pain that simple medication does not relieve quickly.
• You experience abdominal or lower back pain.
• Vaginal swelling or unusually heavy bleeding develops.
• You develop signs of infection: fever, general ill feeling, headache, dizziness or muscle aches.
• New, unexplained symptoms develop. Drugs used in treatment may produce side effects.

Endometrial Biopsy
(Uterine Biopsy)

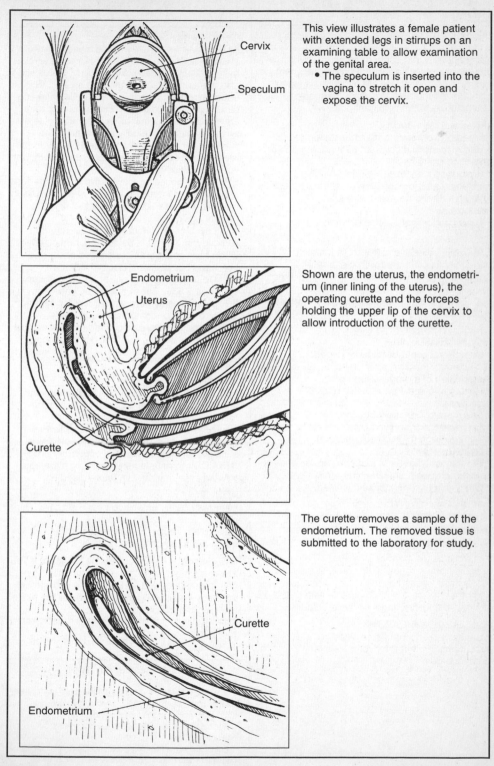

This view illustrates a female patient with extended legs in stirrups on an examining table to allow examination of the genital area.
- The speculum is inserted into the vagina to stretch it open and expose the cervix.

Cervix

Speculum

Shown are the uterus, the endometrium (inner lining of the uterus), the operating curette and the forceps holding the upper lip of the cervix to allow introduction of the curette.

Endometrium

Uterus

Curette

The curette removes a sample of the endometrium. The removed tissue is submitted to the laboratory for study.

Curette

Endometrium

Endometrial Hyperplasia

 GENERAL INFORMATION

DEFINITION—An overgrowth of tissue in the endometrium (inner lining of the uterus). This is not cancerous, but some hyperplasia, even though reversible, is considered premalignant. Terms used to describe the hyperplasia (simple, complex, adenomatous and atypical) help characterize its premalignant potential.

SIGNS & SYMPTOMS
- Bleeding between normal menstrual periods.
- Heavy menstrual flow (saturating a tampon or pad once every hour).
- Prolonged menstrual periods.
- Bleeding after menopause (postmenopausal).
- Vaginal discharge, especially after menopause.
- Lower abdominal cramps occur in some patients.

CAUSES—Excessive estrogen (a female hormone) as compared with the amount of progesterone (another female hormone). This excess is caused internally, or from the use of hormone-containing medications. Endometrial hyperplasia rarely occurs in women who have a normal menstrual cycle.

RISK INCREASES WITH
- Use of oral contraceptives or estrogen replacement therapy (after menopause) without the addition of a progesterone drug.
- History of chronic anovulation (lack of ovulation).
- Early age of first menstruation.
- Polycystic ovarian syndrome.
- Hypertension (high blood pressure).
- Diabetes mellitus.
- Women who have not had children, or who delayed childbirth until the later fertile years.
- Obesity in postmenopausal women.
- Late menopause (over age 55).

HOW TO PREVENT—No specific preventive measures.

PROBABLE OUTCOME
- In most cases, hormonal treatment with a progesterone (progestin) will reverse the hyperplasia caused by the excess estrogen.
- In other cases, it is often curable with D & C (dilatation and curettage) or hysterectomy.

POSSIBLE COMPLICATIONS
- Excessive, uncontrollable bleeding.
- Confirmation that the hyperplasia is precancerous.

HOW TO TREAT

GENERAL MEASURES
- Diagnostic tests may include laboratory studies, such as blood tests of hormone levels; hysteroscopy (visual examination of the cervix and uterus); ultrasound and Pap smear. An endometrial biopsy and a D & C (dilatation and curettage) as a treatment and to obtain tissue for microscopic examination (biopsy) to rule out any malignancy is usually necessary.
- Treatment will be individualized based on the medical test findings, your age, risk factors, and your reproductive desires.
- It may be necessary for your doctor to perform a second endometrial biopsy or D & C following treatment, to see if the endometrial lining is normal again.
- Occasionally a hysterectomy (surgery to remove the uterus) is performed, particularly when hormone therapy has failed and precancerous cells are discovered.
- Try to reduce psychological stress that can complicate your illness and delay your recovery. If you can't resolve the stress, ask for help from family, friends or competent counselors.
- Use heat to relieve pain. Place a heating pad or hot-water bottle on your abdomen or back.
- Take frequent hot baths to relax muscles and relieve discomfort.

MEDICATION
- Progesterone (progestin), a female hormone, is often prescribed. If progestin is prescribed, the following menstrual period may be particularly heavy and may be associated with cramps. You may use nonprescription drugs, such as nonsteroidal anti-inflammatory drugs (NSAIDS), to relieve minor pain from cramps.
- Avoid aspirin; it may increase bleeding.

ACTIVITY
- No restrictions unless you have surgery. Then resume your activities gradually.
- You may resume sexual relations once medical clearance is given.

DIET—Usually, no special diet is required. If you are overweight, a weight reduction plan may help regulate cycles and decrease estrogen in the body and can significantly reduce the risk of recurrent endometriosis.

CALL YOUR DOCTOR IF

- You or a family member has symptoms of endometrial hyperplasia.
- You experience excessive bleeding (saturating more than 1 pad or tampon every hour).
- You develop signs of infection: fever, pain, a general ill feeling, headache, dizziness or muscle aches.
- New, unexplained symptoms develop. Drugs used in treatment may produce side effects.

Endometriosis

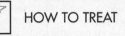

GENERAL INFORMATION

DEFINITION—A disorder in which tissue resembling the inner lining of the uterus (endometrium) appears at unusual locations in the lower abdomen. This tissue may be found on the ovary surfaces; behind the uterus, low in the pelvic cavity; on the intestinal wall and rarely, at distant sites in the body (e.g., lung, arm or leg). Endometriosis can affect females between puberty and menopause but is most common between ages 30 and 40.

SIGNS & SYMPTOMS—The following symptoms may begin abruptly or develop over many years:
• Pelvic pain; pain with sexual intercourse.
• Painful menstruation (much worse than normal menstrual cramps).
• Premenstrual spotting.
• Abnormal menstrual cycles or periods.
• Infertility.
• Lower back pain.
• Blood in the urine; painful urination.
• Blood in the stool; painful defecation.

CAUSES—Unknown, but the following theory is most accepted among medical professionals: Normally during ovulation, the uterus lining thickens to prepare for implantation of a fertilized egg. If fertilization and implantation do not occur, the lining tissue peels away from the uterus and is expelled in the menstrual flow. In some cases, this material builds up and passes backward out of the fallopian tubes into the pelvic cavity, where it floats freely and attaches itself to other tissues and organs. The transplanted tissue reacts each month as if it were still in the uterus, thickening and peeling away. New bits of peeled-off tissue create new implants. The growing endometrial tissue between pelvic organs may cause them to adhere together, producing pain and other symptoms.

RISK INCREASES WITH
• Women who don't become pregnant or delay childbirth.
• Family history of endometriosis.
• Daughters of women who took the drug DES (diethylstilbestrol) during pregnancy.

HOW TO PREVENT—No known preventive steps. Early diagnosis and treatment help prevent the spread of endometriosis.

PROBABLE OUTCOME
• Without treatment, endometriosis becomes increasingly severe.
• Endometriosis is a recurring disorder, but it usually subsides after menopause.
• Symptoms can be relieved with either medication or surgery, or a combination of both.
• Women with severe disease have less success with treatment.

POSSIBLE COMPLICATIONS
• Sterility.
• Chronic, disabling, but never life-threatening, pain.
• Bowel or bladder problems.
• Adhesions (scarring) of pelvic organs.
• Recurrence of endometriosis after medical therapy or surgery.
• Implants on the ovary can lead to large cysts and pelvic masses called endometriomas.

HOW TO TREAT

GENERAL MEASURES
• Diagnosing the disorder may take time, requiring repeated examinations or surgical diagnostic procedures, such as laparoscopy.
• Treatment after diagnosis will vary depending on the stage of the disease and your age and desire to have children.
• If you want children, consider pregnancy as soon as possible. Pregnancy may offer some relief from the disorder. Delaying pregnancy may result in infertility.
• To relieve discomfort, use a heating pad or a hot-water bottle on your abdomen or back, or take warm baths.
• Laser surgery or electrocoagulation may be used to remove the endometriosis.
• Surgery to remove implants, or a hysterectomy to remove the reproductive organs in women who don't want to become pregnant.
• See the Resource section of this book for additional information.

MEDICATION
• You may use nonprescription drugs, such as nonsteroidal anti-inflammatory drugs (NSAIDs), to relieve minor pain.
• Stronger pain relievers may be prescribed.
• Oral contraceptives, progestogens, danazol, and hormones are commonly used for treating endometriosis by suppressing ovarian function.

ACTIVITY
• Exercise helps relieve pain and reduces estrogen levels which may help to slow the growth of endometriosis.

DIET—Avoid caffeine, as it seems to aggravate pain in some women.

CALL YOUR DOCTOR IF

• You or a family member has symptoms of endometriosis.
• Pain becomes intolerable.
• You have excessive vaginal bleeding.
• New, unexplained symptoms develop. Drugs used in treatment may produce side effects.
• Symptoms recur after treatment.

Fibroid Tumor Removal (Myomectomy)

 GENERAL INFORMATION

DEFINITION—Removal of fibroid tumors (leiomyoma, myoma) from the uterus through incisions in the lower abdomen. In the treatment of fibroid tumors, myomectomy is an alternative to hysterectomy and can be an effective method of treatment when drug therapy has been unsuccessful. It is a particularly appealing treatment method to women who wish to retain childbearing capabilities.

REASONS FOR PROCEDURE
• Pelvic pain or back pain.
• Anemia caused by excessive loss of blood.
• Pressure on the bladder.
• Abnormal uterine bleeding.
• Difficulty in becoming pregnant.
• Discomfort with sexual intercourse.
• Very large size of tumors (larger than a cantaloupe).

RISK INCREASES WITH
• Obesity.
• Smoking.
• Poor nutrition, especially inadequate iron intake that has led to anemia.
• Other preexisting medical illness (e.g., diabetes, hypertension).
• Use of drugs such as cortisone, antihypertensives, beta-adrenergic blockers or diuretics.

DESCRIPTION OF PROCEDURE
• A general anesthetic will be administered.
• One or more incisions are made in the lower abdomen.
• The muscles are separated and connective tissues are cut free to expose the uterus.
• There are 3 major types of fibroids: subserous appear on the outside of the uterus; intramural are confined to the wall of the uterus and submucous appear inside the uterus. Rarely, fibroids can involve the cervix.
• Each tumor is removed separately, and each excision is repaired.
• The internal structures are closed in layers.
• The skin is closed with sutures or skin clips, which can be removed 2 to 7 days after surgery.
• For some fibroid growths, the surgery may be done with a hysteroscopic loop cautery, laser myoma resection, or laparoscopic or hysteroscopic surgery.

PROBABLE OUTCOME—The uterus is left intact, and you will still have menstrual periods. Your next period may be heavier than usual but should occur at about the expected time. Allow about 6 weeks for recovery from surgery.

POSSIBLE COMPLICATIONS
• Excessive bleeding
• Perforation of the uterus or bowel during surgery.

• Surgical-wound infection.
• Adhesions (internal scarring) will sometimes develop, and may interfere with future fertility.
• If you become pregnant following a myomectomy, a cesarean birth may be required.
• Recurrence of the tumor, sometimes requiring a hysterectomy.

 FOLLOW-UP CARE

GENERAL MEASURES
• A hard ridge should form along the incision. As it heals, the ridge will gradually recede.
• Use an electric heating pad, a heat lamp or a warm compress to relieve incisional pain.
• Use sanitary napkins or tampons to absorb blood.
• Bathe and shower as usual. You may wash the incision gently with mild unscented soap.
• Don't smoke.

MEDICATION
• Antibiotics are often prescribed to help prevent infection following surgery.
• Prescription pain medication should generally be required for only 2 to 7 days following the procedure.
• You may use nonprescription drugs, such as acetaminophen, for minor pain.
• Vaginal creams or medicated douches, if vaginal discharge develops an unpleasant odor.

ACTIVITY
• To help recovery and aid your well-being, resume daily activities, including work, as soon as you are able.
• Resume driving about 2 weeks following surgery.
• Sexual relations may be resumed after one month, or in accordance with your doctor's orders.

DIET—Clear liquid diet until the gastrointestinal tract functions again. Then eat a well-balanced diet to promote healing.

CALL YOUR DOCTOR IF

• You experience vaginal bleeding that soaks more than 1 pad per hour.
• You develop signs of infection: headache, muscle aches, dizziness or a general ill feeling and fever.
• You have abdominal swelling or severe abdominal pain.
• The urge to urinate frequently persists longer than 1 month.
• Excessive vaginal discharge persists beyond 1 month after surgery.
• Symptoms recur after surgery.
• New, unexplained symptoms develop. Drugs used in treatment may produce side effects.

Fibroid Tumor Removal (Myomectomy)

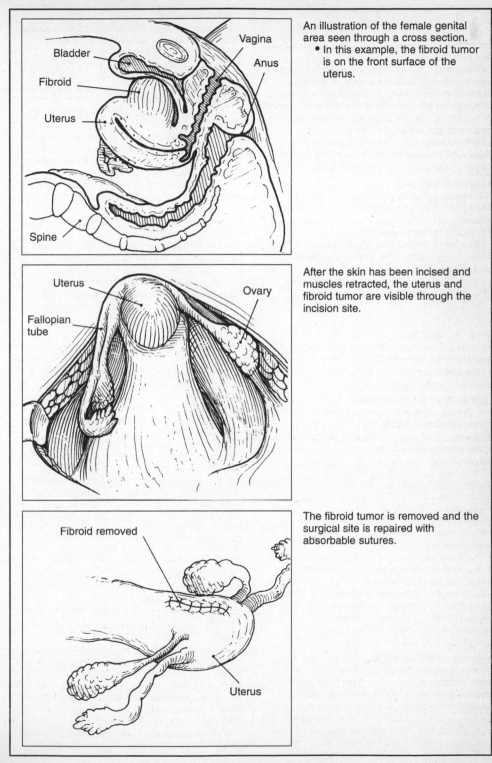

An illustration of the female genital area seen through a cross section.
- In this example, the fibroid tumor is on the front surface of the uterus.

Bladder

Fibroid

Uterus

Vagina

Anus

Spine

After the skin has been incised and muscles retracted, the uterus and fibroid tumor are visible through the incision site.

Uterus

Fallopian tube

Ovary

The fibroid tumor is removed and the surgical site is repaired with absorbable sutures.

Fibroid removed

Uterus

Fibroid Tumor, Uterine (Myoma; Leiomyoma)

 GENERAL INFORMATION

DEFINITION
• An abnormal growth of cells in the muscular wall (myometrium) of the uterus. The term "fibroids" is misleading. The cells are not fibrous; they are composed of abnormal muscle cells. Uterine fibroids are common and almost always benign (not cancerous).
• Fibroids can appear on the outside of the uterus, on the wall of the uterus or inside the uterus. Rarely, fibroids can involve the cervix.

SIGNS & SYMPTOMS
• Often, no symptoms.
• Frequent, heavy or painful menstrual periods.
• Passage of large clots with menstrual periods.
• Bleeding between periods.
• Feelings of pressure on the bladder or rectum.
• Anemia (weakness, fatigue and paleness).
• Increased vaginal discharge (rare).
• Painful sexual intercourse or bleeding after intercourse (rare).
• Pelvic pain.
• Infertility.

CAUSES—Exact cause is unknown. Estrogen is required for their stimulation and growth; as a result, fibroids are rare in prepubertal girls or postmenopausal women.

RISK INCREASES WITH
• Unopposed estrogen replacement therapy may cause excessive growth of fibroids.
• Genetic factors. Fibroid tumors are 3 to 9 times more common in African American women than in Caucasian women.

HOW TO PREVENT—No known way to prevent, but avoiding the use of female hormones may decrease the risk of fibroids.

PROBABLE OUTCOME
• Tumors usually decrease in size without treatment after menopause.
• Hospitalization, if surgery is necessary. Fibroids are generally removed surgically when they cause excessive bleeding, produce symptoms that interfere with conception or pregnancy or if they become malignant (rare).
• Fibroids can often be surgically removed without removing the entire uterus (myomectomy). The ability to conceive will continue as long as the uterus remains intact.

POSSIBLE COMPLICATIONS
• Heavy bleeding and anemia.
• Complications can occur in pregnancy such as spontaneous abortion or premature labor. Placental separation may occur when the placenta overlies the fibroid. With a large fibroid, fetal growth may be at risk because blood flow is diverted from the fetus to the fibroid.
• Fibroids may recur following surgery.
• Malignant change in the fibroid tumor (rare) is usually signaled by very rapid growth.

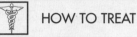 HOW TO TREAT

GENERAL MEASURES
• Diagnostic tests may include blood tests, ultrasound, laparoscopy, hysteroscopy or hysterosalpingogram.
• Treatment will depend on symptoms, location and size of the fibroids, your general health and desire for future pregnancies.
• For minimal symptoms, no treatment may be needed and you will be reexamined in 6 to 12 months.
• Hormonal therapy is often considered as the first step in treatment.
• Surgery may be recommended for certain situations and several different surgical procedures are possible. If surgery is recommended, be sure you understand all aspects of it before making a decision.
• Blood transfusions may be necessary to correct anemia.

MEDICATION
• The estrogen in low-dose oral contraceptive pills does not represent a significant risk. High-dose estrogen may cause fibroids to enlarge. Consider other forms of contraception, such as a diaphragm, cervical cap, intrauterine device (IUD), condom or a contraceptive foam or jelly.
• Progestin supplementation may help minimize uterine bleeding.
• Use nonsteroidal anti-inflammatory drugs (NSAIDs), such as ibuprofen, for pain.
• Take iron supplements if you are anemic.
• A gonadotropin-releasing hormone may be prescribed. It will induce an abrupt, artificial menopause that will stop the bleeding and reduce the size of the fibroid. In general, this therapy is not used for longer than 6 months.

ACTIVITY—No restrictions unless surgery is performed. Then you may need bed rest for a period of time, some restricted activity, and no sexual intercourse for approximately one month.

DIET—No special diet.

 CALL YOUR DOCTOR IF

• You or a family member has symptoms of a fibroid tumor.
• Fibroid tumors have been diagnosed and symptoms become more severe.
• You saturate a pad or tampon more often than once an hour.
• New, unexplained symptoms develop. Drugs used in treatment may produce side effects.

Genital Herpes

GENERAL INFORMATION

DEFINITION—A virus infection of the genitals transmitted by sexual relations (intercourse or oral sex). It can affect both sexes and may involve the vagina, cervix, thighs, buttocks and penis. Genital herpes is often found in the presence of other sexually transmitted diseases.

SIGNS & SYMPTOMS
- Painful blisters, preceded by itching, burning or irritation on the vaginal lips or penis. In women, the blisters may extend into the vagina to the cervix and urethra. After a few days, the blisters rupture and leave painful, shallow ulcers which last 1 to 3 weeks.
- Difficult, painful urination.
- Enlarged lymph glands.
- Fever and a general ill feeling.

CAUSES
- Usually caused by herpes type 2 virus (HSV-2). Herpes type 1 virus (HSV-1) causes common cold sores on the lips and mouth but can sometimes cause genital herpes.
- Genital herpes is usually transmitted by a sexual partner who has active herpes lesions. Lesions may be on the genitals, hands, lips or mouth. However, it may also be transmitted from an infected partner who has no recognizable symptoms of HSV infection. Once transmitted, incubation period is 2 to 7 days.

RISK INCREASES WITH
- Multiple sexual partners.
- Unprotected sexual activity.
- Serious illness that has lowered resistance.
- Use of immunosuppressive or anticancer drugs.
- Stress.
- Smoking.
- Other "triggers" that can cause a recurrence include genital trauma, menstruation, sunbathing and other existing infections.

HOW TO PREVENT
- Avoid sexual intercourse or oral sex if either partner has blisters or sores.
- Have the male use a condom during sexual activity if either sex partner has inactive genital herpes (especially important if the infected partner has frequent recurrences).
- Avoid oral sex with a partner who has cold sores on the mouth.
- If you are pregnant, tell your doctor if you have had herpes or any genital lesions in the past. Precautions will be taken to prevent infection of the baby.
- Avoid stress when possible.

PROBABLE OUTCOME
- Genital herpes is currently considered incurable, but symptoms and recurrence can be relieved with treatment.

- During symptom-free periods, the virus returns to its dormant state. Symptoms recur when the virus is reactivated. Recurrent symptoms are not new infections.
- The discomfort varies from person to person and from episode to episode in the same person. Usually, the first herpes infection is much more uncomfortable than recurrences of the virus.

POSSIBLE COMPLICATIONS
- Generalized disease and possibly death in persons who must take anticancer drugs or immunosuppressive drugs.
- Transmittal of life-threatening systemic herpes to a newborn infant from an infected mother.
- Secondary bacterial infection.

HOW TO TREAT

GENERAL MEASURES
- Confirmation of the diagnosis may be made by a laboratory study of fluid from the lesion.
- Treatment is directed toward relieving symptoms, reducing recurrence pattern and preventing complications.
- Women should wear cotton underpants or pantyhose with a cotton crotch.
- To reduce pain during urination, women may urinate through a toilet-paper roll or plastic cup with the bottom cut out, or pour a cup of luke-warm water over the genitals while urinating.
- Warm baths with a tablespoon of salt added can reduce the pain caused by the blisters.
- Women with genital herpes should have an annual Pap smear and physical examination to rule out any complications.
- See the Resource section of this book for additional information.

MEDICATION
- Acyclovir (an antiviral medication) in oral form is recommended for treatment of initial episodes to reduce the time of infection and the likelihood and frequency of recurrent outbreaks. Acyclovir is also used in the management of recurrent genital herpes. A topical form of acyclovir is available but is not as effective.
- Use mild painkillers, such as acetaminophen.

ACTIVITY—Avoid intercourse until symptoms disappear.

DIET—No special diet.

CALL YOUR DOCTOR IF

- You or a family member has symptoms of genital herpes.
- Symptoms worsen, or don't improve in 1 week, despite treatment.
- Unusual vaginal bleeding or swelling occurs.

Gonorrhea

GENERAL INFORMATION

DEFINITION—An infectious venereal disease of the reproductive organs that is sexually transmitted. Transmission can be by either oral sex or intercourse. In females, it involves the urethra (tube from the bladder to the outside of body) and reproductive system; in males, it involves the urethra; and in both sexes, the rectum, throat, joints and, sometimes, the eyes. It can affect people of all ages (even young children) who have sexual contact with infected persons. The peak incidence is between ages 20 and 30. Although readily treatable, this infection has reached epidemic levels in the U.S. Incubation period is from 2 to 10 days.

SIGNS & SYMPTOMS
- Females often have few or no symptoms. Males usually have more pronounced symptoms.
- Difficult or painful urination.
- Thick green-yellow discharge from the penis or vagina.
- Pelvic inflammatory disease.
- Pain or tenderness with sexual intercourse (sometimes).
- Spotting or bleeding between menstrual periods.
- Rectal discomfort and discharge (sometimes).
- Joint pain.
- Rash, especially on palms.
- Mild sore throat (sometimes).

CAUSES—Infection from gonococcus bacteria that grow well on delicate, moist tissue; the bacteria are usually transmitted sexually. Sexual activity involving the rectum or mouth may transmit infection to those areas if either partner is infected.

RISK INCREASES WITH
- Multiple sexual partners, whether heterosexual or homosexual.
- Unprotected sexual activity (without a barrier condom) with an infected partner.
- Prostitution.
- Child sexual abuse.
- Passage of newborn through the infected birth canal of the mother.

HOW TO PREVENT
- Avoid sexual partners whose health practices and status are uncertain.
- Maintain a mutually monogamous sexual relationship.
- Use a latex condom during sexual activity.
- This condition must be reported to the local health department to prevent its spread. Your cooperation is important, and your confidentiality will be maintained.

PROBABLE OUTCOME—Usually curable in 1 to 2 weeks with treatment.

POSSIBLE COMPLICATIONS
- Gonococcal eye infection and corneal scarring. This may cause blindness.
- Blood poisoning (gonococcal septicemia).
- Meningitis.
- Infectious arthritis.
- Pelvic inflammatory disease.
- Endocarditis (inflammation within the heart) and destruction of cardiac valves.
- Sexual impotence in men, if untreated.
- Infertility in women.
- Death from congestive heart failure or meningitis.

HOW TO TREAT

GENERAL MEASURES
- Diagnostic tests may include blood studies, laboratory culture and microscopic analysis of the discharge from the reproductive organs, urethra, rectum or throat.
- Treatment is with antibiotic medication. Follow-up laboratory cultures will confirm cure.
- Patients should be tested for other sexually transmitted diseases.
- Use separate linens and disposable eating utensils during treatment.
- Wash hands frequently, especially after urination and bowel movements.
- Don't touch eyes with hands.
- Inform all sexual contacts so that they can seek testing and treatment.
- See the Resource section of this book for additional information.

MEDICATION
- Antibiotics will be prescribed to fight the infection. Take all the medicine as prescribed, even if symptoms subside.
- You may take nonprescription drugs, such as acetaminophen or aspirin, to reduce discomfort, but not in place of antibiotics.

ACTIVITY—No restrictions, except don't resume sexual activity until a follow-up culture shows the infection is cured. Sexual partners must also be cured or a reinfection can occur. Treatment failures and resistance to antibiotics can also occur.

DIET—No special diet. Reduce consumption of caffeine and alcohol during treatment. These irritate the urethra.

CALL YOUR DOCTOR IF

- You or a family member has symptoms of gonorrhea.
- Chills, fever, abdominal pain, genital sores or joint pain occur either before or during treatment.
- New, unexplained symptoms develop. Drugs used in treatment may produce side effects.

Granuloma Inguinale (Donovanosis)

GENERAL INFORMATION

DEFINITION—A sexually transmitted disease generally affecting people living in tropical climates. It is becoming more common in the U.S., especially in the south and southwest regions. Incubation period is 8 to 12 weeks.

SIGNS & SYMPTOMS
- Formation of a nonpainful lesion (cyst, papule or nodule) in the genital area that does not readily heal. This lesion ulcerates (becomes open and runny) and may spread so that it involves most of the vulva and sometimes the buttocks and lower abdomen.
- Marked discomfort occurs if the ulceration spreads to the urethra or anal area. Walking, sitting and sexual intercourse become painful.
- Vaginal discharge that has an unpleasant odor.

CAUSES—An organism, Calymmatobacterium granulomatis (also called Donovania granulomatis or Donovanosis), that is spread via sexual intercourse with an infected person.

RISK INCREASES WITH
- Multiple sexual partners.
- Unprotected intercourse.
- Infection with other sexually transmitted diseases.

HOW TO PREVENT
- Maintain a mutually monogamous sexual relationship.
- Have the male partner use a latex condom during sexual activity.
- Cleanse the genital area before and after sex. Douching is usually not effective.
- If there has been possibility of exposure, seek medical care immediately. Early treatment may prevent painful symptoms from developing.

PROBABLE OUTCOME—With treatment, healing should begin within a week, but complete resolution will take up to 3 weeks.

POSSIBLE COMPLICATIONS
- Secondary bacterial infection.
- Relapse may occur if treatment is stopped too soon.
- Scars may form where infection occurred.
- Surgical intervention may be required in cases where the infection has caused advanced tissue destruction.

HOW TO TREAT

GENERAL MEASURES
- Diagnosis is confirmed with laboratory studies of scrapings or biopsies of the lesions.
- Testing (screening) for other sexually transmitted diseases is often recommended.
- Treatment is with antibiotics.
- Sitz baths frequently relieve discomfort caused by the lesions. Sit in a tub of hot water for 10 to 15 minutes. Repeat baths as often as 3 or 4 times a day.
- Sexual partners should be examined and, if necessary, treated for infection.
- A follow-up medical examination after treatment is important to verify that healing is complete.
- See the Resource section of this book for additional information.

MEDICATION—An antibiotic, such as tetracycline, will be prescribed. Take all the medication as prescribed, even if symptoms subside. Antibiotics may reduce the effectiveness of oral contraceptives. If you are currently using oral contraceptives for birth control, discuss this with your doctor

ACTIVITY—Avoid sexual intercourse during the active phase of the infection.

DIET—No special diet. If taking tetracycline, avoid dairy products within 3 hours of taking the medicine.

CALL YOUR DOCTOR IF

- You or a family member has symptoms of granuloma inguinale.
- Symptoms worsen despite treatment.
- New, unexplained symptoms develop. Drugs used in treatment may produce side effects.

Growth & Development in Adolescents (Puberty in Females)

GENERAL INFORMATION

DEFINITION—Puberty is the time of hormone changes in both sexes. It begins nearly 2 years earlier in females than males. In females, it usually takes place anywhere between the ages of 8 to 14 and may last for 2 to 3 years. At puberty, the hypothalamus and the pituitary glands produce hormones that stimulate the ovaries to increase production of female sex hormones (estrogen hormones). This causes the reproductive organs to mature in both size and function, allowing reproduction to become possible. Adolescence is the period of transition from childhood to adulthood and is generally considered to last from the beginning of puberty to age 18 or 20.

CHARACTERISTICS
• Breast budding. It is usually the first sign (at around age 11). The breasts often grow at uneven rates, which is completely normal, and the difference usually disappears by the time full maturity is reached.
• Growth of pubic hair (in some females, this is the first sign of puberty).
• Growth of hair under the arms starts about 1 year after the pubic hair appears.
• A significant growth spurt and increase in weight. During adolescence, body weight may double due to increased fat and height increases by 15% to 20%. Some girls attain their adult physique by age 13; others do not do so until age 18.
• Widening of the pelvis; fat deposits on the hips; enlargement of the uterus.
• Development of sweat glands under the arm and in the groin.
• Menstruation occurs at an average age of 12-1/2 years. Girls who are overweight tend to start menstruating earlier than the average. Menstruation may be delayed in girls who are malnourished, involved in strenuous sports or other physical activities (e.g., dancing) or have a chronic health disorder. The first few menstrual periods are usually sporadic and can continue to be irregular for the first 2 years.
• Other aspects of puberty include an increased appetite, changes in the sleep-wake cycle and temperament fluctuations. Intense emotions and mood swings are typical (which are probably attributable to hormone changes).

PROBABLE OUTCOME
• The age at the time of puberty is variable and the onset can be especially troublesome in girls. There are physical, mental and emotional changes that make adolescence a particularly difficult time.
• Early puberty and development toward physical maturity is normally not a cause for concern. However, you should consult your doctor if your daughter shows signs of precocious puberty (before age 8).

POSSIBLE COMPLICATIONS
• Delayed puberty. The age varies but may be first considered if a girl has no signs of sexual development by age 13. Usually no extensive medical work-up to look for causes is recommended until after age 16.
• Severe acne.
• Eating disorders (anorexia nervosa or bulimia nervosa).
• Emotional disorders.

PROMOTING WELL-BEING

GENERAL MEASURES
• A parent should prepare a prepubescent child for the experience. If unsure about how to communicate, seek help from educational reference materials on parenting, the family doctor or other resources in the community.
• As a daughter goes through puberty and adolescence, parents should try to keep the lines of communication open and keep discussions nonjudgmental and honest. There is no easy answer to the adolescent's complex problems dealing with family, friends, society and the additional life stresses on teenagers.
• Tampons or sanitary pads are acceptable for use during menstrual periods. With good hygiene, there should be no problems with menstrual odor.
• A girl's first pelvic examination should be at age 16 to 18 (if not done previously) to ensure normal reproductive anatomy and for Pap smear testing.
• Seek professional help if an adolescent girl appears to have an eating disorder (anorexia nervosa or bulimia nervosa).
• See the Resource section of this book for additional information.

MEDICATION—If there is a problem with cramps during menstrual periods, a mild nonprescription pain medicine may be used.

OTHER—Adolescent girls should be encouraged to eat well, maintain a normal weight and develop a routine exercise program.

CALL YOUR DOCTOR IF

• You have concerns about your daughter's physical or sexual development.
• Any unusual vaginal bleeding or discharge occurs, or there is excessive pain during menstruation.
• Your daughter develops any psychological or behavioral problems.

Hirsutism

GENERAL INFORMATION

DEFINITION—Excessive growth of hair on the face and body of a woman, in places where hair growth is ordinarily absent. It usually occurs gradually over an extended period of time.

SIGNS & SYMPTOMS
• Hair thickens and darkens and grows in a male pattern (beard, moustache, chest).
• Irregular or no menstruation.
• Acne.
• Sometimes accompanied by deepening of the voice, increased muscle mass and enlargement of the clitoris. When these symptoms occur, the complex is known as "virilization."
• Infertility problems (sometimes).

CAUSES
• Usually due to excessive production of androgens (male hormones) from the ovary or adrenal gland caused by some conditions, such as polycystic ovarian syndrome or congenital adrenal hyperplasia.
• Adrenal or ovarian tumor (uncommon).
• Hormonal imbalance can be induced by significant stress.
• Idiopathic (no apparent cause).

RISK INCREASES WITH
• Family history of hirsutism.
• Dark-haired individuals, especially those of Hispanic, African-American, Mediterranean or Indian ancestry.
• Use of male hormones (androgens) or corticosteroid medications, birth control pills, hormones and some antihypertensive drugs.
• Stress.
• Menopause or anovulation (failure to ovulate).

HOW TO PREVENT—No specific preventive measures.

PROBABLE OUTCOME
• Diagnosis and treatment of any underlying cause can frequently halt further hair growth. Response to treatment may take 6 to 12 months.
• Excess hair may be eliminated by various methods.

POSSIBLE COMPLICATIONS
• Poor self image; may feel unattractive and find social interaction with other people difficult.
• Infertility.
• Abnormal uterine bleeding and anemia.
• Increased risk of diabetes mellitus if the cause of hirsutism is polycystic ovarian disease.
• Hirsutism may be unresponsive to initial treatment.

HOW TO TREAT

GENERAL MEASURES
• A physical examination, laboratory studies and possibly some imaging studies (CT scan or MRI) will aid in diagnosing any underlying cause of the hirsutism.
• The specific type of treatment will depend on the cause of the hirsutism. A mild case of hirsutism with no menstrual irregularities may require no treatment. For others, treatment sometimes depends on the patient's desire for future childbearing.
• Ovarian or adrenal tumors should be surgically removed.
• Cosmetic treatment choices include shaving, plucking, bleaching or waxing. Chemical depilatories may also be used but are not always effective on thick or coarse hair. Shaving and plucking can cause infection or scarring. Electrolysis will remove hair permanently but should be done by a licensed professional.
• See the Resource section of this book for additional information.

MEDICATION
• There are no medicines specifically approved for the purpose of treating hirsutism.
• Medicines that may be recommended for hirsutism caused by excess androgen production include dexamethasone, oral contraceptives, leuprolide, spirinolactone (a mild diuretuc) and other antiandrogens. They vary in effectiveness and take 3 to 6 months for results. They may help decrease new hair growth but will usually not change the amount of hair you already have.
• Additional medications may be prescribed for any underlying disorder.
• If skin becomes irritated from shaving, use nonprescription 1% hydrocortisone cream.
• Depilatories or creams to remove hair are often recommended. Use with caution as they may irritate the skin.

ACTIVITY—Usually no restrictions.

DIET
• No special diet.
• If overweight, a weight loss diet is usually recommended.

CALL YOUR DOCTOR IF

• You or a family member has symptoms of hirsutism.
• New, unexplained symptoms develop. Drugs used in treatment may produce side effects.
• You become pregnant. Some medicines used to treat hirsutism will need to be discontinued.

HIV & AIDS
(Human Immunodeficiency Virus & Acquired Immunodeficiency Syndrome)

 GENERAL INFORMATION

DEFINITION—AIDS (or acquired immune deficiency syndrome) is caused by a virus called HIV (human immunodeficiency virus), which weakens the body's natural abilities to fight infections and cancer. HIV is transmitted through the body fluids (blood, semen, breast milk and, possibly, urine, feces and saliva) of infected persons. Once thought to be transmitted only between homosexual males, HIV is now known to affect people of all ages, gender and sexual preferences. Today, in the U.S., women and adolescents are the two fastest growing groups of people with AIDS.

SIGNS & SYMPTOMS—Initial infection with HIV may produce no symptoms. Once AIDS develops, the following symptoms may occur:
• Unexplained fever.
• Skin rash.
• Weakness or fatigue.
• Unexplained weight loss.
• Recurrent respiratory and skin infections.
• Swollen lymph glands throughout the body.
• Swollen joints.
• Enlarged spleen.
• Frequent yeast infections.
• Diarrhea.
• Mouth sores.
• Night sweats.

CAUSES—HIV (human immunodeficiency virus), a virus (retrovirus) that invades and destroys cells of the immune system. HIV infection results in lowered resistance to other infections and some cancers.

RISK INCREASES WITH
• Sexual contact with infected persons.
• Multiple sexual partners.
• Use of contaminated needles for intravenous drug use.
• Transfusions of blood or blood products from a person who is HIV positive. Due to stringent donor screening and laboratory testing, transfusion of HIV-tainted blood products is extremely rare in the U.S. (1:400,000).
• Children born to an HIV-infected mother.
• Exposure of hospital workers and laboratory technicians to blood, feces and urine of HIV-positive patients. Greatest risk is with an accidental needle injury.
• Note: Usual, nonsexual contact does not transmit the disease, so a person with HIV infection is not a risk to the general population.

HOW TO PREVENT
• Avoid sexual contact with affected persons or known intravenous drug users.
• Sexual activity should be restricted to partners whose sexual histories are known.
• Use condoms for vaginal, oral and anal intercourse (effectiveness is not proven, but their consistent use may reduce transmission).
• Avoid intravenous self-administered drugs. Do not share unsterilized needles.
• Avoid unscreened blood products (some foreign countries may not test the blood for HIV as strenuously as the U.S. does).
• Women who have tested positive for HIV should not breast-feed, to avoid passing HIV on to their infant.
• Infected people or those in risk groups are advised not to donate blood, sperm, organs or tissue.

PROBABLE OUTCOME—This condition is currently considered incurable. However, symptoms can be relieved or controlled, and scientific research into causes and treatment continues. AIDS may not develop for years following a positive HIV test. Once ill, survival averages vary.

POSSIBLE COMPLICATIONS—Serious infection in various body systems, cancer, death.

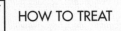 HOW TO TREAT

GENERAL MEASURES
• Laboratory blood studies of blood cells and HIV-antibodies test (may not become positive for 6 months after contact) can confirm the diagnosis. Newly diagnosed patients should be checked for other sexually transmitted diseases, as well as infections such as TB.
• Obtain psychotherapy or counseling to cope with anxiety and depression about having the disease and the likelihood of death.
• Hospitalization may be required when there are complications.
• Some patients join in research programs (working to find improved treatments or vaccines) which may provide free care.
• Early diagnosis is helpful. If you are at risk, obtain a medical evaluation even if you feel well.
• If you are pregnant, or plan to become pregnant, HIV testing can be helpful. If infected, special treatment during pregnancy can reduce risks of infecting the newborn.
• Avoid exposure to people with infections (e.g., colds or flu).
• Contact social agencies in your area about AIDS support groups.
• See the Resource section of this book for additional information.

HIV & AIDS
(Human Immunodeficiency Virus & Acquired Immunodeficiency Syndrome) (cont.)

MEDICATION

• Drugs are currently not effective in curing HIV or AIDS. A variety of drugs are used to prevent infections or control them as they develop.
• Antiretroviral drugs (didanosine, stavudine, zalcitabine, zidovudine) and protease inhibitor drugs are used to treat HIV infection and AIDS, and may slow the progression of the disease. Expert consultation on their use is advised. In an HIV-infected pregnant woman, these drugs (e.g., zidovudine) reduce the risk of HIV infection in the newborn.
• Research continues into new drugs and vaccines for HIV. Many new drugs are in the research and clinical trial stages and, as such, have not been approved by the FDA for widespread use among HIV-infected individuals. However, if you are HIV positive, it may be possible to become an active participant in the research studies for one or more new drugs. Often, the drugs are provided to the research participants free of charge, or at a significantly reduced price. If you are HIV positive and are interested in participating in clinical trials, you should discuss this with your physician, who may be able to refer you to the appropriate clinic or organization for enrollment in drug studies.

ACTIVITY

• Activities will depend on the state of health of each individual. Symptoms, such as fatigue or infections, can limit some activities.
• Rest is important, but an exercise routine is also recommended.

DIET

• Maintain good nutrition. Malabsorption, altered metabolism and weight loss are common among AIDS patients.
• Avoid raw eggs, unpasteurized milk or other potentially contaminated foods.

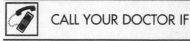 CALL YOUR DOCTOR IF

• You or a family member has symptoms of HIV infection.
• Infection occurs after diagnosis. Symptoms of infection include fever, headache, muscle aches, dizziness, a general ill feeling, cough and diarrhea.
• Other new symptoms develop. Drugs used in treatment have many side effects.

Hormone Replacement Therapy

 GENERAL INFORMATION

DEFINITION—Estrogens are the hormones responsible for female sex characteristics. Estrogen deficiency usually begins in the premenopausal years and progresses as a woman goes through menopause. Most of the signs and symptoms of menopause result from the decrease in estrogen production. Hormone replacement therapy (HRT) or just estrogen replacement therapy (ERT) is used to diminish menopausal signs and symptoms and help prevent other medical problems.

MEDICATION
• HRT usually consists of an estrogen hormone plus a progestogen (progestin) hormone. The two hormones combined protect against endometrial cancer, a risk with estrogen taken alone. Estrogen therapy alone may be used for women who have had a hysterectomy.
• The dose, form and regimen for the medications depend on the individual patient's requirements, age and reason for the replacement therapy. Most frequently, patients take both medications daily on a continual basis, while others may take them on a cyclic schedule during the month.
• Doses or schedules may need to be adjusted to completely resolve the symptoms of menopause.
• The medications can be supplied in oral form or skin patch (for estrogen). Also, an estrogen cream is available that can be prescribed to relieve vaginal symptoms.
• For long-term protection from osteoporosis and cardiovascular disease, HRT must be taken indefinitely.
• If a scheduled dose is missed, take it as soon as possible. If it is almost time for the next dose, skip the missed one. Don't double the dose and never wear more than one patch at a time.
• If nausea is a problem, take the tablets with food or immediately after a meal. The nausea usually disappears with continued use.

EFFECTS OF THERAPY
• Relieves hot flashes (sweating episodes).
• Relieves vaginal symptoms of irritation and dryness that can cause pain and discomfort during sexual intercourse.
• Prevents osteoporosis.
• Helps prevent cardiovascular diseases.

• The therapy may ease the emotional and nervous symptoms of menopause (e.g., depression, irritability or insomnia), which can be associated with other postmenopausal symptoms such as hot flashes.
• Medical evidence is uncertain as to whether or not HRT will keep a woman feeling young or promote soft or unwrinkled skin.

PRECAUTIONS—A woman and her doctor should discuss the benefits and risks associated with hormone therapy in terms of her individual medical history, general health, age and other circumstances. Precautions may need to be taken when the following factors exist in a woman being considered for HRT:
• Previous reaction or allergic response to estrogens or other medications or food.
• Past or current history of smoking.
• Current use of other prescription or nonprescription medications.
• Family history of bone disease, cancer, hypertension (high blood pressure), endometriosis, epilepsy, fibroids, gallbladder disease, heart or circulatory disease, stroke, kidney or liver disease, diabetes mellitus, migraine headaches or excess calcium in the blood.

CONTRAINDICATIONS
• History of breast cancer (depending on when the diagnosis was made).
• Past history or active blood-clotting disorder (thrombophlebitis) is generally not a contraindication but should always be discussed with the doctor.
• Known or suspected pregnancy.
• History of endometrial cancer (depending on when the diagnosis was made).
• Undiagnosed vaginal bleeding needs to be evaluated before hormone treatment is initiated.

RISKS, POSSIBLE SIDE EFFECTS OR ADVERSE REACTIONS
• HRT is generally well tolerated. The most common undesirable side effect is abnormal uterine bleeding, which usually diminishes in time. Notify your doctor if it does occur.
• Swollen feet or legs.
• Mood changes.
• Dry skin, rashes or permanent brown spots on skin (known as hyperpigmentosis).
• Mood changes.
• Breast tenderness or pain.

Hormone Replacement Therapy (cont.)

- Pelvic cramping.
- Fatigue.
- Depression.
- Irritability.
- Headaches.
- When estrogen is taken alone (without progestin), there is a significant increase in the risk of endometrial cancer in women who have a uterus.
- Medical studies show conflicting results regarding a possible increased risk of breast cancer in women taking HRT. Discuss with your doctor whether or not the benefits of HRT outweigh any possible increased risk to you.
- Note: The usual dosages of hormone replacement therapy for menopausal symptoms are kept low and are less likely to cause side effects or adverse reactions than the higher doses used in oral contraceptives or used to treat some cancers.

FOLLOW-UP EXAMINATIONS—Women taking hormones should have an annual pelvic examination, including a Pap smear test, and a mammogram.

 CALL YOUR DOCTOR IF

- You or a family member has symptoms of menopause and is interested in hormone replacement therapy.
- You develop symptoms of a blood clot: sudden or severe headache; sudden loss of coordination; sudden loss or change in vision; pains in the chest, groin, or leg (especially the calf); sudden unexplained shortness of breath; sudden slurring of speech; weakness or numbness in arm or leg.
- New, unexplained symptoms develop. Drugs used in treatment may produce side effects.

Hysterectomy, Abdominal (Salpingo-Oophorectomy)

GENERAL INFORMATION

DEFINITION—Removal of the uterus, cervix, and often the fallopian tubes and ovaries, through an incision in the abdomen. Be sure you understand all aspects of this surgical procedure, its risks and benefits and any possible alternative therapies. With removal of the ovaries, sudden surgical menopause occurs.

REASONS FOR PROCEDURE
• Uterus: Cancer or suspected cancer, fibroid tumors, chronic bleeding, prolapsed (dropped) uterus, endometriosis, chronic pelvic infection, severe menstrual pain or voluntary sterilization.
• Fallopian tubes and ovaries: Cancer or suspected cancer of the ovaries, precancerous or twisted ovarian cysts, ovarian pregnancy, ovarian abscess, damage to the ovaries from severe endometriosis.

RISK INCREASES WITH
• Obesity.
• Smoking.
• Conditions resulting in excessive estrogen exposure, such as estrogen drugs, delayed childbirth, chronic anovulation (see Glossary).
• Iron-deficiency anemia, heart or lung disease, or diabetes mellitus.
• Use of drugs such as cortisone, diuretics, antihypertensives or beta-adrenergic blockers.

DESCRIPTION OF PROCEDURE
• A general or regional anesthetic is given.
• A urinary catheter is placed.
• An incision is made in the abdomen (horizontal or vertical depending on the condition).
• The abdominal organs are examined.
• In a simple hysterectomy, only the uterus and cervix are removed along with visible tumors. In a total hysterectomy, the fallopian tubes and ovaries are cut free and removed as well (salpingo-oophorectomy).
• Any stretched ligaments are repaired.
• The vagina is often closed with sutures at its deeper end; the surgical wound is closed.
• The catheter may remain for hours to days.

PROBABLE OUTCOME
• Relief from symptoms caused by benign uterine conditions.
• Cancer prognosis is good when treated early.
• Expect permanent sterility (see Glossary).

POSSIBLE COMPLICATIONS
• Risk of infection or bleeding.
• Inadvertent injury to the bowel, bladder or ureters (see Glossary).
• Anesthetic problems.
• Urinary tract infection.
• Respiratory infection, particularly pneumonia.

FOLLOW-UP CARE

GENERAL MEASURES
• Hospital stay may be 2 to 5 days.
• To keep lungs clear, cough frequently while using appropriate support. Deep breathing aids are frequently available.
• Once home, someone should be available to help care for you for the first few days.
• Use an electric heating pad, a heat lamp or a warm compress to relieve incisional or gas pain.
• Shower as usual. You may wash the incision gently with mild unscented soap.
• Use sanitary napkins—not tampons—to absorb blood or drainage (discharge is normal but has an unpleasant odor).
• Surgery aftereffects may include constipation, fatigue, urinary symptoms and weight gain.
• The psychological aftermath of a hysterectomy will depend on the individual. Some women feel only relief, others experience frequent and unexpected crying episodes (may be due to hormonal changes) and a few suffer from depression. Seek help from your doctor and support from family and friends.

MEDICATION
• After surgery, medicines for pain, gas, nausea or constipation may be prescribed.
• Antibiotics if infection develops.
• Hormone replacement is recommended unless there are reasons why they should not be taken.

ACTIVITY
• To help recovery and aid your well-being, resume daily activities and work as soon as you are able. Recovery at home takes 1 to 3 weeks, with full activities resumed in 6 to 8 weeks.
• Resume driving 2 weeks after returning home.
• Sexual relations may be resumed in 4 to 6 weeks (or when advised). Most women experience no change in sexual function, some report improvement, while others have a worsening sexual function, specifically, loss of libido (sexual desire).

DIET—Clear liquid diet until the gastrointestinal tract functions again. Then eat a well-balanced diet to promote healing.

CALL YOUR DOCTOR IF

• Vaginal bleeding soaks more than 1 pad per hour.
• Frequent urge to urinate or excessive vaginal discharge persists longer than 1 month.
• You experience increased pain or swelling in the surgical area.
• You develop signs of infection: headache, muscle aches, dizziness or a general ill feeling and fever.

Hysterectomy, Abdominal
(Salpingo-Oophorectomy)

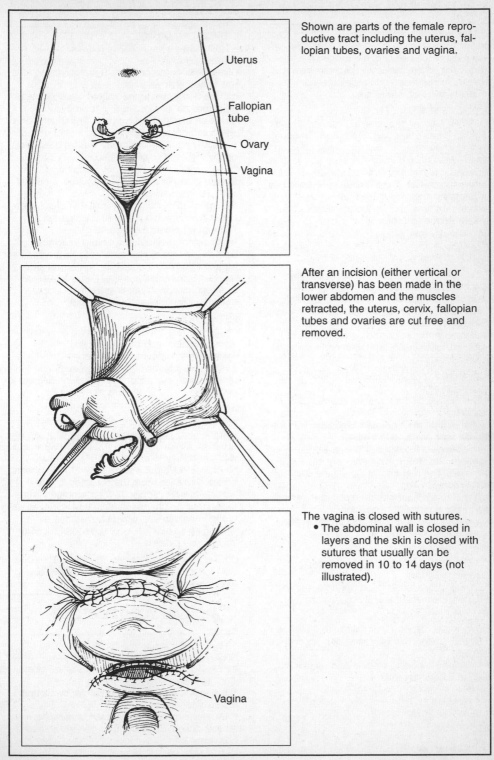

Shown are parts of the female reproductive tract including the uterus, fallopian tubes, ovaries and vagina.

Uterus

Fallopian tube

Ovary

Vagina

After an incision (either vertical or transverse) has been made in the lower abdomen and the muscles retracted, the uterus, cervix, fallopian tubes and ovaries are cut free and removed.

The vagina is closed with sutures.
- The abdominal wall is closed in layers and the skin is closed with sutures that usually can be removed in 10 to 14 days (not illustrated).

Vagina

Hysterectomy, Vaginal

 GENERAL INFORMATION

DEFINITION—Removal of the uterus, including cervix, through an incision made in the deepest recesses of the vagina. This surgery is frequently accompanied by reconstructive surgery (colporrhaphy) to repair bladder muscles and rectal muscles.

REASONS FOR PROCEDURE
• Uterus: Cancer or suspected cancer, fibroid tumors, chronic bleeding, prolapsed (dropped) uterus, endometriosis, chronic pelvic infection, severe menstrual pain or voluntary sterilization.
• Fallopian tubes and ovaries: Cancer or suspected cancer of the ovaries, precancerous or twisted ovarian cysts, ovarian pregnancy, ovarian abscess, damage to the ovaries from severe endometriosis.

RISK INCREASES WITH
• Obesity.
• Smoking.
• Conditions resulting in excessive estrogen exposure, such as estrogen drugs, delayed childbirth, chronic anovulation (see Glossary).
• Iron-deficiency anemia, heart or lung disease, or diabetes mellitus.
• Use of drugs such as cortisone, diuretics, antihypertensives or beta-adrenergic blockers.

DESCRIPTION OF PROCEDURE
• A general or regional anesthetic is administered.
• The urinary bladder may be drained by catheter.
• The vaginal walls are carefully separated from the bladder and rectal muscles.
• The deepest recesses of the vagina are opened. The uterus and cervix are cut free and removed. The rear part of the vagina is closed with sutures.
• The bladder muscles and rectal muscles are sewn into their proper position.
• A small catheter (Foley) may be left in the bladder for a few days.

PROBABLE OUTCOME
• Relief from symptoms caused by benign uterine conditions.
• Cancer prognosis is good when treated early.
• Expect permanent sterility (see Glossary).

POSSIBLE COMPLICATIONS
• Excessive bleeding; surgical-wound infection.
• Rectal, ureter (see Glossary) or bladder damage.
• Muscles supporting bladder and rectum may require a second repair.

 FOLLOW-UP CARE

GENERAL MEASURES
• Hospital stay may be 2 to 5 days.
• To keep lungs clear, cough frequently while using appropriate support. Deep breathing aids are frequently available.
• Once home, someone should be available to help care for you for the first few days.
• Use an electric heating pad, a heat lamp or a warm compress to relieve incisional or gas pain.
• Shower as usual. You may wash the incision gently with mild unscented soap.
• Use sanitary napkins—not tampons—to absorb blood or drainage (discharge is normal but has an unpleasant odor).
• Surgery aftereffects may include constipation, fatigue, urinary symptoms and weight gain.
• The psychological aftermath of a hysterectomy will depend on the individual. Some women feel only relief, others experience frequent and unexpected crying episodes (may be due to hormonal changes), and a few suffer from depression. Seek help from your doctor and support from family and friends.

MEDICATION
• After surgery, medicines for pain, gas, nausea or constipation may be prescribed.
• Antibiotics if infection develops.
• Hormone replacement is recommended unless there are reasons why they should not be taken.

ACTIVITY
• To help recovery and aid your well-being, resume daily activities and work as soon as you are able. Recovery at home takes 1 to 3 weeks, with full activities resumed in 6 to 8 weeks.
• Resume driving 2 weeks after returning home.
• Sexual relations may be resumed in 4 to 6 weeks (or when advised). Most women experience no change in sexual function, some report improvement, while others have a worsening sexual function, specifically, loss of libido (sexual desire).

DIET—Clear liquid diet until the gastrointestinal tract functions again. Then eat a well-balanced diet to promote healing.

CALL YOUR DOCTOR IF

• Vaginal bleeding soaks more than 1 pad per hour.
• Frequent urge to urinate or excessive vaginal discharge persists longer than 1 month.
• You experience increased pain or swelling in the surgical area.
• You develop signs of infection: headache, muscle aches, dizziness or a general ill feeling and fever.

Hysterectomy, Vaginal

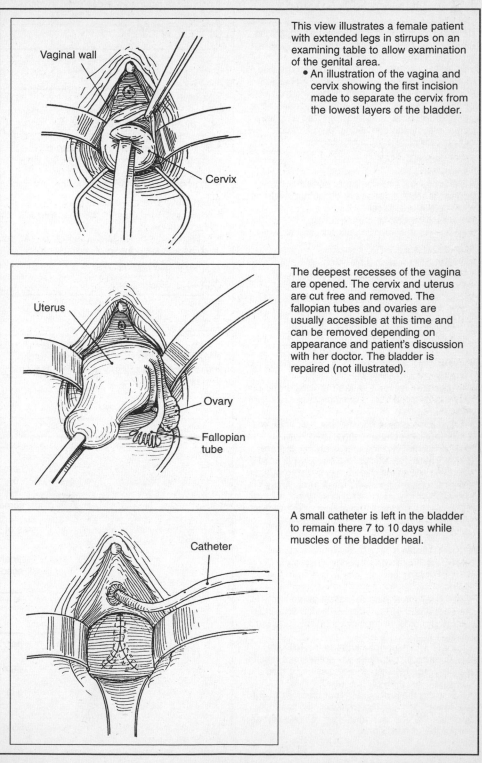

Vaginal wall

Cervix

This view illustrates a female patient with extended legs in stirrups on an examining table to allow examination of the genital area.
- An illustration of the vagina and cervix showing the first incision made to separate the cervix from the lowest layers of the bladder.

Uterus

Ovary

Fallopian tube

The deepest recesses of the vagina are opened. The cervix and uterus are cut free and removed. The fallopian tubes and ovaries are usually accessible at this time and can be removed depending on appearance and patient's discussion with her doctor. The bladder is repaired (not illustrated).

Catheter

A small catheter is left in the bladder to remain there 7 to 10 days while muscles of the bladder heal.

Hysterosalpingography

GENERAL INFORMATION

DEFINITION—Hysterosalpingography (HSG) is an x-ray examination used to help diagnose a suspected intrauterine tumor, mass or congenital malformation, or suspected blockage in the fallopian tubes. HSG is often necessary in cases of infertility to help determine the problems involved. Ultrasound techniques have been improved so that they can also diagnose some intrauterine conditions, but ultrasound cannot diagnose a tubal blockage.

REASONS FOR PROCEDURE
• Infertility.
• Confirm tubal and uterine abnormalities, congenital malformations and traumatic injuries.
• Multiple miscarriages.
• Excessively painful menstruation.
• Follow-up to some surgical procedures.

RISK INCREASES WITH
• Undiagnosed vaginal bleeding.
• Pelvic inflammatory disease (PID).
• Pregnancy.

DESCRIPTION OF PROCEDURE
• The procedure is usually performed early in the menstrual cycle, after the menstrual flow has ended but before ovulation (and any possible pregnancy) has occurred.
• The procedure may be done in a hospital or in the office of a radiologist.
• A speculum is inserted into the vagina and the cervix is grasped with a tenaculum (a hook-like instrument).
• A dye apparatus is attached to the cervix and a dye (a radio-opaque contrast medium) is slowly inserted into the uterus and x-rays are taken. There may be some discomfort or mild cramping felt as the dye is injected. You may be asked to change positions for different x-ray views.
• The x-rays will show the outline of the uterus and fallopian tubes as the dye fills them.

PROBABLE OUTCOME
• Normal findings reveal a symmetrical uterine cavity, the dye flowing through unblocked fallopian tubes, and no leak of dye from the uterus.
• The x-rays may help reveal an abnormality in the shape/size of the uterine interior, scarring, tumors (fibroids) or a blockage in the fallopian tubes.
• If there is a minor blockage in the fallopian tubes, the contrast agent will sometimes resolve the blockage by removing or dissolving it as the contrast flows through the tube.
• Following the procedure, your chances of becoming pregnant increase slightly, possibly because the contrast agent has removed small blockages or adhesions.

POSSIBLE COMPLICATIONS
• Allergic reaction to the dye used in the test (hives, itching, low blood pressure).
• Uterine perforation.
• Infection.

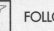

FOLLOW-UP CARE

GENERAL MEASURES
• Some symptoms, such as mild cramping, a slow pulse, nausea or dizziness may occur following the procedure. These are temporary.
• Conditions detected by the hysterosalpingogram may require further testing for confirmation, usually a laparoscopy or hysteroscopy (see Glossary for these terms).

MEDICATION
• A mild sedative may be administered prior to the procedure.
• Following the procedure, use mild painkillers, such as acetaminophen, if necessary.

ACTIVITY—No restrictions.

DIET—No special diet.

CALL YOUR DOCTOR IF

• Pain or swelling increases in the genital area.
• You develop signs of infection: headache, muscle aches, dizziness or a general ill feeling and fever.

Hysterosalpingography

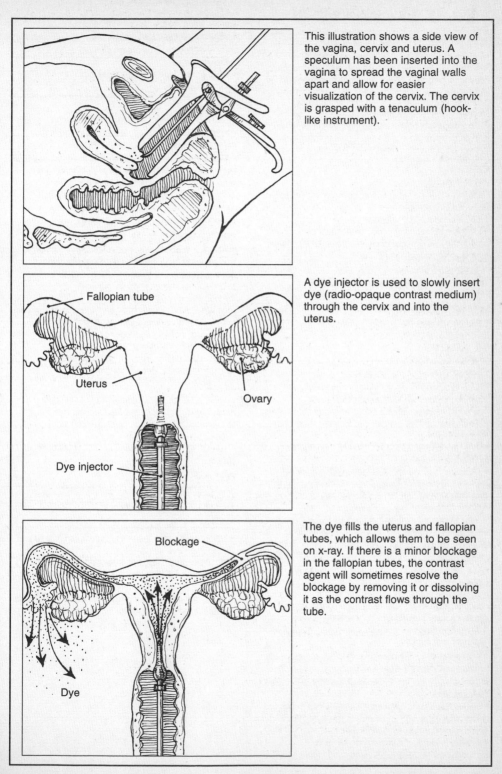

This illustration shows a side view of the vagina, cervix and uterus. A speculum has been inserted into the vagina to spread the vaginal walls apart and allow for easier visualization of the cervix. The cervix is grasped with a tenaculum (hook-like instrument).

A dye injector is used to slowly insert dye (radio-opaque contrast medium) through the cervix and into the uterus.

Fallopian tube

Uterus

Ovary

Dye injector

The dye fills the uterus and fallopian tubes, which allows them to be seen on x-ray. If there is a minor blockage in the fallopian tubes, the contrast agent will sometimes resolve the blockage by removing it or dissolving it as the contrast flows through the tube.

Blockage

Dye

Hysteroscopy

GENERAL INFORMATION

DEFINITION—A procedure in which a hysteroscope (a small lighted telescopic instrument) is inserted through the vagina and cervix to help diagnose and treat abnormalities within the uterus and genital tract.

REASONS FOR PROCEDURE
• Evaluation and treatment of abnormal uterine bleeding.
• To view the status or location of an IUD (intrauterine device).
• Infertility.
• Habitual abortion.
• Uterine polyps, fibroids or adhesions (e.g., Asherman's syndrome).
• Obstructed fallopian tubes.
• Detection, monitoring or treatment of endometrial hyperplasia (abnormal cell growth).
• Congenital malformations.
• Staging of cancer.
• Placement of silicone plugs for tubal sterilization.

RISK INCREASES WITH
• Active uterine bleeding.
• Current infection.
• Pregnancy.
• Uterine cancer.

DESCRIPTION OF PROCEDURE
• The procedure may be performed in the doctor's office, an outpatient facility or a hospital. A general or a local anesthetic is used.
• The woman lies on her back and places her feet into stirrups.
• The urinary bladder is drained and the cervix is gradually dilated.
• Fluid or carbon dioxide gas (CO_2) may be used to distend (enlarge) the uterine cavity to improve visualization and allow any operative manipulations to be achieved.
• The hysteroscope is passed through the vagina and cervix into the uterine cavity for viewing. Video monitoring is often used at the same time.
• A variety of instruments are available for use in hysteroscope procedures, including microscissors, special clamps with electrocautery attachment, wire loops for excision and lasers when needed.
• The examination and any surgical measures will be performed.
• The hysteroscope is withdrawn.

PROBABLE OUTCOME
• There may be some discomfort following the procedure.
• Hysteroscopic diagnostic studies may rule out a medical problem or indicate the need for further evaluation and treatment.
• Hysteroscopic treatment or surgical procedures have a high success rate.

POSSIBLE COMPLICATIONS
• Uterine perforation.
• Excessive bleeding.
• Gas embolism caused by the carbon dioxide used to distend the uterine cavity (rare).
• Pelvic infection.
• Allergic reaction to the fluid used to distend the uterus (rare).

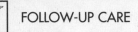

FOLLOW-UP CARE

GENERAL MEASURES
• Following the procedure, the medical staff will monitor your vital signs for a period of time. Have someone drive you home.
• There may be some slight bleeding and cramping. Use sanitary napkins for the bleeding.

MEDICATION
• Medicine is usually not necessary following the procedure. In some surgical procedures, estrogen may be prescribed to promote regrowth of the uterine lining.
• Antibiotics may be prescribed to fight or treat infection. Antibiotics may reduce the effectiveness of oral contraceptives. If you are currently using oral contraceptives for birth control, discuss this with your doctor.
• You may use nonprescription drugs, such as acetaminophen, for minor pain.

ACTIVITY
• Rest at home the remainder of the day. Additional restrictions may be required, depending on the extent of the surgical procedure.
• Avoid sexual intercourse for 2 weeks or as directed.

DIET—No special diet.

CALL YOUR DOCTOR IF

• Vaginal bleeding soaks more than 1 pad per hour.
• You develop signs of infection: headache, muscle aches, dizziness or a general ill feeling or fever.
• New, unexplained symptoms develop. Drugs used in treatment may produce side effects.

Hysteroscopy

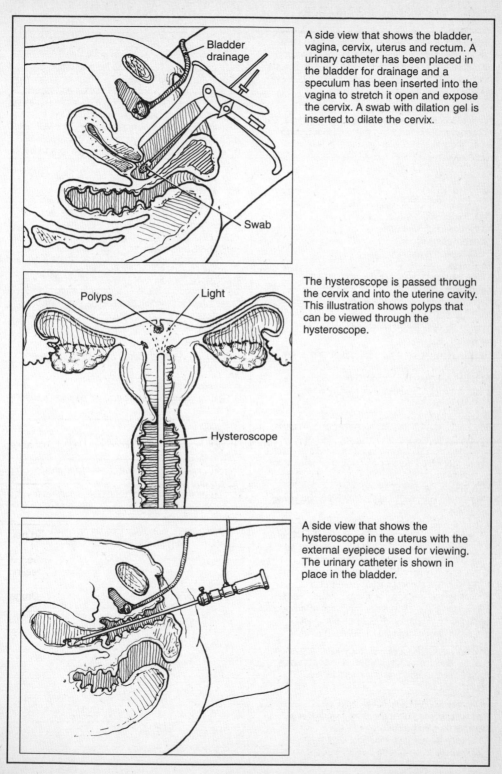

A side view that shows the bladder, vagina, cervix, uterus and rectum. A urinary catheter has been placed in the bladder for drainage and a speculum has been inserted into the vagina to stretch it open and expose the cervix. A swab with dilation gel is inserted to dilate the cervix.

Bladder drainage

Swab

The hysteroscope is passed through the cervix and into the uterine cavity. This illustration shows polyps that can be viewed through the hysteroscope.

Polyps

Light

Hysteroscope

A side view that shows the hysteroscope in the uterus with the external eyepiece used for viewing. The urinary catheter is shown in place in the bladder.

Incontinence, Functional

 GENERAL INFORMATION

DEFINITION—An involuntary loss of urine from the bladder that occurs infrequently (transient), or the failure to comprehend the need to urinate (functional).

SIGNS & SYMPTOMS
• Forgetting to urinate.
• Urinating at inappropriate times or places.
• Occasional problems in getting from bed to toilet in time.

CAUSES
• Dementia.
• Depression.
• Mobility disorders.

RISK INCREASES WITH
• Urinary tract infection.
• Diabetes mellitus.
• Increasing age.
• Arthritis.
• Use of diuretics or antidepressants.
• Estrogen deficiency.
• History of many pregnancies.
• Spinal cord injury.
• General debilitated condition.

HOW TO PREVENT
• Eat a normal, well-balanced diet and exercise regularly to build and maintain muscle strength.
• Learn and practice Kegel exercises before symptoms of functional incontinence begin.
Kegel exercises:
The purpose is to recognize, control and develop the muscles of the pelvic floor. These are the muscles used to interrupt urination in mid-stream. The following exercises strengthen these muscles so you can control or relax them completely:
• To identify which muscles are involved, alternately start and stop urinating when using the toilet.
• Practice tightening and releasing these muscles while sitting, driving, watching TV, etc.
• Tighten the muscles a small amount at a time, "like an elevator going up to the 10th floor." Then release very slowly, "one floor at a time."
• Tighten the muscles from front to back, including the anus, as in the previous exercise.
• Practice exercises every morning, afternoon and evening. Start with 5 times each and gradually work up to 20 or 30 each time.

PROBABLE OUTCOME—If the underlying cause can be determined and treated, incontinence problems can be cured or significantly improved.

POSSIBLE COMPLICATIONS
• Most likely to continue unless underlying causes can be treated.
• Urinary tract infections.
• Social isolation due to fear of embarrassment.

 HOW TO TREAT

GENERAL MEASURES
• Urinalysis, physical examination and ultrasound may be used to help identify the underlying cause of the incontinence.
• Following treatment of the underlying cause, it may be necessary to rely on external devices or superabsorbent pads.
• Specially trained nurses or therapists will help a patient learn how to cope with the problem, through scheduled voiding, prompting and habit training.
• In some cases, incontinence will require caregiver assistance for management.
• Absorbent pads or diapers may be worn.
• Learn and practice Kegel exercises (see instructions in How to Prevent).
• See the Resource section of this book for additional information.

MEDICATION—Medicine is usually not necessary for this disorder, but antibiotics may be prescribed if there is a complicating urinary tract infection. Antibiotics may reduce the effectiveness of oral contraceptives. If you are currently using oral contraceptives for birth control, discuss this with your doctor.

ACTIVITY—As tolerated by physical condition.

DIET
• No diet restrictions.
• Start a weight loss program if excess weight is a problem.

 CALL YOUR DOCTOR IF

• You or a family member has symptoms of functional incontinence.
• You develop signs of infection, such as fever, pain on urination, frequent urination or a general ill feeling.
• New, unexplained symptoms develop. Drugs used in treatment may produce side effects.

Incontinence, Stress

GENERAL INFORMATION

DEFINITION—An involuntary loss of urine that accompanies any action that suddenly increases pressure in the abdomen. It can affect both sexes (males rarely) and all ages. It is the most common type of incontinence in women.

SIGNS & SYMPTOMS—Unintentional loss of urine with lifting, exercising, sneezing, singing, coughing, laughing, crying or straining to have a bowel movement.

CAUSES—A change in the relationship of the uterus to the bladder resulting in shortening of the urethra (tube from the bladder to the outside), and loss of the normal muscular support for the bladder and floor of the pelvis. These changes occur as a result of injury to the pelvic floor from repeated vaginal childbirth. Obesity and aging may also be factors.

RISK INCREASES WITH
• Repeated vaginal childbirth.
• Vaginal birth of large children.
• Post-menopausal women.
• Obesity.
• Chronic lung disease with a cough.

HOW TO PREVENT
• Eat a normal, well-balanced diet and exercise regularly to build and maintain muscle strength.
• Obtain regular physical exams to detect early problems.
• Learn and practice Kegel exercises after childbirth, before symptoms of stress incontinence begin.
Kegel exercises:
The purpose is to recognize, control and develop the muscles of the pelvic floor. These are the muscles used to interrupt urination in mid-stream. The following exercises can be used to help strengthen these muscles:
• To identify which muscles are involved, alternately start and stop urinating when using the toilet.
• Practice tightening and releasing these muscles while sitting, walking, watching TV, etc.
• Tighten the muscles a small amount at a time, "like an elevator going up to the 10th floor." Then release very slowly, "one floor at a time."
• Tighten the muscles from front to back, including the anus, as in the previous exercise.
• Practice exercises every morning, afternoon and evening. Start with 5 times each and gradually work up to 20 or 30 each time.

PROBABLE OUTCOME—If the stress incontinence is not severe, exercise can improve the muscle function. If it is severe, it can often be cured with surgery.

POSSIBLE COMPLICATIONS
• Complete loss of urinary control. This requires surgery.

• Urinary tract infections.
• Social isolation due to fear of embarrassment.
• Kidney failure.

HOW TO TREAT

GENERAL MEASURES
• Urinalysis and other laboratory studies will help diagnose a urinary tract infection.
• Treatment as needed for any infections or tumors.
• Weight loss, smoking cessation or cough suppression may be indicated.
• Collagen injections in the tissue surrounding the urethra may help minimize urine leakage.
• Other therapy possibilities include biofeedback, electrical stimulation or special weights to strengthen pelvic muscles.
• Learn and practice Kegel exercises (see instructions in How to Prevent).
• Wear absorbent underpants or incontinence pads if needed.
• A pessary (support device) made of rubber or other material to fit inside the vagina to support the uterus and lower muscular layer of the bladder is helpful for some.
• Frequently, it is necessary to have urodynamic testing (studies of the actual urine flow), either in the doctor's office or at a special clinic, to evaluate the incontinence and confirm it is stress related and not a combination of stress and urge incontinence.
• Surgery to tighten relaxed or damaged muscles that support the bladder may help.
• See the Resource section of this book for additional information.

MEDICATION
• Antibiotics for any complicating urinary tract infection.
• Sympathomimetic drug therapy, which helps urethral muscles, may be prescribed.
• Estrogen therapy may be prescribed.

ACTIVITY—No restrictions.

DIET
• Start a weight loss program if overweight.
• Decrease intake of caffeine and alcohol.
• Fluid intake may need to be adjusted.

CALL YOUR DOCTOR IF

• You or a family member has symptoms of stress incontinence.
• You develop signs of infection, such as fever, frequent or painful urination, or a general ill feeling.
• Symptoms don't improve after 3 months of Kegel exercises, or symptoms become intolerable and you wish to consider surgery.
• New, unexplained symptoms develop. Drugs used in treatment may produce side effects.

Incontinence, Urge

 GENERAL INFORMATION

DEFINITION—Inability to control the bladder once the urge to urinate occurs. It may occur alone or sometimes with stress incontinence (involuntary loss of urine on coughing, straining, sneezing, etc.). The prevalence of urinary incontinence increases with age and affects women more often than it does men.

SIGNS & SYMPTOMS—Involuntary loss of urine almost immediately after feeling a slight urge to urinate. The volume of lost urine may range from a few drops to complete bladder emptying. There may also be an excessive need to urinate at night (nocturia).

CAUSES
• Overactive muscles that cause bladder to contract and empty.
• Stone, cancer or obstruction in the urinary tract.

RISK INCREASES WITH
• Central nervous system disorders (stroke, Parkinson's).
• Obesity.
• Surgery that may traumatize the urethra.
• Injury of the urethra from any cause.

HOW TO PREVENT
• Eat a normal, well-balanced diet and exercise regularly to build and maintain muscle strength.
• Learn and practice Kegel exercises before symptoms of urge incontinence begin.
Kegel exercises:
• The purpose is to recognize, control and develop the muscles of the pelvic floor. These are the muscles you use to interrupt urination in mid-stream. The following exercises (Kegel exercises) strengthen these muscles so you can control or relax them completely:
• To identify which muscles are involved, alternately start and stop urinating when using the toilet.
• Practice tightening and releasing these muscles while sitting, standing, walking, driving, watching TV or listening to music.
• Tighten the muscles a small amount at a time, "like an elevator going up to the 10th floor." Then release very slowly, "one floor at a time."
• Tighten the muscles from front to back, including the anus, as in the previous exercise.
• Practice exercises every morning, afternoon and evening. Start with 5 times each and gradually work up to 20 or 30 each time.

PROBABLE OUTCOME—There are several different forms of treatment available, some still experimental. If the first treatment techniques don't work, get medical advice about alternatives.

POSSIBLE COMPLICATIONS
• Urinary tract infections.
• Social isolation due to fear of embarrassment.
• Skin irritation.

 HOW TO TREAT

GENERAL MEASURES
• Any underlying cause should be identified and treated.
• Treatment may involve bladder training techniques, medication, surgery, exercises and use of special aids to ease discomfort.
• Wear absorbent underpants or superabsorbent pads if necessary.
• A planned schedule for emptying the bladder is helpful. Prompting by a caregiver will help.
• Keep a daily diary of fluid intake and urination frequency. This will help assess progress.
• Learn and practice Kegel exercises (see instructions in How to Prevent).
• Use bedside commodes, urinals or bedpans if necessary.
• A pessary (support device) made of rubber or other material to fit inside the vagina to support the uterus and lower muscular layer of the bladder is helpful for some.
• Frequently, it is necessary to have urodynamic testing (studies of the actual urine flow), either in the doctor's office or a special clinic, to evaluate the incontinence and confirm it is urge related and not a combination of stress and urge incontinence.
• Surgery to tighten relaxed or damaged muscles that support the bladder.
• Biofeedback/behavioral training may be recommended.
• See the Resource section of this book for additional information.

MEDICATION
• Anticholinergic drugs to stimulate muscle contractions may be prescribed.
• Antibiotics may be prescribed if there is a complicating urinary tract infection. Antibiotics may reduce the effectiveness of some oral contraceptives. Discuss this with your doctor.

ACTIVITY—No restrictions.

DIET
• Start a weight loss program if you are overweight.
• Decrease intake of alcohol and caffeine.
• Fluid intake may need to be adjusted.

📞 CALL YOUR DOCTOR IF

• Any sign of infection develops, such as fever, pain on urination, frequent urination or a general ill feeling.
• Symptoms don't improve after 3 months of Kegel exercises and medicines, or symptoms become intolerable and you wish to consider surgery.
• New, unexplained symptoms develop. Drugs used in treatment may produce side effects.

Interstitial Cystitis

GENERAL INFORMATION

DEFINITION—A chronic inflammation of the interstitium (the area between the bladder lining and the bladder muscle). Interstitial cystitis has symptoms similar to cystitis (bacterial infection of the bladder), but urine cultures are negative for bacteria and antibiotics usually do not help. The average age of onset is 40, but it affects women of all ages. Symptoms range from mild to severe and can come and go over a period of months or years.

SIGNS & SYMPTOMS
• Pelvic pain and pressure.
• Urgent need to urinate (sometimes 60 to 80 times a day in severe cases).
• Sensation of incomplete emptying of the bladder.
• Frequent, excessive need to urinate at night (nocturia).
• Pain during sexual intercourse.
• Burning when urinating.
• Vaginal and rectal pain (sometimes).

CAUSES—Exact cause is unknown. Studies suggest that it is a syndrome of bladder inflammation possibly initiated by bacterial infection, autoimmune process (misdirected immune response in which the body's defenses become self-destructive) or contact irritants. It is probably not an infectious disease.

RISK INCREASES WITH
• A history of sensitivities or allergies to medications, food or other substances; hay fever or asthma.
• Rheumatoid arthritis.
• Previous hysterectomy.

HOW TO PREVENT—None known.

PROBABLE OUTCOME
• Treatments are available that may control or minimize the symptoms but do not cure the disorder. Medical studies are ongoing to help determine the cause, more beneficial treatments and a possible cure.
• Women with the disorder may have flare-ups and remissions; also, different women respond to different treatment. In some women, a treatment may work initially and then later lose its effectiveness.

POSSIBLE COMPLICATIONS—Unrelieved symptoms that come and go and may vary in intensity from mild to severe.

HOW TO TREAT

GENERAL MEASURES
• Initial diagnostic tests will include urine studies (which are usually normal) and a pelvic examination. Conditions that have similar symptoms (bladder infection, kidney problems,

vaginal infections, endometriosis and sexually transmitted diseases) will need to be excluded.
• If other tests are negative, a cystoscopy (use of a small lighted telescope to view the inside of the bladder) is often recommended. A biopsy is taken at this time to rule out a malignancy. As an added benefit, cystoscopy often helps relieve symptoms. It involves distention of the bladder by filling it with water, thereby stretching the bladder and increasing its capacity.
• There is no consistently effective treatment for the disorder. Options include various oral medications, medication instilled into the bladder, special routines for stretching the bladder, diet changes, bladder retraining, relaxation training, and transcutaneous electrical nerve stimulation (TENS).
• Counseling, biofeedback or self-hypnosis or self-relaxation therapy is recommended to help manage the stress, anger, anxiety and, sometimes, depression that accompanies disorders of chronic pain.
• Surgical measures are rarely used (only as a last resort when other methods of treatment have failed and quality of life warrants drastic steps).
• See the Resource section of this book for additional information.

MEDICATION
• Antihistamines, anticholinergics, nonsteroidal anti-inflammatory drugs (NSAIDs) and antidepressants all have limited success with decreasing the symptoms.
• Sodium pentosanpolysulfate has demonstrated effectiveness in relieving symptoms for some women.
• DMSO (dimethyl sulfoxide) or other medications may be instilled (placed directly) into the bladder. The DMSO is left in for about 15 minutes and then expelled. The treatment is repeated every 2 weeks or until symptoms are relieved. DMSO use produces a garlic-like smell to the skin and breath lasting up to 72 hours.

ACTIVITY—No restrictions other than those caused by the symptoms.

DIET
• Elimination of caffeine-containing beverages, alcohol, artificial sweeteners, spicy foods, brewer's yeast, citrus fruits and tomatoes in the diet may help relieve symptoms.
• A bland diet helps some patients.

CALL YOUR DOCTOR IF

• You or a family member has symptoms of interstitial cystitis.
• Intolerable pain occurs during treatment.
• New, unexplained symptoms develop. Drugs used in treatment may produce side effects.
• Symptoms recur after treatment.

Kegel Exercises

GENERAL INFORMATION

DEFINITION
• Kegel exercises (named for the individual who invented them) are designed to strengthen the muscles that surround part of the vagina, urethra and rectum, and will increase your ability to control and relax these muscles completely. The pelvic floor muscles are important in women because they support the organs in the pelvis (uterus, bowel and bladder). Keeping these muscles strong can help prevent a prolapsed uterus or poor bladder control and may add pleasure to sexual intercourse.

• Over time, weakness develops in the pelvic floor muscles due to normal wear and tear and childbirth. The bladder, uterus and rectum begin to slip down and get squeezed into the lower regions of the pelvis. Stress incontinence may develop (urine is released during lifting, sneezing or exercising). Performing Kegel exercises can help many women relieve these symptoms.

• Pregnant women will benefit from Kegel exercises. They may be performed while on your back only, through the fourth month of pregnancy, and then should be done only while standing or sitting during subsequent months. After the fourth month, the growing uterus could put excessive weight on major blood vessels. Following childbirth, the exercises are helpful and can be started almost immediately.

INSTRUCTIONS

LEARNING THE TECHNIQUE
• To get the feel of the muscles, alternately start and stop urinating while using the toilet. Practice this tightening and releasing action while sitting, standing, walking, driving, and watching TV.

• Kegel exercises can be performed while lying on the floor, sitting or standing. On the floor, lie on your back with knees bent and about 12 inches apart with feet flat on the floor. Arms should be resting at your sides.

• Try to tighten the muscles a small amount at a time, "like an elevator going up to the tenth floor." Then, release very slowly one "floor" at a time.

• Be careful not to contract or squeeze other muscles when you do Kegel exercises. If you are on your back on the floor, keep knees apart as you squeeze, don't squeeze buttock muscles, and particularly, don't tighten the abdominal muscles. They can increase pressure on the pelvic floor muscles.

EXERCISE ROUTINE
• Do these exercises every morning, afternoon and evening (3 times a day). Try to maintain a daily schedule. They can be done before or after meals, while in the shower or while brushing your teeth at the sink.

• Start with 5 times each and gradually work up to 10 and then 20 to 30 each time.

• In addition to the daily routine, try to think about the pelvic muscles when you are lifting something heavy, sneezing, coughing or laughing. Do the pelvic muscle contraction whenever you anticipate extra pressure on your pelvis. Practice is required, but eventually it will become a habit.

KEGEL AIDS
• Weighted vaginal cones can be used to help strengthen the pelvic muscles. The cones come in a set of 5 that vary in weight. The tapered end of the cone is inserted into the vagina and the pelvic muscle is contracted to try and hold it in so that it doesn't slip out of the vagina. As the muscles get stronger, you progress to a heavier cone.

• A perineometer (or Kegelometer) is a device that is placed in the vagina and has a numbered gauge that will show the strength of the muscle contraction.

Note: These devices are not inexpensive. Talk to your doctor about their possible usefulness in your situation.

• Training on Kegel exercises may also be provided by your doctor, nurse, physical therapist or midwife.

• Computer-assisted biofeedback technique is available in some medical offices. It measures the strength of muscle contractions and determines if the correct muscles are being used.

• See the Resource section of this book for additional information.

OTHER SUGGESTIONS TO KEEP PELVIC FLOOR STRONG
• If you are overweight, try to lose the excess pounds. Pelvic floor problems are more likely to occur in overweight women.

• Don't smoke. There appears to be a predisposition to pelvic weakness among smokers.

• Always lift heavy objects with care, or get help with the lifting if needed.

• Keep aerobic exercises low impact. It is not known for sure if high impact aerobics affect the pelvic floor, but the trauma of repetitive jolting may lead to damage of the pelvic nerves and muscles.

• Avoid constipation. Straining may cause damage to pelvic muscles or nerves. Eat a high fiber diet and drink at least 8 to 10 glasses of water daily.

CALL YOUR DOCTOR IF

You want additional information about Kegel exercises.

Kegel Exercises

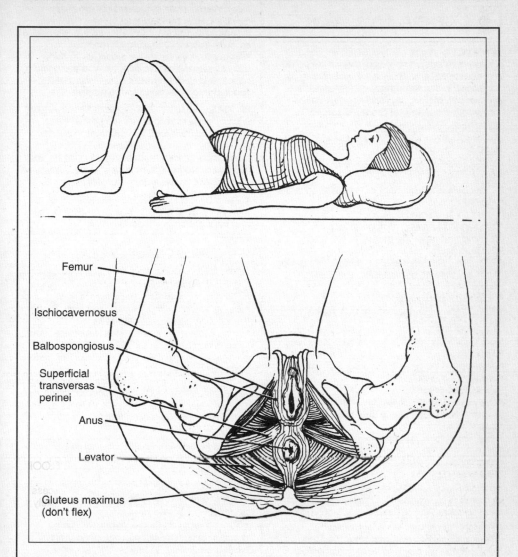

Femur

Ischiocavernosus

Balbospongiosus

Superficial
transversas
perinei

Anus

Levator

Gluteus maximus
(don't flex)

The top illustration shows a woman lying on the floor while performing Kegel exercises.
The woman is on her back with her knees bent and about 12 inches apart; her feet are flat on
the floor; her arms are resting at her side.

The lower illustration shows the muscles that surround part of the vagina, urethra and rectum;
these are the muscles that are used to perform Kegel exercises.

Laparoscopy

GENERAL INFORMATION

DEFINITION—A procedure that allows visual examination and some treatments of the pelvic and abdominal organs. The procedure is performed with a laparoscope, a small lighted telescope. Laporoscopy is sometimes called "belly-button surgery" or "bandaid surgery."

REASONS FOR PROCEDURE
• Evaluation and treatment of infertility in women.
• Evaluation of known or suspected endometriosis.
• Diagnosis and treatment of ectopic pregnancy.
• Complications from pelvic disease.
• Masses or cysts in the pelvis.
• Undiagnosed pelvic or abdominal pain.
• Fibroid tumors of the uterus.
• Hysterectomy.
• Location and removal of an intrauterine device (IUD) which has perforated the lining of the uterus.
• Voluntary sterilization.
• For diagnosis and treatment of a variety of abdominal disorders.

RISK INCREASES WITH
• Obesity.
• Smoking.
• Heart or lung disease.
• Advanced pregnancy.
• Previous abdominal surgery, especially for intra-abdominal infections (such as ruptured appendicitis).
• Previous bowel surgery.
• Use of drugs such as antihypertensives, antiarrhythmics, diuretics or beta-adrenergic blockers.

DESCRIPTION OF PROCEDURE
• Laparoscopy is performed in an outpatient surgical facility or hospital.
• General anesthetic is administered by injection and inhalation with an airway tube placed in the windpipe (a local anesthetic is sometimes used).
• It is often necessary to place an instrument (tenaculum) on the cervix in order to help move the uterus around.
• A small incision (half an inch to an inch long) is made in or below the patient's navel. A needle is inserted to inflate the abdomen with carbon dioxide.
• The operating table is tilted to allow the bowel and carbon dioxide to float up toward the chest. The laparoscope is then inserted through the incision and is used to examine the abdomen visually. Occasionally, other small incisions are made in order to insert other surgical instruments.
• The laparoscope can also be used to perform surgeries, including gallbladder removal, tubal ligation, aspiration and excision of ovarian cyst,

and multiple other gynecological procedures.
• The laparoscope and any other instruments inserted are removed, and the carbon dioxide is allowed to escape from the abdomen.
• Small sutures under the skin and an adhesive bandage are used to close the wound. In some cases, a long-acting local anesthetic can be injected into the wound for pain relief.

PROBABLE OUTCOME—Expect full recovery without complications. You may experience slight discomfort for 24 to 48 hours. You may have aches in your shoulders and chest from the carbon dioxide that was used to inflate your abdomen. No treatment is necessary. Allow 6 days for full recovery from surgery.

POSSIBLE COMPLICATIONS—Perforation of the intra-abdominal organs (bowel, bladder or liver) and intra-abdominal blood vessels.

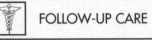

FOLLOW-UP CARE

GENERAL MEASURES
• Change the adhesive bandage daily.
• Bathe and shower as usual. You may wash the incision gently with mild soap.
• If the procedure was for sterilization and you were taking birth control pills, finish your present package; then you will no longer need birth control methods.
• Use sanitary pads (not tampons) to stop slight vaginal bleeding which may occur after surgery.
• Sit in a warm tub of water for 10 to 15 minutes at a time to relieve discomfort.

MEDICATION
• Prescription pain medication should generally be required for only 2 to 7 days following the procedure.
• You may use nonprescription drugs, such as acetaminophen, for minor pain.

ACTIVITY
• To help recovery and aid your well-being, resume daily activities as soon as you are able.
• Resume driving 24 hours after surgery.
• Sexual relations may be resumed in 2 or 3 days after recovery from surgery.

DIET
• Avoid carbonated beverages for 48 hours after surgery.
• No special diet.

CALL YOUR DOCTOR IF

• You develop signs of infection: headache, muscle aches, dizziness or a general ill feeling and fever.
• You have excessive bleeding or discharge from either the surgical area or the vagina.
• You experience abdominal swelling or pain.
• New, unexplained symptoms develop. Drugs used in treatment may produce side effects.

Laparoscopy

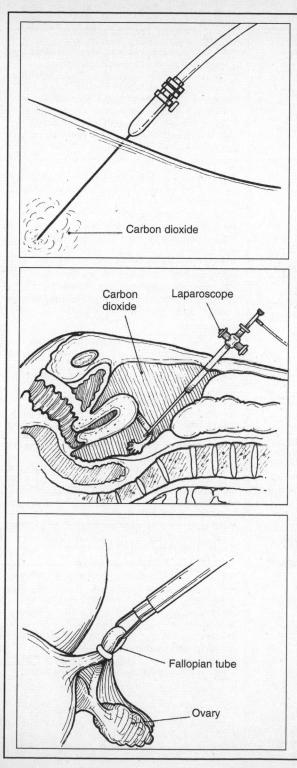

A hollow needle is inserted through the abdominal wall to inflate the abdomen with carbon dioxide.
- The operating table is tilted to allow the bowel and carbon dioxide to flow upward toward the chest.

Carbon dioxide

Carbon dioxide   Laparoscope

The laparoscope is inserted through the incision area to allow examination of the abdominal contents under direct vision.

The laparoscope may be used to provide passage of other instruments for doctors to perform surgical procedures if necessary.
- After the laparoscope is removed, carbon dioxide is allowed to escape from the abdomen. The small amount remaining will be readily absorbed by the body.
- Sutures under the skin and adhesive bandages are used to close the wound (not illustrated).

Fallopian tube

Ovary

Laparotomy

 GENERAL INFORMATION

DEFINITION—Abdominal surgery to identify, diagnose or treat a variety of conditions in women.

REASONS FOR PROCEDURE
- Diagnostic examination of the abdominal organs.
- Collection of tissue samples for diagnosis.
- Closure of hernias in the abdominal wall.
- Repair or removal of abnormal tissue.
- Removal of diseased organs.
- Correction of unsightly or disfiguring abnormalities.

RISK INCREASES WITH
- Stress; obesity; smoking.
- Excess alcohol consumption.
- Poor nutrition.
- Recent acute respiratory infection.
- Chronic illness.
- History of prior abdominal surgery, particularly if it occurred at the site of the current surgery.
- Use of drugs such as antihypertensives, muscle relaxants, tranquilizers, sleep inducers, insulin, sedatives, beta-adrenergic blockers or cortisone.

DESCRIPTION OF PROCEDURE
- Spinal or general anesthesia is administered by injection and inhalation with an airway tube placed in the windpipe.
- An incision (usually four to six inches long) is made in the abdomen. The abdominal muscles are separated, and the peritoneum (inner lining of the abdomen) is opened.
- Blood vessels cut during the surgery are cauterized, clamped and tied.
- Wound edges are retracted with a special instrument.
- Fluid in the abdominal cavity is often removed for laboratory examination.
- The abdominal organs are examined. Other surgeries may be performed at this time.
- Samples of suspicious tissue are gathered or diseased areas are treated.
- The peritoneum is closed, and the muscles are reconstructed with heavy sutures.
- The skin is closed with sutures or clips, which usually can be removed about 3 to 7 days after surgery.

PROBABLE OUTCOME—Expect complete healing without complications. Allow about 4 weeks for recovery from surgery.

POSSIBLE COMPLICATIONS
- Excessive bleeding.
- Surgical-wound infection.
- Incisional hernia.
- Abscess or excessive scar (keloid) formation.
- Complications related to the anesthetic.
- On rare occasions, injury to bowel, bladder, pelvic organs and blood vessels.

FOLLOW-UP CARE

GENERAL MEASURES
- A hard ridge should form along the incision. As it heals, the ridge will recede gradually.
- Use an electric heating pad, a heat lamp or a warm compress to relieve incisional pain.
- Bathe and shower as usual. You may wash the incision gently with mild unscented soap.
- Move and elevate legs often while resting in bed to decrease the chance of deep-vein blood clots.

MEDICATION
- Prescription pain medication should generally be required for only 2 to 7 days following the procedure.
- You may use nonprescription drugs, such as acetaminophen, for minor pain.
- Stool softener laxative, if needed to prevent constipation.
- Antibiotics, if needed to fight or prevent infection. Antibiotics may reduce the effectiveness of some oral contraceptives. If you are currently taking oral contraceptives for birth control, discuss this with your doctor.

ACTIVITY
- To help recovery and aid your well-being, resume daily activities, including work, as soon as you are able.
- Avoid vigorous exercise for 6 weeks after surgery.
- Resume sexual relations when follow-up medical examination reveals complete healing.
- Resume driving about 3 weeks after returning home.

DIET—Nasogastric suction is frequently required, followed by a clear liquid diet until the gastrointestinal tract functions again. Then eat a well-balanced diet to promote healing. Another diet may be prescribed depending on any special condition.

 CALL YOUR DOCTOR IF

- Pain, swelling, redness, drainage or bleeding increases in the surgical area.
- You develop signs of infection: headache, muscle aches, dizziness or a general ill feeling and fever.
- You experience nausea, vomiting, abdominal swelling, constipation or severe pain.
- New, unexplained symptoms develop. Drugs used in treatment may produce side effects.

Laparotomy

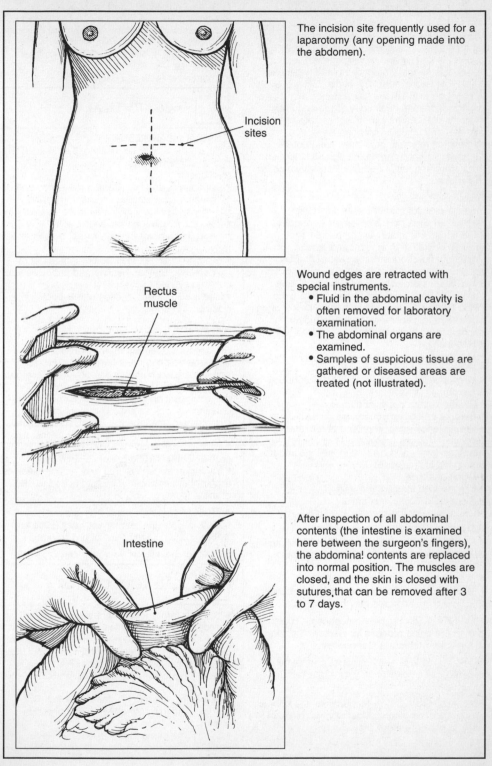

The incision site frequently used for a laparotomy (any opening made into the abdomen).

Incision sites

Rectus muscle

Wound edges are retracted with special instruments.
- Fluid in the abdominal cavity is often removed for laboratory examination.
- The abdominal organs are examined.
- Samples of suspicious tissue are gathered or diseased areas are treated (not illustrated).

Intestine

After inspection of all abdominal contents (the intestine is examined here between the surgeon's fingers), the abdominal contents are replaced into normal position. The muscles are closed, and the skin is closed with sutures that can be removed after 3 to 7 days.

Menopause

GENERAL INFORMATION

DEFINITION—The permanent cessation of menstruation. This occurs as early as age 40 or as late as age 55 and usually spans 1 to 2 years. It is normally diagnosed in females after 1 year of absent menstrual periods. Menopause is only one event in the "climacteric," a biological change in all body tissue and body systems that occurs in both sexes between the mid-40s and mid-60s. Menopause is sometimes referred to as "the change of life." Menopause occurring before age 40 is termed premature and may need medical evaluation for the cause.

SIGNS & SYMPTOMS
Physical changes (directly associated with decreased blood levels of female hormones):
• Menstrual irregularity accompanied by a gradual decrease in amount and duration of menstrual flow. Menstruation usually tapers to spotting only, and then to complete cessation.
• Hot flashes or flushes—sensations of heat spreading from the waist or chest toward the neck, face and upper arms (symptoms are often referred to as vasomotor instability), often accompanied by sweating.
• Headaches.
• Dizziness.
• Rapid or irregular heartbeat.
• Vaginal itching, burning or discomfort during intercourse.
• Bloating in the upper abdomen.
• Bladder irritability; urinary incontinence.
• Breast tenderness; shrinking of breasts.
Emotional changes (associated with lower hormone levels and conflicting feelings about aging and loss of fertility):
• Mood changes.
• Pronounced tension and anxiety.
• Sleeping difficulty; insomnia.
• Depression or melancholy and fatigue.

CAUSES
• A normal decline in ovary function, resulting in decreased levels of the female hormones, estrogen and progesterone.
• Surgical removal of both ovaries.
• May occur following chemotherapy for cancer; this type of menopause may be reversible.

RISK INCREASES WITH—Menopause is a natural part of the aging process for women. Smoking is a risk for premature menopause.

HOW TO PREVENT—Menopause cannot be avoided, but its effects may be controlled or moderated.

PROBABLE OUTCOME—Menopause is a normal process, not an illness. Most women make an easy transition without crisis.

POSSIBLE COMPLICATIONS
• Increased irritability and susceptibility to infection in the urinary tract.
• Decreased skin elasticity and vaginal moisture.
• Increased risk of hardening of the arteries, heart disease, stroke and osteoporosis after menopause.
• Changes in feelings of self-worth.

HOW TO TREAT

GENERAL MEASURES
• Psychotherapy or counseling, if emotional changes interfere with work or personal relationships.
• Continue to use birth control measures until 12 months after your last menstrual period.
• Reduce stress in your life as much as possible.
• If you take estrogen-replacement therapy, have a Pap smear annually or as recommended by your doctor.
• Lifestyle changes may be brought about by menopause. Stay as healthy and happy as you can and live life to the fullest.
• See the Resource section of this book for additional information.

MEDICATION
• Hormone replacement therapy (HRT) or estrogen replacement therapy (ERT). Because hormone treatment has benefits as well as some risks, learn all you can about replacement therapy before deciding on treatment. HRT helps prevent osteoporosis and coronary heart disease, as well as providing relief from symptoms of menopause (hot flashes, vaginal dryness, insomnia and sleep disturbances).
• Calcium supplements if your diet does not provide at least 1000 mg of calcium a day.
• Vaginal estrogen creams may help dryness by replenishing estrogen losses that lead to the dryness.

ACTIVITY—No restrictions. Active exercise is beneficial. Weight-bearing activities (such as walking) can help maintain bone strength.

DIET—No special diet. Increase calcium intake.

CALL YOUR DOCTOR IF

• You or a family member has symptoms of menopause. Other causes should be ruled out.
• You experience excessive bleeding, prolonged periods or spotting between your periods. These may be signs of other disorders.
• Bleeding appears 6 months or more after your last period.
• New unexplained symptoms develop. Hormones used in treatment may produce side effects.
• Symptoms of menopause return while undergoing estrogen replacement therapy.

Menorrhagia (Hypermenorrhea)

 GENERAL INFORMATION

DEFINITION—A fairly common disorder that is characterized by an unusually heavy or prolonged period of menstrual flow. The average amount of blood loss during a normal menstrual period is about two ounces. With menorrhagia, a woman may lose three ounces or more. It rarely signifies a serious underlying disorder.

SIGNS & SYMPTOMS
• Excessive menstrual flow (varies greatly from woman to woman, but flow is generally considered to be excessive when it fully saturates a large pad or tampon in 1 hour).
• Menstrual period lasts for more than 7 days.
• Passing of large clots of blood.
• Paleness and fatigue (anemia).

CAUSES
• Anovulation (failure to release an egg each month).
• Imbalance of female hormones (estrogen and progesterone).
• Fibroids (benign uterine tumors).
• Pelvic infection.
• Endometrial disorder.
• Intrauterine device (IUD).
• Ovarian tumor.
• Hypothyroidism.

RISK INCREASES WITH
• Obesity.
• Estrogen administration (without progestin).
• Young women who have not established a regular ovulation cycle.
• Women approaching menopause.

HOW TO PREVENT—Annual pelvic examinations with a cervical smear test (Pap smear).

PROBABLE OUTCOME
• Varies with cause of bleeding.
• Patients whose menorrhagia is caused by hormonal imbalances usually respond well to treatment.

POSSIBLE COMPLICATIONS
• Anemia due to excessive blood loss.
• Surgery may be required.

 HOW TO TREAT

GENERAL MEASURES
• Special medical diagnostic tests (e.g., Pap smear, pregnancy test, endometrial biopsy, blood test) may be performed to help determine the cause of the bleeding.
• Ultrasound of pelvic regions to evaluate possible fibroids.
• Treatment usually depends on the age of the woman, whether or not she desires future pregnancy, and any underlying disorder.
• Wear extra sanitary pads during excessive flow to prevent embarrassment.
• If using an IUD, consider a change to another method of contraception.
• Dilatation and curettage, often referred to as D & C (dilatation of the cervix and scraping out of the uterus with a curette), may be performed. Hysteroscopic evaluation with ablation (surgical removal) of the uterine lining may be considered in women who have completed childbearing.
• Hysterectomy may be considered in persistent cases when fertility is not desired.

MEDICATION
• Hormone therapy may be prescribed to control bleeding.
• If hormones cannot be taken for some reason, other medications to control the bleeding may be recommended.
• Iron replacement therapy may be prescribed for anemia.

ACTIVITY—Resting with feet up may be helpful.

DIET—No special diet.

 CALL YOUR DOCTOR IF

• You or a family member has signs or symptoms of menorrhagia.
• You have excessive vaginal bleeding that soaks more than one tampon or pad per hour.
• Symptoms worsen after treatment begins.
• New, unexplained symptoms develop. Drugs used in treatment may cause side effects.

Menstruation & Menstrual Cycle

 GENERAL INFORMATION

DEFINITION

• In the U.S., the average age of a girl's first period is 12 years, although it is normal to start as early as age 10 or as late as age 16. Menopause (when periods stop) usually occurs around age 50, although that, too, can vary by several years. Except perhaps for the first two years of menstruation, and barring pregnancy, nursing and certain illnesses or other problems, the reproductive cycle repeats with predictable regularity every month.

• Exercise, diet and stress can delay the onset of menstruation or alter cycles once they've been established. Athletes and others who exercise strenuously can sometimes delay the onset of their periods, so a 16- or 17-year-old in that group may not have started menstruating. The connection between exercise and amenorrhea (absence of menstrual periods) may be related to body fat content, because fat affects estrogen. Young women who are very thin from malnourishment may not start menstruating until they gain weight, with a certain portion of that weight being fat.

• Young women with eating disorders such as anorexia or bulimia often do not menstruate. A girl should see her doctor if she hasn't started menstruating by age 16, or if by age 13 or 14 she hasn't begun to develop breasts or pubic and underarm hair.

SCHEDULE

• Many young women have very irregular periods during the first few years of menstruating and may even skip some months.

• In addition, young women don't always ovulate every month when they first get their periods. There's no sure way for a young woman to know which month she is ovulating and which she is not. So, from the time her periods begin, a young woman should assume she can get pregnant each and every month, even if her periods are irregular.

• Eventually, periods become regular, but even when they do, a missed or late period once a year, especially at a stressful time, is normal.

• Periods usually last from 3 to 5 days, but anywhere from 2 to 7 days is normal. The amount of blood varies, usually starting out light, then heavy, then light again. Use pads or tampons to absorb the flow.

• Menstruation is just one part of the menstrual cycle, in which a woman's body prepares for pregnancy each month. A cycle is counted from the first day of one period to the first day of the next. An average cycle is 28 days, but anywhere from 23 to 35 days is normal.

SIGNS & SYMPTOMS

• The menstrual cycle has its ups and downs of hormones, and different people react differently to hormonal swings. Just before and during menstruation, levels of the female hormones estrogen and progesterone are low. That's when some women feel bloated, irritable or blue, and many experience cramps, sore breasts, backache, nausea, headache or fatigue.

• A day or two after your period starts, you begin to feel better. Hormone levels go back on the upswing and discomfort usually decreases.

• Some 20% to 40% of menstruating women have PMS, or premenstrual syndrome. Starting anywhere from mid-cycle to a few days before menstruation begins, women with PMS may have one or all of a virtual laundry list of physical and emotional symptoms: breast swelling and tenderness, fluid retention, increased thirst or appetite, craving for sweets and/or salty foods, headaches, anxiety, hostility, restlessness, irritability, depression and loss of self-confidence. PMS doesn't usually affect teenagers, though. It increases with age and is more prevalent in women in their 30s and 40s.

OTHER MONTHLY CHANGES

• Estrogen and progesterone levels are very low at the beginning of the cycle. During menstruation, levels of estrogen, made by the ovaries, start to rise and cause the lining of the uterus to grow and thicken. In the meantime, an egg (ovum) in one of the ovaries starts to mature. It is encased in a sac called the Graafian follicle, which continues to produce estrogen as the egg grows.

• At about day 14 of a typical 28-day cycle, the sac bursts and the egg leaves the ovary, traveling through one of the fallopian tubes to the uterus. The release of the egg from the ovary is called ovulation.

• Some women know when they're ovulating, because at mid-cycle they have some pain, typically a dull ache on either side of the lower abdomen lasting a few hours. Some women also have very light bleeding during ovulation.

• After the egg is expelled, the sac (now called a corpus luteum) remains in the ovary, where it starts producing progesterone. The rising levels of estrogen and progesterone help build up the uterine lining to prepare for pregnancy.

• The few days before, during and after ovulation are a woman's "fertile period," the time when she can become pregnant. Because the length of menstrual cycles varies, many women ovulate earlier or later than day 14. It's even possible for a woman to ovulate while she is still bleeding, simulating a normal period. (Stress or other problems can sometimes cause a cycle to be shorter or longer.) If a woman has sex with a man during this time and conception occurs, she becomes pregnant.

Menstruation & Menstrual Cycle (cont.)

• The fertilized egg attaches to the uterus, and the corpus luteum makes all the progesterone needed to keep it implanted and growing until a placenta (an organ connecting the fetus to the mother) develops. The placenta then provides nourishment for the baby.

• If an egg is not fertilized that month and the woman doesn't get pregnant, the corpus luteum stops making hormones and gets reabsorbed in the ovary. Hormone levels drop again, the lining of the uterus breaks down, menstruation begins and the cycle repeats.

CRAMPS

• More than half of menstruating women have cramp-like pain during their periods. The medical term for menstrual pain is dysmenorrhea.

• Cramps are usually felt in the pelvic area and lower abdomen but can radiate to the lower back or down the legs.

• Many girls have cramps severe enough to keep them home from school. Among younger women, dysmenorrhea is the most frequent cause of absenteeism from school.

• Many women go through phases when cramps are severe, then get better for several years, and then worsen again.

• Mechanically, cramps are like labor pains. Just as the uterus contracts to open up the cervix (neck of the uterus) and push out a baby, it contracts to expel menstrual blood. Often, after several years of menstruating or after childbirth, the cervical opening enlarges. The uterus doesn't have to contract as much to discharge the menstrual flow, so there is less cramping.

• Menstrual pain may also come from the bleeding process itself. When the uterine lining separates from the wall, it releases chemicals called prostaglandins. Prostaglandins cause blood vessels to narrow, impeding the supply of oxygen to the uterus. Just as the pain of a heart attack comes from insufficient blood to the muscles of the heart, too little blood to the uterine muscle might cause the pain of menstrual cramps. Menstrual pain can have other causes, including tumors, fallopian tube infection and endometriosis, a condition in which fragments of the lining of the uterus become embedded elsewhere in the body.

NONDRUG TREATMENT FOR CRAMPS

• Cutting down on salt might help reduce fluid buildup, and support hose may alleviate swelling in the legs or ankles. Extra rest is one way to deal with fatigue, and a heating pad or hot water bottle can ease cramps.

• Exercising during menstruation can help reduce pain because it causes release of brain chemicals called endorphins, which are natural painkillers. Exercise may also decrease pain by affecting prostaglandin metabolism, and by increasing blood flow within the body.

MEDICATIONS FOR CRAMPS

• Ibuprofen, the active ingredient in some non-steroidal anti-inflammatory drugs (NSAIDs) such as Advil, Nuprin and Motrin IB, inhibits prostaglandin production, thus easing the discomfort of cramps. Aspirin also suppresses prostaglandins, but it's often not as effective for menstrual pain. Avoid aspirin for children or teenagers who have chickenpox or flu symptoms because Reye's syndrome, a rare but sometimes deadly illness, may develop.

• Several nonprescription NSAIDs, such as Midol and Pamprin, are specifically formulated for menstrual symptoms. Read the labels of these medicines before you buy them, because different formulations often contain different ingredients or strengths of ingredients. For example, Teen Formula Midol contains acetaminophen for pain and pamabrom (a mild diuretic) for fluid retention. Pamprin contains acetaminophen, pamabrom and pyrilamine maleate (an antihistamine) for tension and irritability. Cramp Relief Formula Midol IB contains only ibuprofen. Manufacturers may change their product's ingredients, so it's a good idea to check the label each time you buy the product.

• Plain acetaminophen products like Tylenol and Aspirin-Free Anacin also may help menstrual pain. It takes time for pain relievers to work, so it's best to take them at the onset of pain.

• If needed, your doctor may prescribe stronger painkillers, diuretics or oral contraceptives. One side effect of birth control pills is relief of menstrual cramps. They prevent the lining of the uterus from building up as much, so there is less bleeding. This means less prostaglandin production and blood-vessel narrowing, because there is less lining to separate, and fewer contractions, because there is less tissue to push out. In severe cases, hormones (e.g., gonadotropin-releasing hormone [Gn-RH]) can stop ovary function and relieve pain.

 CALL YOUR DOCTOR IF

• You or a family member has questions about the monthly menstrual cycle.

• Menstrual bleeding becomes excessive (soaking 1 or more pads or tampons an hour).

• You use tampons and develop signs of toxic shock syndrome (TSS): sudden fever over 102°F, vomiting, diarrhea, dizziness, fainting or sunburn-like rash. TSS is a rare, but sometimes fatal, disorder. Seek medical help immediately. Note: This information was adapted in part from the *FDA Consumer* (magazine of the U.S. Food & Drug Administration).

Molluscum Contagiosum

 GENERAL INFORMATION

DEFINITION—A contagious viral infection of the skin anywhere on the body. The virus usually occurs on the face, trunk and extremities in children. In adults, it usually occurs on the inner thighs, abdomen or genitals.

SIGNS & SYMPTOMS—Papules (small raised bumps on the skin) with the following characteristics:
• Bumps are firm, smooth, domed with a central pit and skin-colored or white. The overlying skin is transparent and thin.
• Bumps are usually 2 mm to 6 mm in diameter. A few may be as large as 10 mm.
• Bumps cause eye irritation if they are on the eyelids.
• Bumps can be painful or cause itching.

CAUSES—DNA virus of the pox group. This virus may be transmitted sexually. The incubation is 2 weeks to 2 months.

RISK INCREASES WITH
• Previous allergies or family history of allergy.
• Multiple sex partners.
• Unprotected sexual activity.
• HIV infection.
• Close, personal contact with infected person.
• Use of immunosuppressive drugs.
• Transmission can occur from swimming pools.

HOW TO PREVENT
• To prevent spread to other parts of the body or to other people, don't scratch bumps.
• Avoid sexual contact with infected persons.
• Maintain a mutually monogamous sexual relationship with your partner.
• Have your partner use a condom for sexual activity.

PROBABLE OUTCOME—If untreated, a few papules may increase to 20 to 50 lesions in several weeks. They will disappear sponta- neously in 6 to 12 months. However, they should be treated to prevent their spread to other persons.

POSSIBLE COMPLICATIONS
• Scarring or disfigurement.
• Immunocompromised individuals may have extensive infections.

 HOW TO TREAT

GENERAL MEASURES
• Medical treatment to remove the papules with liquid nitrogen or curettage (scraping).
• After treatment with liquid nitrogen, leave the blisters alone. The tops will come off spontaneously in 7 to 14 days.
• Keep blisters dry. Use small adhesive bandages to cover any blisters that may be irritated by clothing.
• Testing (screening) for other sexually transmitted diseases is often recommended.
• Your sexual contacts should be examined and, if necessary, treated for infection.

MEDICATION—Medicine usually is not necessary for this disorder. However, in some cases, a topical medication to kill the virus may be prescribed.

ACTIVITY—Avoid sexual relations until bumps disappear.

DIET—No special diet.

CALL YOUR DOCTOR IF

• You or a family member has symptoms of molluscum contagiosum.
• The following occur after treatment:
  Fever.
  Signs of infection (swelling, redness, pain, tenderness or warmth) at the treatment site.

Ovarian Cancer

 GENERAL INFORMATION

DEFINITION—A malignant growth in the ovary that is likely to spread to other body parts and threaten life. It affects females of all ages but is most common after age 50. There are many different types of ovarian cancer. Epithelial tumors account for the majority and are the most aggressive. Other ovarian cancers are slow growing or metastasized from other cancer in the body.

SIGNS & SYMPTOMS—Frequently no symptoms occur until the tumor becomes large.
Early symptoms:
• Vague discomfort in the lower abdomen.
• Abdominal swelling or bloating.
• Gastrointestinal upsets.
• Irregular menstrual periods.
Later symptoms:
• Nausea, vomiting or constipation.
• Deep voice.
• Excessive hair growth.
• Unexplained weight loss.
• An enlarged, hard and sometimes tender mass in the lower abdomen.
• Pain with intercourse.
• Anemia.

CAUSES—Unknown.

RISK INCREASES WITH
• Family history of ovarian cancer.
• Late pregnancies (over age 30).
• Never having had children.
• High-fat diet.
• Women who have previously been diagnosed with cancers of the breast, uterus, colon or rectum.

HOW TO PREVENT
• Have yearly pelvic examinations which may aid in earlier detection and treatment. If your mother or sister had ovarian cancer, additional screening tests, such as ultrasound, may be recommended.
• Oral contraceptives help to reduce risk.
• Preventive oophorectomy (removal of the ovaries) has been suggested for some women who have a mother or sister with ovarian cancer.

PROBABLE OUTCOME—25% to 50% of women with ovarian cancer survive at least 5 years after treatment. The prognosis is related closely to the stage of the disease when it is first diagnosed. With aggressive treatment, the long-term survival rate is improving.

POSSIBLE COMPLICATIONS
• Reaction to radiation and/or anticancer drug therapy.
• Pleural effusion (excess of fluid in the lining of the lungs).
• Ascites (excess fluid in the peritoneal cavity).
• Bowel or urinary tract obstruction.
• Fatal spread of cancer to other body parts.

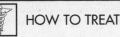 HOW TO TREAT

GENERAL MEASURES
• Diagnostic tests may include pelvic examination, laboratory blood studies, ultrasound of the abdomen, x-rays of the abdomen and CT or MRI.
• Laboratory blood studies will include tests for tumor markers or antigens; the most common of these tests is for a marker called CA-125. Additional tests may be performed to determine if the cancer has spread to other body parts.
• Specific treatment will vary, depending on the stage of the disease, the type of cancer cell and the patient's age.
• Surgery is usually performed to remove the cancerous ovary and other affected areas, including fallopian tubes, uterus and the other ovary (sometimes). The goal of surgery is to remove as many of the cancer cells as possible so chemotherapy will be more effective. In young patients who want to retain reproductive capacity, it may be possible to remove only the ovary and the tube. In some cases, follow up surgery is required to determine the effectiveness of the treatment.
• Chemotherapy, depending on cell type and stage of disease, is usually recommended along with surgery for the best outcome. Radiation therapy is less commonly used.
• Counseling and joining in a support group are recommended to learn to accept and cope with cancer.
• See the Resource section of this book for additional information.

MEDICATION
• Anticancer drugs (chemotherapy); usually a combination of drugs is recommended.
• Pain relievers, as needed.

ACTIVITY—No restrictions after recovery from surgery.

DIET—Eat a normal, well-balanced diet that is high in protein to promote repair of body tissues.

 CALL YOUR DOCTOR IF

• You or a family member has symptoms of an ovarian tumor.
• The following occur after surgery:
    Increased pain, swelling, redness or drainage from the surgical wound.
    Pain or swelling in the leg.
    Signs of infection, such as fever, chills, muscle aches or headache.
• New, unexplained symptoms develop. Drugs used in treatment may produce side effects.

Ovarian Cyst or Tumor Removal

GENERAL INFORMATION

DEFINITION—Removal of cysts or tumors on an ovary.

REASONS FOR PROCEDURE
• Cancer or suspected cancer in the ovaries.
• Rupture or twisting of an ovarian cyst.

RISK INCREASES WITH
• Adults over 60.
• Stress.
• Obesity.
• Smoking.
• Poor nutrition.
• Alcoholism.
• Recent or chronic illness.
• Use of drugs such as antihypertensives, muscle relaxants, tranquilizers, sleep inducers, insulin, sedatives, beta-adrenergic blockers or cortisone.

DESCRIPTION OF PROCEDURE
• Diagnostic tests performed before surgery may include blood and urine studies; CT scan of pelvic organs; laparoscopy or culdoscopy; ultrasound; x-rays of chest, lower abdomen and lower intestinal tract; culdocentesis (see Glossary for all).
• Surgery is usually performed by an obstetrician-gynecologist or general surgeon, in a hospital.
• General anesthesia is administered by injection and inhalation with an airway tube placed in the windpipe.
• An incision is made in the abdomen. The abdominal muscles are separated and the peritoneum is opened.
• Blood vessels supplying the ovaries are located, clamped and tied.
• The tumor or cyst in the ovary is located, cut free and removed, or the cyst may be destroyed by electrocauterization (see Glossary).
• During surgery, the tissue removed may be sent to the laboratory for examination by frozen section (see Glossary).
• If examination reveals signs of cancer, the ovary is removed.
• The peritoneum is closed, and the abdominal muscles are sewn together with heavy sutures.
• The skin is closed with sutures or clips, which can usually be removed about 10 days after surgery.
• This surgery, under many conditions, can be performed laparoscopically; several small incisions are made and different instruments are used to remove the cyst or tumor. Your doctor can determine which approach is best for your circumstances.

PROBABLE OUTCOME
• Expect complete healing of surgical wound.
• If cancer is detected, your doctor will prescribe treatment with radiation or anticancer drugs.
• Allow about 4 weeks for recovery from surgery.

POSSIBLE COMPLICATIONS
• Excessive bleeding.
• Surgical-wound infection.
• Excessive scarring (keloid).
• Recurrent cancer.

FOLLOW-UP CARE

GENERAL MEASURES
• Average hospital stay is 5 to 7 days. However, if surgery is performed laparoscopically, patients are often not admitted at all or go home the next day.
• A hard ridge should form along the incision. As it heals, the ridge will gradually recede.
• Use an electric heating pad, a heat lamp or a warm compress to relieve incisional pain.
• Bathe and shower as usual. You may wash the incision gently with mild unscented soap.
• Move and elevate legs often while resting in bed to decrease the likelihood of deep-vein blood clots.

MEDICATION
• Prescription pain relievers should be required for no longer than 4 to 7 days. Use only as much as you need.
• Stool softeners to prevent constipation.
• Hormone supplements.
• Antibiotics to fight or prevent infection. Antibiotics may reduce the effectiveness of some oral contraceptives. If you are taking oral contraceptives for birth control, discuss this with your doctor.
• You may use nonprescription drugs, such as acetaminophen, for minor pain. Avoid aspirin.

ACTIVITY
• To help recovery and aid your well-being, resume daily activities, including work, as soon as you are able.
• Avoid vigorous exercise for 6 weeks after surgery.
• Resume sexual relations when your doctor has determined that healing is complete.

DIET—Clear liquid diet until the gastrointestinal tract functions again. Then eat a well-balanced diet to promote healing.

CALL YOUR DOCTOR IF

• Pain, swelling, redness, drainage or bleeding increases in the surgical area.
• You develop signs of infection: headache, muscle aches, dizziness or a general ill feeling and fever.
• You experience nausea, vomiting, constipation, abdominal swelling or hot flashes.
• New, unexplained symptoms develop. Drugs used in treatment may produce side effects.

Ovarian Cyst or Tumor Removal

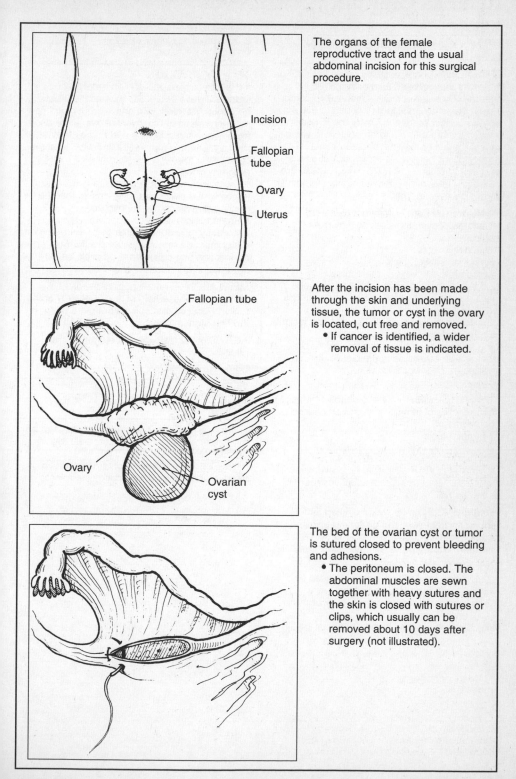

The organs of the female reproductive tract and the usual abdominal incision for this surgical procedure.

Incision

Fallopian tube

Ovary

Uterus

Fallopian tube

Ovary

Ovarian cyst

After the incision has been made through the skin and underlying tissue, the tumor or cyst in the ovary is located, cut free and removed.
- If cancer is identified, a wider removal of tissue is indicated.

The bed of the ovarian cyst or tumor is sutured closed to prevent bleeding and adhesions.
- The peritoneum is closed. The abdominal muscles are sewn together with heavy sutures and the skin is closed with sutures or clips, which usually can be removed about 10 days after surgery (not illustrated).

Ovarian Tumor, Benign (Ovarian Growth)

 GENERAL INFORMATION

DEFINITION—A benign, cystic (saclike) tumor on the ovary that contains fluid or semisolid material. These are usually small but, in some cases, they may grow large enough to make a woman appear pregnant. Often, the largest ovarian tumors turn out to be benign. In some cases, the tumor may have features that suggest it will behave as a cancer, but over a long period of time (10 to 20 years). These are called low malignant-potential ovarian tumors or borderline ovarian tumors.

SIGNS & SYMPTOMS—May not cause symptoms. If symptoms occur, they may include:
• Mild pelvic pain.
• Pain in the lower back.
• Discomfort with sexual intercourse.
• Abnormal menstruation, including changes in menstrual flow, length of periods and intervals between periods.
• Excessive hair growth, deep voice and weight gain (sometimes).
• If a large ovarian tumor twists or ruptures, there will be severe pain, rigid muscles and swelling in the lower abdomen.

CAUSES
• Usually unknown, but it is probably related to abnormalities of female hormone production and secretion.
• Endometriosis.

RISK INCREASES WITH—Unknown.

HOW TO PREVENT—No specific preventive measures. Use of oral contraceptives may decrease risk.

PROBABLE OUTCOME—Most ovarian tumors require no treatment and disappear spontaneously within 2 months. In most other cases, treatment usually provides a complete cure.

POSSIBLE COMPLICATIONS
• Emergency abdominal surgery caused by twisting, rupture or bleeding of the ovary.
• Some types of ovarian tumors may become malignant (cancerous).
• Ascites (excess fluid in the peritoneal cavity).

 HOW TO TREAT

GENERAL MEASURES
• Diagnostic tests include laboratory blood studies, x-rays and pelvic examination. Usually, ultrasound studies, with and without blood flow measurements of the involved ovary, are used for diagnosis and to help determine the best therapy. Laparoscopy (see Glossary), in some cases, and, rarely, a CT scan or MRI may be recommended.
• Treatment may not be necessary, except to have regular pelvic examinations so that the tumor's growth can be monitored.
• Some tumors require surgery to diagnose accurately, rule out malignancy or to treat. If one ovary must be removed (oophorectomy), normal conception and childbirth is possible as long as a normal ovary remains on the other side.

MEDICATION—Female hormones may be prescribed. These help shrink or destroy some tumors. Oral contraceptives are often used as the first step in treatment.

ACTIVITY—No restrictions if surgery is not necessary.

DIET—No special diet.

 CALL YOUR DOCTOR IF

• You or a family member has symptoms of an ovarian tumor, especially severe pain, rigidity and abdominal distention.
• New, unexplained symptoms develop. Drugs used in treatment may produce side effects.

Pediculosis
(Head Lice; Body Lice; Crab Lice)

GENERAL INFORMATION

DEFINITION—Skin inflammation caused by tiny parasites (lice) which live on the body or in clothing. They affect hairy areas anywhere, especially the scalp, eyebrows or genital area and areas in which clothing is in close contact with skin, such as the shoulders, waist, back of the neck, genital area or buttocks.

SIGNS & SYMPTOMS
• Itching and scratching, sometimes intense and usually in hair-covered areas.
• Eggs ("nits") on hair shafts. The nits look like tiny white spheres, approximately 0.8 mm long, that appear "cemented to the hair" and cannot be easily moved.
• Scalp inflammation and matted hair.
• Enlarged lymph glands at the back of the scalp or in the groin (sometimes).
• Red bite marks and hives.

CAUSES—Tiny (1 mm to 3 mm) parasites that bite through skin to obtain nourishment (blood). The bites cause itching and inflammation. Some lice live on skin, although they are difficult to see. Others live in clothing near skin. Eggs (nits) adhere to hairs.

RISK INCREASES WITH
• Crowded living conditions.
• Family history of lice.
• Sexual intercourse with an infected person.
• Contact with infected objects such as combs, hats, clothing.
• Contact with an infected person.

HOW TO PREVENT
• Bathe and shampoo often.
• Change or wash your clothes daily.
• Change bed linens often.
• Don't share combs, brushes or hats with others.
• Careful follow-up in schools and day care centers where episodes have occurred.

PROBABLE OUTCOME—Usually curable with medicated creams, lotions and shampoos. Allow 5 days after treatment for symptoms to disappear. Lice often recur.

POSSIBLE COMPLICATIONS
• Infection at the site of deep scratching.
• Persistent itching and skin irritation caused by too-frequent use of the pediculicide (antilice medication).

HOW TO TREAT

GENERAL MEASURES—The following measures apply to all members of the household, and to any sexual partners of household members:

• Use the prescribed medicated shampoo, cream or lotion.
• Machine-wash all clothing and linen in hot water. Dry in the dryer's hot-air cycle. Iron the clothing and linen, if possible. Washing removes the lice, and ironing destroys nits.
• If you don't have a washing machine, iron the clothes and linen, or seal for 3 weeks in a plastic bag to kill lice and nits.
• Dry-clean nonwashable items, including pillows and stuffed animals, or seal in a plastic bag for 3 weeks.
• Boil articles such as combs, curlers, hairbrushes and barrettes. Hair does not have to be shaved.
• Spray (with Lysol or similar product) all furniture that comes in contact with infected body areas.
• See the Resource section of this book for additional information.

MEDICATION—Antilice (pediculicide) cream, lotion or shampoo. Various commercial treatments are available over the counter, including NIX (permethrin), Kwell (lindane) and RID (pyrethrin butoxide). Infants and pregnant women may need a pediculicide that is less toxic than that prescribed for other family members. Apply creams or lotions to infected body parts according to instructions. To use the shampoo:
• Wet the hair. Apply 1 tablespoon of shampoo. Lather for 4 minutes, working the lather well into the scalp.
• If the shampoo gets into the eyes, wash out right away with water.
• Rinse hair thoroughly and towel dry. Don't use the same towel again without laundering.
• Comb the hair with a fine comb dipped in hot vinegar to remove the lice. The comb must run through the hair repeatedly, from the scalp outward, until the hair is completely free of nits.
• A single application of shampoo is effective in more than 90% of cases. Don't use more frequently than recommended, because the shampoo may cause skin irritation or be absorbed into the body. A repeat application may be necessary in 10 to 14 days.
• If the lice infect eyelashes, the lice must be removed carefully by the doctor. The prescribed medications should not be applied to the eye or eyelashes. You may apply petroleum jelly to the eyelashes for 1 week after removal of the lice.

ACTIVITY—No restrictions.

DIET—No special diet.

CALL YOUR DOCTOR IF

You or anyone in your household has symptoms of lice, or symptoms recur after treatment.

Pelvic Examination & Pap Smear

GENERAL INFORMATION

DEFINITION—Examination of the female external and internal genitalia. The Pap smear (cervical smear), carried out during the pelvic examination, is a laboratory study used to detect cancerous or precancerous cells on the cervix. It can also detect some uterine cancers, as well as some other tumors of the female reproductive organs. Annual pelvic examination with a Pap smear is recommended for most women, and more often for those in high-risk categories. Regular, annual pelvic examinations with a Pap smear can detect many cancerous and precancerous cells in their early stages, when they are most likely to be cured.

REASONS FOR PROCEDURE
• Routine diagnostic check.
• Investigate the cause of abdominal or pelvic pain.
• Unexpected vaginal bleeding or discharge.
• Bladder problems.
• A general check before prescribing any form of contraception.
• Pain during intercourse.
• Suspected sexually transmitted disease.
• In pregnancy, to assess the position of the baby.
• As a part of infertility studies.
• Screening test for cancer.

RISK INCREASES WITH—None expected.

DESCRIPTION OF PROCEDURE
• Do not douche before the examination.
• It is usually recommended that you urinate just before the examination; this may make it easier for your doctor to detect any abnormalities.
• The examination is performed in the examiner's office.
• On the examining table, you will lie on your back with knees bent and legs apart (legs are usually placed in stirrups for support).
• The external genital organs (vulva) will be examined visually for lumps, sores, skin discoloration, inflammation and qualities suggesting the general hormonal status.
• A speculum is placed inside the vagina and opened. The speculum is an instrument that holds the vaginal walls apart and allows the examiner to see the cervix and vagina and check for inflammation, infection, scars or growths. There may be some feeling of pressure on the bladder or rectum with the speculum in place. Because most lubricants will interfere with the Pap smear results, warm water is generally used to decrease the friction as the speculum is inserted.

• With a swab, a sampling of cells is taken from the cervix and placed on a glass slide for the Pap smear test. If you have an infection or there are signs of infection present, a sample of vaginal or cervical discharge may be taken for laboratory analysis also.
• After the speculum is removed, the examiner will place two fingers in the vagina and the other hand on top of the abdomen to check placement of uterus and ovaries and to assess their size, shape, consistency and tenderness. This procedure may cause some discomfort.
• Usually there is a rectal examination, in which the examiner places one finger in the rectum (often, one finger is placed in the vagina at the same time) to check the rectum itself and other nearby structures.

PROBABLE OUTCOME—There are no aftereffects expected from the examination. In routine examinations, the results are usually normal.

POSSIBLE COMPLICATIONS—None expected from the examination. The findings may indicate a disorder to be treated or a condition requiring further diagnostic testing.

FOLLOW-UP CARE

GENERAL MEASURES
• There may be some slight vaginal discharge following the examination. Use a tissue to wipe, or place one in your underpants temporarily. If there is bleeding (rare), a sanitary pad may be necessary.
• Any findings from the physical examination, as well as any recommendations for further diagnostic testing, will be discussed with you by the examiner.
• The results of the Pap smear testing may take several days or more. They will be reported to you by phone or mail. Be sure you and the doctor follow up on any abnormalities that are detected.

MEDICATION—Medicine is not necessary.

ACTIVITY—No restrictions.

DIET—No special diet.

CALL YOUR DOCTOR IF

You have not had a routine pelvic examination as recommended.

Pelvic Examination & Pap Smear

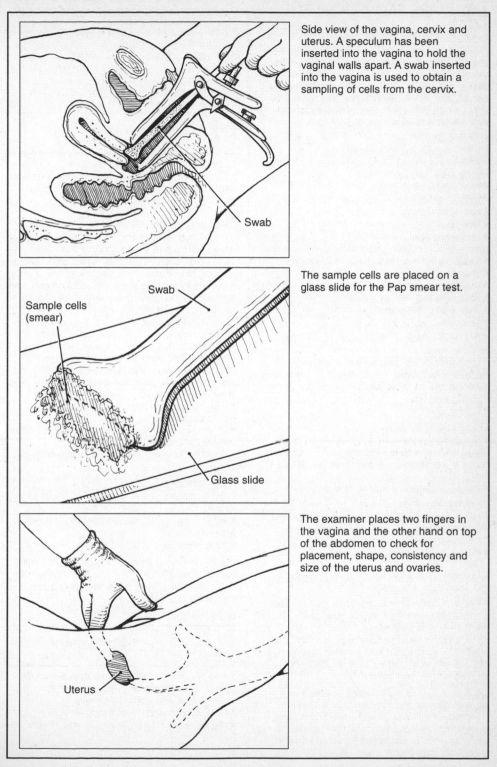

Side view of the vagina, cervix and uterus. A speculum has been inserted into the vagina to hold the vaginal walls apart. A swab inserted into the vagina is used to obtain a sampling of cells from the cervix.

Swab

The sample cells are placed on a glass slide for the Pap smear test.

Swab

Sample cells (smear)

Glass slide

The examiner places two fingers in the vagina and the other hand on top of the abdomen to check for placement, shape, consistency and size of the uterus and ovaries.

Uterus

Pelvic Inflammatory Disease (PID; Salpingitis)

 GENERAL INFORMATION

DEFINITION—Infection of the female internal reproductive organs. It is contagious if it is caused by a sexually transmitted organism. PID can involve the fallopian tubes, cervix, uterus, ovaries and urinary bladder. It usually affects sexually active females after puberty.

SIGNS & SYMPTOMS
Early symptoms (up to 1 week):
• Pain in the lower pelvis, usually on both sides.
• Irregular bleeding.
• Pain with intercourse.
• Vaginal discharge.
• General ill feeling.
• Low fever.
• Frequent, painful urination.
Later symptoms (1 to 3 weeks later):
• Severe pain and tenderness in the lower abdomen.
• High fever.
• Foul-smelling vaginal discharge.
• Pain with cervical manipulation.

CAUSES
• Bacterial infection (chlamydial, gonorrheal or mycoplasmal) or a virus. This may be transmitted by an infected sexual partner.
• Abortion (spontaneous or induced), particularly if not performed by a medical professional.
• Pelvic surgery.
• Rarely, childbirth.

RISK INCREASES WITH
• Multiple sexual partners, or exposure to a single partner who is infected.
• Use of an intrauterine contraceptive device (IUD).
• Previous history of PID or cervicitis.

HOW TO PREVENT
• Use rubber condoms, spermicidal creams or sponges to help prevent sexually transmitted infections.
• Oral contraceptives appear to decrease the risk.
• Maintain a mutually monogamous relationship with your sexual partner.
• Seek routine medical checkups for sexually transmitted diseases if you or your partner have multiple sexual partners.
• Have your sexual partner evaluated and treated if necessary. Don't resume sexual activity with your partner until his tests show no infection, or he has been treated.

PROBABLE OUTCOME—Usually curable with early treatment and avoidance of further infection. The illness lasts from 1 to 6 weeks, depending on its severity and the organisms involved. Poorer prognosis if treated late and unsafe lifestyle continues.

POSSIBLE COMPLICATIONS
• Pelvic abscess and rupture. This can be life-threatening.
• Adhesions (bands of scar tissue) inside the pelvis.
• Infertility.
• Ectopic pregnancy.
• Recurrence, or chronic infection.

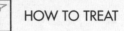 HOW TO TREAT

GENERAL MEASURES
• Diagnostic tests may include laboratory blood studies and culture of the vaginal discharge, pelvic ultrasound and surgical diagnostic procedures, such as laparoscopy or culdocentesis (see Glossary for these terms).
• If infection is mild, treatment may be done on an outpatient basis. It is important to adhere to your treatment and medication schedule. Close medical follow-up care is necessary.
• Use heat, such as warm baths, to relieve pain and discomfort. Sit in a tub of warm water for 10 to 15 minutes as often as needed.
• Use sanitary pads to absorb the discharge or menstrual flow; don't douche during treatment.
• Hospitalization may be required for severe illness, further diagnostic studies, suspected abscess, patient's failure to comply or to respond to outpatient therapy or in case of pregnancy.
• Surgery is sometimes necessary to drain a pelvic abscess.
• Hysterectomy may be recommended for older patients who desire no more children.
• Psychotherapy or counseling, if infertility occurs.

MEDICATION
• Intravenous or intramuscular antibiotics to fight infection.
• Early or mild PID may be treated with oral antibiotics.
• Pain relievers.

ACTIVITY—Avoid sexual intercourse, and the use of tampons, until healing is complete. Rest in bed until any fever subsides. Allow several weeks for recovery.

DIET—No special diet.

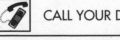 CALL YOUR DOCTOR IF

• You or a family member has symptoms of pelvic inflammatory disease.
• Symptoms recur after treatment.
• New, unexplained symptoms develop. Drugs used in treatment may produce side effects.

Polycystic Ovarian Syndrome
(Stein-Leventhal Syndrome)

 GENERAL INFORMATION

DEFINITION—Ovary enlargement from many small cysts. The hormonal regulation of the ovary malfunctions, resulting in a reduction or absence of ovulation (the monthly release of the egg from the ovary). Women with this condition are often infertile.

SIGNS & SYMPTOMS
• Irregular menstrual bleeding resulting in alternating periods of light and heavy flow.
• Increased time between periods, often up to several months.
• Increased hair growth (hirsutism) on the face, arms, legs and from pubic area to navel.
• Hypertension (high blood pressure).
• Deepening of the voice.
• Enlarged ovaries or clitoris.
• Infertility.
• Higher energy level.
• Obesity.
• Acne.

CAUSES—An imbalance between the pituitary gonadotropin luteinizing hormone (LH) and follicle-stimulating hormone (FSH), resulting in a lack of ovulation and increased testosterone production.

RISK INCREASES WITH
• Endometrial hyperplasia or carcinoma.
• Obesity.
• High blood pressure.
• Diabetes mellitus.
• Breast cancer.

HOW TO PREVENT—Cannot be prevented at present. Women should receive appropriate cancer screening tests to reduce the risk factors of uterine cancer and breast cancer.

PROBABLE OUTCOME—Hormone therapy can be used to decrease masculine characteristics and other hormonal therapy can be used to restore fertility. Some signs and symptoms may never disappear completely.

POSSIBLE COMPLICATIONS
• Permanent hormone imbalance.
• Infertility.
• Increased likelihood of uterine cancer and breast cancer.

 HOW TO TREAT

GENERAL MEASURES
• Diagnostic tests may include laboratory studies of blood hormone levels, pelvic ultrasound, laparoscopy or endometrial biopsy (see Glossary for these terms) to rule out hyperplasia or cancer.
• No ideal medical treatment exists. Drugs may be prescribed to help relieve the symptoms of the disorder; these drugs will be determined by the severity of symptoms and whether there is a desire for pregnancy.
• You may need professional help if you want to remove excess hair from your face, arms and legs. Drugs may be prescribed. Other methods of hair removal include bleaching, electrolysis, plucking, waxing and depilation.
• See the Resource section of this book for additional information on hirsutism and infertility.

MEDICATION
• Progestin or oral contraceptives for patients not desiring pregnancy.
• Clomiphene citrate or other drugs for those patients who desire pregnancy.
• A few drugs have been tried for the excess hair (hirsutism), but the success rate is not high, and side effects are numerous.

ACTIVITY—No restrictions on activity, including sexual intercourse.

DIET—No special diet. Weight loss is recommended if you are overweight.

 CALL YOUR DOCTOR IF

• You or a family member has symptoms of polycystic ovarian syndrome.
• Your periods become profuse or more frequent than usual.
• You develop a lump or swelling in the breast.
• Symptoms recur after treatment or surgery.
• You want a referral to remove excess body hair.
• New, unexplained symptoms develop. Drugs used in treatment may produce side effects.

Premenstrual Syndrome (PMS; Premenstrual Tension)

GENERAL INFORMATION

DEFINITION—Symptoms that begin 7 to 14 days prior to a menstrual period and usually stop when menstruation begins. About half of all women experience PMS at some time, some very frequently. The peak incidence occurs between ages 25 and 40.

SIGNS & SYMPTOMS
- Nervousness and irritability.
- Dizziness or fainting.
- Depression or mood swings.
- Increased or decreased sex drive.
- Headaches.
- Tender, swollen breasts.
- Bloating, constipation, diarrhea.
- Fluid retention which causes weight gain and puffiness in ankles, hands and face.
- Fatigue.
- Acne outbreaks.
- Decreased urination.
- Over 150 other symptoms have been attributed to PMS.

CAUSES—Unknown, but may be due to fluctuations in the circulating level of hormones (especially estrogen and progesterone). These fluctuations cause retention of sodium in the bloodstream, resulting in edema in body tissues including the brain. Increased levels of prostaglandin (a chemical) in the bloodstream may be a factor. Additional theories about the basis of PMS include psychiatric, endocrinologic, diet, endorphin, serotonin, prostaglandin, fluid retention, vitamin and other factors.

RISK INCREASES WITH
- Increased levels of stress.
- Caffeine, high fluid intake, and smoking all seem to intensify or increase symptoms.
- PMS is exacerbated with age.
- PMS can occur with other disorders such as depression.

HOW TO PREVENT—No specific preventive measures, but try to avoid stressful situations at the expected time of PMS. Also share your feelings and needs with a friend or spouse.

PROBABLE OUTCOME—Present treatments may or may not be effective. Medication can relieve some symptoms. However, many new treatments are in the experimental stage, offering hope for the future.

POSSIBLE COMPLICATIONS—Emotional stress severe enough to disrupt a woman's life.

HOW TO TREAT

GENERAL MEASURES
- A physical examination will be done to rule out other disorders. Diagnosis usually depends on a history of symptoms and their relationship to the menstrual cycle. Keeping a menstrual diary helps monitor and record symptoms.
- Treatment steps involve education, diet, exercise and lifestyle changes. There are no medications clearly indicated for PMS, however, a number of medications or vitamin supplements may help to reduce the symptoms.
- Reduce stress where possible. Learn relaxation techniques.
- Stop smoking.
- Join a support group. Talking about your PMS problems with others can help.
- Get individual or conjoint (couple) counseling.
- See the Resource section of this book for additional information.

MEDICATION—These are used with varying degrees of success:
- Nonsteroidal anti-inflammatory drugs (NSAIDs) to decrease prostaglandin levels.
- Diuretics to reduce fluid retention.
- Pain medications such as acetaminophen or ibuprofen.
- Vitamin B-6; vitamin E; magnesium.
- Antianxiety drugs or antidepressants.
- Danazol for total symptom complex; leuprolide (Lupron) or Gn-Rh (gonadotropin-releasing hormone) when complete ovarian suppression is deemed appropriate.
- Oral contraceptives may help.
- Tranquilizers or sedatives to relieve tension.
- Other medications are undergoing study and may be found to be more effective.

ACTIVITY
- Begin a regular, aerobic exercise program. Exercise can help relieve symptoms of PMS.
- Get regular sleep.

DIET
- Decrease salt intake during the premenstrual phase.
- Eat a low-fat, high-complex carbohydrate diet.
- Eat frequent small meals.
- Limit intake of caffeine and alcohol.

CALL YOUR DOCTOR IF

- You or a family member has symptoms of PMS that interfere with normal activities or relationships.
- Symptoms don't improve, despite treatment.
- New, unexplained symptoms develop. Drugs used in treatment may produce side effects.

Pruritus Vulvae

 GENERAL INFORMATION

DEFINITION—An acute or chronic disorder of the skin around the vulva (the vaginal lips) and anus. This disorder is characterized by severe itching or burning of the vulva. It is not contagious. It affects female adolescents and adults, especially after menopause.

SIGNS & SYMPTOMS
- Intense itching, sensitivity and irritation in the genital area. The skin may be dry.
- Thin, white vaginal discharge (sometimes).
- Discomfort during sexual intercourse.

CAUSES
- Skin disease, such as psoriasis or lichen planus.
- Systemic disease, such as diabetes mellitus.
- Atrophy and dryness caused by estrogen deficiency.
- Skin reaction to irritants, such as toilet tissue, sanitary pads, soap, douches, deodorants, powders, perfume and fabric.
- Systemic allergies, including food allergies.
- Human papillomavirus.
- Disorder of the vagina or rectum, such as vaginitis or hemorrhoids.
- Urinary tract infections will occasionally produce vulvar burning.

RISK INCREASES WITH
- Stress.
- Days prior to menstruation.
- Hot, humid weather.
- Diabetes mellitus.
- Lack of urinary control.

HOW TO PREVENT
- Wear cotton underpants rather than nylon or other synthetic material.
- Avoid wearing tight-fitting clothes or nylon pantyhose.
- Avoid contact with irritants listed in Causes.
- Obtain medical treatment for underlying disorders.

PROBABLE OUTCOME—Treatment usually provides relief in 1 to 2 weeks.

POSSIBLE COMPLICATIONS
- Secondary bacterial infection of the inflamed skin.
- Chronic course.
- Development of malignancies of the vulva (rare).

 HOW TO TREAT

GENERAL MEASURES
- Diagnostic tests may include laboratory study of vaginal secretions and, if needed, a biopsy (see Glossary) of the vulva.
- Treatment of any underlying cause.
- Wear cotton underclothes.
- Do not use vaginal deodorants, douches or perfumes.
- Keep the area as dry and cool as possible. Wear loose clothing.
- Don't scratch the itchy area. Scratching will aggravate soreness and irritation.
- Wash the genital area once a day, using water and unscented soap only. Pat, do not rub, the area dry with a clean cotton towel.
- Use a lubricant, such as K-Y Lubricating Jelly, during intercourse.
- After urinating or having a bowel movement, clean the genital area gently with absorbent cotton or antiseptic wipes. Wipe from front to back (vagina to anus).
- During menstruation, use tampons rather than sanitary napkins until the disorder heals.
- Sit in bathtub of warm (tepid, not hot) water several times a day to help relieve itching.

MEDICATION
- Treatment for any infectious cause found.
- Use low-potency, nonprescription steroid creams or ointments.
- Your doctor may prescribe more potent, prescription-strength steroid creams or lotions to reduce inflammation. These require 24 to 36 hours to provide relief.
- Ointments that contain hormones are sometimes recommended.
- Benzodiazepines or antihistamines at night to ensure rest.

ACTIVITY—Avoid overexertion, heat and excessive sweating.

DIET—No special diet, except to avoid foods to which you may be allergic. Avoid coffee or other caffeinated beverages. Also avoid tomatoes and peanuts, as they can aggravate the condition.

CALL YOUR DOCTOR IF

- You or a family member has symptoms of pruritus vulvae.
- Symptoms don't improve in 2 weeks, despite treatment.
- Scratching leads to skin infection.
- New, unexplained symptoms develop. Drugs used in treatment may produce side effects.

Rape Trauma Syndrome

 GENERAL INFORMATION

DEFINITION—The physical and emotional aftereffects of rape. Rape refers to any sexual act committed by one person on another, without that person's consent, using either force or the threat of force. Rape involves varying degrees of physical and psychological trauma. In most cases the rapist is a man and the victim is a woman.

SIGNS & SYMPTOMS
Immediately following rape:
• Physical injuries such as cuts, bruises or other injuries, including vaginal and rectal tears.
• Fear, anger, crying or unusual behavior such as laughter.
• No outward emotional signs (sometimes).
Aftereffects (may be weeks to months):
• Feelings of self-blame and guilt.
• Depression and withdrawal, even from family and friends.
• Mood swings; feelings of grief, shame, revenge.
• Loss of appetite.
• Fear of intercourse; fear of men.
• Nightmares; sleep disorders.
• Loss of self-esteem.
• Fear of being alone.
• Anxiety.
• Sense of hopelessness about the future.

CAUSES—Rape is extremely traumatizing. All rape victims will suffer physical and psychological aftereffects.

RISK INCREASES WITH—Any victim of rape or attempted rape.

HOW TO PREVENT
• There is no prevention for rape trauma syndrome.
• The scope of rape prevention is complex and involves individuals, society and government.

PROBABLE OUTCOME
• It takes most rape victims a long time to feel like they are back in a normal existence; some never do, and some say that they are a completely changed person.
• Length of recovery time may vary depending on the individual and previous life experiences.
Recovery generally involves 3 stages:
Acute stage (dealing with the immediate physical and emotional effects).
Outward adjustment stage (may seem to be doing well, but may be suppressing feelings).
Integration stage (facing the problem; resolution of the rape experience takes place).

POSSIBLE COMPLICATIONS
• Sexually transmitted diseases.
• Emotional trauma that may last years.
• Significant pelvic injury.
• Pregnancy (rare).

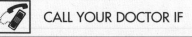 **HOW TO TREAT**

GENERAL MEASURES
Immediate care:
• Emergency medical assessment and care will be provided for your physical injuries.
• A general physical examination and pelvic examination will be conducted according to specific medical guidelines. A report is normally made to local law enforcement personnel.
• Ask for assistance from a Rape Crisis Center (or similar agency). These organizations can provide immediate support and help you through the urgent medical, emotional and legal necessities.
• Medical personnel will discuss with you the risks of pregnancy, sexually transmitted diseases, HIV/AIDS, hepatitis B and other infections, what preventive measures are available and what follow-up tests may be required. There may be need for consideration of immediate hormonal contraception (morning-after pill) if risk of pregnancy exists.
Aftereffects care:
• Arrange for counseling or psychological help. This is important for your emotional recovery. Don't just try to put the matter out of your mind, and don't try to "go it alone." Suppressing your feelings can increase distress.
• It may be helpful to keep a journal or diary about your feelings, thoughts and reactions. Talk over your feelings with trusted friends and family.
• Prepare yourself as much as possible for legal proceedings that force you to relive the trauma and may cause additional emotional upsets.

MEDICATION
• Antibiotics, if venereal infection is suspected or diagnosed. Antibiotics may reduce the effectiveness of some oral contraceptives. If you are currently using oral contraceptives for birth control, discuss this with your doctor.
• Hormones to prevent pregnancy ("morning-after pill") may be recommended.
• Sedatives or tranquilizers for a short time to reduce anxiety.
• Tetanus prophylaxis may be recommended.

ACTIVITY—Resume your normal life as quickly as possible. Regaining control of your life is a major step to healing and recovery.

DIET—No special diet.

📞 **CALL YOUR DOCTOR IF**

• You or someone you know has been raped.
• Emotional and/or physical problems worsen or are not improved with treatment.
• You experience any side effects from medications prescribed following a rape.

Scabies

GENERAL INFORMATION

DEFINITION—A highly contagious disease caused by infestation of the skin by a parasitic mite called Sarcoptes scabiei. Scabies can be transmitted from person to person (by shared clothing or bed linen) and from one site to another in the same person. They usually infect the skin of the finger webs, and folds under the arms, breasts, elbows, hands, feet, waist, genitals and buttocks.

SIGNS & SYMPTOMS
• Small, itchy blisters (usually in a thin line) on several parts of the body; itching is usually more intense at night. The blisters break easily when scratched.
• Broken blisters leave scratch marks and thickened skin, crisscrossed by grooves and scaling.

CAUSES—A mite that burrows into deep skin layers, where the female mite deposits eggs. Eggs mature into adult mites in 3 weeks. Mites are 0.1 mm in diameter and can only be seen under a microscope. Scratching collects mites and eggs under the fingernails, so they spread to other parts of the body.

RISK INCREASES WITH
• Crowded or unsanitary living conditions.
• Contact with an infested person (usually by physical contact, but mites can pass by just standing close to an infected person).
• Multiple sexual partners.
• Serious illness that has lowered resistance.
• Use of immunosuppresive or anticancer drugs.

HOW TO PREVENT
• Avoid contact with persons or linen and clothing that you suspect may be infected with scabies.
• Maintain personal cleanliness:
  Bathe daily, or at least 2 to 3 times a week.
  Wash hands before eating.
  Launder clothes often.
• Maintain a mutually monogamous sexual relationship.

PROBABLE OUTCOME
• Itching usually disappears quickly, and evidence of the disease is gone in 1 to 2 weeks with treatment. In 20% of cases, symptoms recur and retreatment is necessary in 20 days. If skin irritation persists longer than this, oral antihistamines or topical steroids may be necessary to break the itch-scratch cycle.
• Scabies may occur in a community in a 7-year cycle (the "seven-year itch").

POSSIBLE COMPLICATIONS—Secondary bacterial infection of mite-infested areas of inflammation.

HOW TO TREAT

GENERAL MEASURES
• Diagnosis is confirmed by discovering the mite, lifting it from its burrow and identifying it under a microscope.
• Treatment is with topical medication.
• Carefully wash all clothes, bedding and toys used prior to or during treatment. Use hot water and machine-dry for at least 20 minutes, or dry-clean. It is not necessary to clean furniture or floors with special care.

MEDICATION—An insecticide lotion (e.g., permethrin, lindane, crotamiton or 5% sulfur ointment) will usually be prescribed. Infants and pregnant women may need a pediculicide that is less toxic than that prescribed for other family members.
• Bathe thoroughly before applying the prescribed medicine.
• Apply from the neck down and cover the entire body.
• Wait 15 minutes before dressing.
• Leave medicine on the skin for a minimum of 8 hours before bathing.
• Your family or other close contacts should be treated at the same time.
• You may need to repeat in 1 week.

ACTIVITY—No restrictions.

DIET—No special diet.

CALL YOUR DOCTOR IF

• You or a family member has symptoms of scabies.
• After treatment, the lesions show signs of infection (redness, pus, swelling or pain).
• New, unexplained symptoms develop. Drugs used in treatment may produce side effects.

Sexual Dysfunction, Female

GENERAL INFORMATION

DEFINITION—Female sexual dysfunction may involve a lack of desire (disorder of desire), an inability to experience sexual pleasure (arousal dysfunction) or an inability to achieve orgasm (orgasmic dysfunction).

SIGNS & SYMPTOMS
- Lack of sexual desire.
- Inability to enjoy sex.
- Lack of vaginal lubrication.
- Failure to achieve orgasm, even when sexually aroused.

CAUSES
- Inadequate or ineffective foreplay.
- Poor communication, or lack of intimacy, between partners.
- Psychological problems, including depression, poor self-esteem, sexual abuse or incest.
- Feelings of shame or guilt about sex.
- Fear of pregnancy.
- Hormonal imbalance (rare).
- Stress and fatigue.
- Acute illness or chronic illness, especially of the central nervous system or endocrine system, as with multiple sclerosis or hypothyroidism.
- Inexperience or inadequate information about sexuality on the part of either partner.
- Repressed anger toward the sexual partner that may result from feelings of being used as a sexual object, physical or emotional abuse, jealousy or fears of disloyalty, or lack of true intimacy.
- Drug or alcohol abuse.
- Gynecologic factors (including vaginal dryness, infection or other disorders).
- Diabetes mellitus can cause orgasmic dysfunction.

RISK INCREASES WITH
- Use of some medications, such as MAO inhibitors, antidepressants, beta-adrenergic blockers.
- Couple discrepancies in expectations and attitudes toward sex.
- Proximity of other people in the home (e.g., children, mother-in-law).
- Previous sexual trauma.

HOW TO PREVENT
- Maintain good communication with your partner. Don't be hesitant about discussing the problem, exploring your needs and asking for help. Your partner's understanding can be important to solving the problem.
- Seek counseling to resolve feelings about past sexual trauma or abuse.

PROBABLE OUTCOME—Best predictors of positive outcome are the desire to change and an overall healthy relationship. Arousal dysfunction is difficult to treat and outcome may vary. Admit the problem and try to establish open communication with your partner. Pretending that you are aroused or have orgasms leaves the problem unsolved.

POSSIBLE COMPLICATIONS
- Permanent inability to enjoy sex.
- Damage to interpersonal relationships.

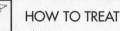

HOW TO TREAT

GENERAL MEASURES
- Diagnostic tests may include laboratory blood tests and other studies to rule out physical causes of arousal or orgasmic dysfunction.
- If no physical problems are found, a detailed sexual history is the most important tool for determining an appropriate treatment program. Possible treatment methods:
- For childhood sexual abuse problems—psychotherapy or counseling.
- For arousal dysfunction—relaxation techniques, sensate focus exercises (see Glossary) or counseling (usually with a sex therapist).
- For orgasmic problems—self-stimulation, new behavior patterns and sexual homework with partner (usually in conjunction with treatment from a sex therapist).
- For medication-caused problems—change in dosage, discontinuance or a change to a different medication.
- Other problems—family therapy, sensate focus exercises (see Glossary) or referral to a specialized sex therapist.
- For all types of sexual dysfunction—open communication, trust, commitment and honesty are all important factors in successful treatment.

MEDICATION—Medication is not necessary unless the sexual problem is due to some underlying medical condition. There is no known aphrodisiac that is effective and safe.

ACTIVITY—No restrictions. Exercise regularly to reduce stress and improve your self-image. A healthy body and mind make enjoyable sex more likely.

DIET—Eat a well-balanced diet. Vitamin and mineral supplements may be helpful. Weight loss program may be recommended if either partner is overweight.

CALL YOUR DOCTOR IF

You have sexual problems and you want help in resolving them.

Sexual Dysfunction, Male Impotence (Erectile Dysfunction)

 GENERAL INFORMATION

DEFINITION
• A consistent inability to achieve or maintain an erection of the penis necessary to have sexual intercourse. (The occasional periods of impotence that occur in just about all adult males are not considered dysfunctional.)
• Impotence is not inevitable with aging. The capacity for erection is retained, though a man may need more stimulation to achieve erection and more time between erections as he ages.

SIGNS & SYMPTOMS
• Inability to achieve an erection.
• Inability to maintain an erection for the normal duration of intercourse.

CAUSES
Psychological causes:
• Guilt feelings.
• A poor relationship with the sexual partner.
• Psychological disorders, including depression, anxiety, stress and psychosis.
• Lack of sexual information, including an understanding of the emotional aspects of sexuality and female anatomy and physiology.
Physical causes:
• Diabetes mellitus.
• Atherosclerosis (hardening of the arteries).
• Use of some antihypertensive medications.
• Disorders of the central nervous system, such as spinal cord injury, stroke or syphilis.
• Endocrine disorders that involve the pituitary, thyroid, adrenal or sexual glands.
• Alcoholism.
• Drug abuse, especially of marijuana, cocaine, narcotics, sedatives, hypnotics or hallucinogens.
• Decreased circulation to the penis from any cause.
Situational causes:
• Presence of other people in the home (such as mother-in-law).

RISK INCREASES WITH
• Recent illness that has lowered strength.
• Recent major surgery.

HOW TO PREVENT
• Maintain good communication with your partner. Encourage him to be open about discussing the problem, exploring his needs and asking for help. Your understanding is critical to solving the problem.
• He should avoid alcohol and drugs that can be abused.
• If he has diabetes, he should adhere closely to his treatment program.
• Your partner should maintain overall good health.

PROBABLE OUTCOME
• In cases with psychological origins, recovery frequently occurs after counseling.

• For cases with physical origins, treatment of the underlying disorder or changes in a medication therapy may improve sexual performance.
• Many patients can benefit from the prescription medication Viagra (sildenafil citrate), which can improve their ability to achieve and maintain a penile erection.

POSSIBLE COMPLICATIONS
• Depression and loss of self-esteem.
• Marital problems or breakdown of close personal relationships.

 HOW TO TREAT

GENERAL MEASURES
• Medical tests or studies to diagnose any underlying disorder or measure nocturnal erections.
• Counseling (alone or with his partner) from a qualified, professional sex therapist.
• If medication is the cause, a change in type or dosage may be helpful.
• Depending on the underlying cause, medication may be prescribed which can improve the ability to achieve and maintain an erection.
• Self-administered penile injection therapy may be prescribed, or use of a vacuum erectile device may be recommended for some patients.
• Surgery to implant a penile prosthesis will help in some cases.
• See the Resource section of this book for additional information.

MEDICATION
• Medication such as Viagra (sildenafil citrate) may be prescribed. This drug does not directly cause penile erections but can increase the body's ability to achieve and maintain an erection in response to sexual stimulation. Not all causes of erectile dysfunction can be treated with Viagra, and not all men respond to the drug. Viagra can have potentially fatal interactions with nitrates, such as those used in nitroglyceride, and should be taken only under the advice of a physician.
• Medication, as needed, to treat any underlying medical condition.
• Medication for self-administered penile injections may be prescribed.

ACTIVITY—No restrictions.

DIET—Eat a well-balanced diet.

 CALL YOUR DOCTOR IF

• Your partner or family member has symptoms of impotence, especially if taking medications.
• New, unexplained symptoms develop. Drugs used in treatment may produce side effects.

Sexual Dysfunction, Male Premature Ejaculation

 GENERAL INFORMATION

DEFINITION—Male orgasm and ejaculation following brief sexual stimulation and prior to satisfactory arousal and orgasm in the sexual partner. This is a common disorder affecting all age groups and usually caused by psychological problems. In adolescent males, ejaculatory control is an acquired behavior that usually increases with experience.

SIGNS & SYMPTOMS
• Repeated episodes of premature ejaculation.
• Feelings of self-doubt, inadequacy and guilt.

CAUSES
• Poor relationship or communication with the sexual partner.
• Fear of impregnating the partner.
• Fear of contracting a sexually transmitted disease.
• Anxiety about sexual performance.
• Cultural or religious conflicts.
• History of furtive sexual encounters (backseat intercourse, masturbation, etc.) which may condition a male to rapid ejaculation.
• Belief that sex is sinful or dirty.
• Rarely may be due to underlying neurological disorder (e.g., prostatitis).

RISK INCREASES WITH—Listed with Causes.

HOW TO PREVENT—No specific preventive measures.

PROBABLE OUTCOME—Usually curable in most people within 6 months after recognition and treatment.

POSSIBLE COMPLICATIONS
• Low self-esteem, anxiety or guilt.
• Damage to marital or interpersonal relationships.

 HOW TO TREAT

GENERAL MEASURES
• Laboratory test results are usually normal, since most males with this problem are healthy individuals.
• You and your partner should work to improve communication.
• Your partner should try to reduce his performance anxiety.

The following methods are recommended by sex researchers and therapists Masters and Johnson. These methods will usually lead to ejaculatory control for 5 to 10 minutes or longer:
• Sensate-focus exercises, in which each partner caresses the other's body without intercourse, to learn the relaxed, pleasurable aspects of touching.
• Mutual physical examination of each other's bodies to acquaint both partners thoroughly with anatomy. This helps reduce shameful feelings about sex.
• Stop-and-start technique, in which the man is stimulated through controlled intercourse or masturbation until he feels an impending ejaculation. Stimulation is stopped, then resumed in 20 to 30 seconds.
• Squeeze technique, in which the woman squeezes her partner's penis with her thumb and forefinger when he feels an impending ejaculation. When ejaculatory feelings pass, intercourse is resumed. This is repeated as often as necessary until the man can control ejaculation to the satisfaction of both partners.
• Individual psychotherapy may be recommended for some men, and marital therapy for couples may be helpful.
• Counseling from a qualified sex therapist if other methods are not successful.

MEDICATION—Medicine usually is not necessary for this disorder.

ACTIVITY—No restrictions. Regular exercise is always beneficial to a healthy lifestyle and personal well-being.

DIET—No special diet.

CALL YOUR DOCTOR IF

Your partner has repeated episodes of premature ejaculation after trying recommended methods.

Sexually Transmitted Diseases (STDs)

GENERAL INFORMATION

STD FACTS:
- Sexually transmitted diseases affect more than 12 million men and women in the United States each year. Many are teenagers or young adults.
- Sexually transmitted diseases are infectious diseases that are transmitted primarily through sexual contact and the exchange between sexual partners of semen, fluid or blood. Some STDs, however, can be transmitted through kissing or other casual contact.
- Sexually transmitted diseases include HIV (the virus that causes AIDS), chancroid, chlamydial infections, trichomoniasis, genital herpes, pubic lice, human papillomavirus, gonorrhea, lymphogranuloma venereum, syphilis, viral hepatitis, scabies, bacterial vaginosis, molluscum contagiosum and others.
- Using drugs or alcohol increases your chances of getting STDs because these substances can interfere with your judgment and your ability to use a condom properly.
- Intravenous (IV) drug use puts a person at higher risk for HIV and hepatitis B because IV drug users often share needles.
- The more sexual partners you have, the higher your chance of being exposed to HIV or other STDs. This is because it is difficult to know whether a person is infected or has had sex with people who are more likely to be infected due to intravenous drug use or other risk factors.
- Sometimes, early in the infection, a person may be asymptomatic (have no symptoms), or symptoms may be easily confused with other illnesses.
- You cannot tell by looking at someone whether he or she is infected with HIV or another STD.

STDs CAN CAUSE:
- Pelvic inflammatory disease (PID), which can damage a woman's fallopian tubes and result in pelvic pain and infertility.
- Ectopic, or tubal, pregnancies (where the pregnancy grows outside of the uterus, often in the fallopian tube). This condition does not result in a viable pregnancy and can be fatal to the woman.
- Death or severe damage to babies born to infected women.
- Sterility (the inability to have children) in both men and women.
- Cancer of the cervix in women.
- Damage to major organs, such as the heart, kidney and brain, if STDs go untreated.
- Chronic disease.
- Death, especially with HIV, hepatitis or syphillis.

RISKS—High-risk behaviors include having vaginal, anal or oral sex with:
- A person who has an STD. This is the riskiest behavior. If you know your partner is infected, avoid intercourse (including oral or anal sex). If you do decide to have sex with an infected person, always be sure to use a new condom from start to finish, every time.
- A male or female prostitute.
- Someone who has shared needles to inject drugs with an infected person.
- Someone whose past partner(s) were infected. Because HIV can be in the body a long time before a person feels sick or develops AIDS, a partner who has had intercourse with a person infected with HIV could pass it on to you, even if the sexual contact was a long time ago (even as long as 10 years), and even if your partner seems perfectly healthy.

PREVENTION:
- Maintain a mutually monogamous sexual relationship.
- Avoid sexual activity with partners who are at risk (see Risks above).
- To lessen the chance of being infected with AIDS or other STDs, people who take part in risky sexual behavior should always use a latex or polyurethane condom. Condoms do not make sex 100 percent safe but, if used properly, can reduce the risk of contracting a sexually transmitted disease, including AIDS.
- In addition to a condom, use of a spermicide called nonoxynol-9 can kill many organisms that cause STDs.
- Pregnant women generally aren't susceptible to uterine infections but are just as likely to contract vaginal or cervical infections (e.g., gonococcus, chlamydia).
- See "Condom Usage" in this book for information on the most effective use of a condom.
- See the Resource section of this book for additional infomation.

CALL YOUR DOCTOR IF

You experience any of the following STD symptoms:
- Discharge from the vagina, penis or rectum.
- Pain or burning during urination or intercourse.
- Pain in the abdomen (women), testicles (men), or buttocks and legs (men and women).
- Blisters, open sores, warts, rash or swelling in the genital or anal area, or the mouth.
- Persistent flu-like symptoms, including fever, headache, aching muscles, or swollen glands.
- You or a family member has questions or concerns about STDs.

Syllabus

GENERAL INFORMATION

DEFINITION—A contagious, sexually transmitted disease that causes widespread tissue destruction. Syphilis is known as the "great mimic," because its symptoms resemble those of many other diseases. It involves the genitals, skin and central nervous system. There are two types of syphilis: the congenital form, which affects newborn infants (0-2 weeks) born to mothers who are infected with syphilis, and the infectious form of syphilis, which affects persons of all ages and both sexes who acquire it through sexual contact.

SIGNS & SYMPTOMS
First or primary stage (Individuals are contagious at this stage; symptoms appear 3 to 6 days after contact.):
• A painless, red sore (chancre) on the genitals, mouth or rectum. The sore usually affects the penis in males and vagina or cervix in females.
Secondary stage (Individuals are also contagious during this stage, which begins 6 or more weeks after the chancre appears.):
• Enlarged lymph glands in the neck, armpit or groin.
• Headache.
• Rash on skin and mucous membranes of the penis, vagina or mouth. The rash has small, red, scaly bumps.
• Fever (sometimes).
Latent stage (Individuals are not infectious at this stage, which begins after one year, but the disease can relapse to the secondary, infectious stage if left untreated.):
• Blood tests will show positive but there are usually no signs or symptoms during the latent stage.
Third or tertiary stage (Noncontagious; may appear years after the first and second stages):
• Mental deterioration; dementia.
• Sexual impotence.
• Loss of balance.
• Loss of feeling or shooting pain in the legs.
• Blindness.
• Meningitis; encephalitis.
• Nephrosis (kidney disease).
• Heart disease.
• Tertiary stage is rare today, as most cases are treated long before the tertiary stage develops.

CAUSES—The infecting germ for both forms is Treponema pallidum.
• The congenital form is spread to the fetus through the bloodstream.
• The contagious form is spread by intimate sexual contact with someone who has syphilis in the first or second stages.

RISK INCREASES WITH
• Multiple sexual partners.
• Sexual activity between homosexual males.

HOW TO PREVENT
• Obtain blood serum test for syphilis early in pregnancy. If infected, get immediate treatment.
• Use latex (rubber) condoms during sexual activity.
• Avoid any sexual contact with a partner who you know, or suspect, is infected.

PROBABLE OUTCOME—Usually curable in 3 months with treatment. In spite of treatment, syphilis returns within 1 year in 10% of patients. If this happens, retreatment is necessary.

POSSIBLE COMPLICATIONS—Widespread tissue destruction and death without treatment.

HOW TO TREAT

GENERAL MEASURES
• Diagnostic tests may include laboratory studies, such as a blood serum test for syphilis, a microscopic exam of discharge from the chancre and a study of spinal fluid. Tests are repeated after treatment.
• Testing (screening) for other sexually transmitted diseases is usually recommended.
• Ensure that all your sexual partners obtain treatment. The public health department will work with you to notify contacts confidentially and help them obtain treatment.
• After treatment, have blood studies done each month for 6 months to check for recurrence. Then repeat blood studies every 3 months for 2 years.
• See the Resource section of this book for additional information.

MEDICATION
• Penicillin by injection unless you are allergic to it. If penicillin cannot be used, other antibiotics will be equally effective.
• Topical medications as needed for skin symptoms.

ACTIVITY—Avoid sexual activity until cure is complete. Then use latex (rubber) condoms during sexual activity.

DIET—No special diet.

CALL YOUR DOCTOR IF

• You or a family member has symptoms of syphilis.
• The following occur during or after treatment:
  Fever.
  Skin rash, sore throat or swelling in any joint, such as the ankle or knee.
• You once had syphilis and have not had a medical checkup in the past year.
• You have had sexual contact with someone who has syphilis.
• New, unexplained symptoms develop. Drugs used in treatment may produce side effects.

Thromboembolic Disorders

GENERAL INFORMATION

DEFINITION—A group of disorders characterized by inflammation of the veins and formation of blood clots (thrombus).
• Superficial thrombophlebitis or phlebitis is inflammation of the wall of a vein located close to the skin surface. It may be accompanied by blood clot formation and may be uncomfortable but usually is not dangerous.
• Phlebothrombosis involves blood clot formation without the vein inflammation.
• Deep vein thrombosis involves formation of a blood clot in the deep veins of calves, legs or pelvis. If part of the blood clot breaks away (an embolus) and passes into the bloodstream, it may cause damage elsewhere in the body.
• Pulmonary embolism occurs when an embolus reaches the lungs and blocks an artery. This is frequently life-threatening.

SIGNS & SYMPTOMS
• Sometimes no symptoms are present.
• Swollen, warm and deeply tender calf or leg.
• Redness in the affected area.
• Weakness, fever, chills, severe pain.

CAUSES—The disorders develop as a result of changes in the venous blood flow due to infection, damage or increased coagulation (clotting) of the blood. Thromboembolic disease can be a serious complication of surgery.

RISK INCREASES WITH
• Obesity.
• Labor and childbirth.
• Immobility in bedridden or elderly persons.
• Oral contraceptive use (with high doses).
• Long airplane flights or automobile trips.
• Systemic disease, including heart problems, cancer and AIDS.
• Intravenous drug abuse.
• Surgery, especially of the hip or knee.
• Complication of varicose veins.
• Cigarette smoking.
• Certain autoimmune and congenital conditions, which lead to blood vessel injuries and clot formation.

HOW TO PREVENT
• Identification of high risk patients and preventive steps such as starting anticoagulant medications.
• A quick return to mobility after surgery or childbirth.
• Take brief, but regular, walks during long trips.
• Avoid risk factors when possible.

PROBABLE OUTCOME—With treatment, expect to return to normal health and activity within 3 to 6 weeks. The prognosis is good once the risk of pulmonary embolism has passed.

POSSIBLE COMPLICATIONS
• The problem may recur or become chronic.
• Pulmonary embolism that may be fatal.
• Excessive bleeding due to anticoagulants.

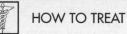

HOW TO TREAT

GENERAL MEASURES
• Diagnostic tests may include ultrasound studies, plethysmography or venography (see Glossary for these terms).
• For thrombophlebitis, treatment usually consists of rest with the legs slightly elevated. Compression (support) stockings, warm moist soaks and medications may be recommended.
• With deep vein thrombosis, hospitalization is usually necessary for intravenous medication; treatment steps involve bed rest or compression stockings. Outpatient care may be permitted.
• Pregnant women with deep vein thrombosis will continue anticoagulant treatment for 6 to 12 weeks following delivery. Medication may be administered through an implanted intravenous catheter.
• If a clot is life-threatening, surgical removal may be required. Surgery may also be necessary to place a filter in the large vein (vena cava) going to the lungs to prevent pulmonary embolism.

MEDICATION
• An anticoagulant (heparin) to reduce blood clotting time is usually started intravenously, then may be changed to an oral anticoagulant (warfarin) for maintenance. Intravenous anticoagulation is used during pregnancy, as oral anticoagulation is associated with birth defects. Anticoagulant level must be monitored to keep it in a safe range.
• Pain medicine as needed.
• Nonsteroidal anti-inflammatory drugs (except in pregnancy) to help prevent formation of clots.
• Discontinue oral contraceptives. Hormonal replacement therapy (HRT) may be continued.

ACTIVITY—Rest in bed until healing is complete. While resting, move legs and feet as much as possible.

DIET—No special diet. If overweight, a weight loss diet is usually recommended.

CALL YOUR DOCTOR IF

• You or a family member has symptoms of thrombophlebitis or deep vein thrombosis.
• Despite treatment, there is increased swelling, redness or pain in the affected area.
• Any unexpected bleeding occurs, or you develop chest pain or shortness of breath. Call immediately! This can be a sign of life-threatening problems!
• New, unexplained symptoms develop. Drugs used in treatment may produce side effects.

Toxic Shock Syndrome (TSS)

 GENERAL INFORMATION

DEFINITION—An acute form of blood poisoning caused by poisons (toxins) released by staphylococcal bacteria. Menstrual toxic shock involves the female reproductive system and respiratory system. Nonmenstrual toxic shock can affect all ages and both sexes (up to 15% of cases occur in males).

SIGNS & SYMPTOMS
- Sudden high fever in a previously healthy person.
- Nausea, vomiting or watery diarrhea.
- Rash that resembles sunburn.
- Low blood pressure.
- Red, watery eyes.
- Vaginal discharge or itching.
- Abdominal pain.
- Difficulty in breathing.
- Dizziness; fainting.
- Muscle aches or pains.
- Excessive thirst.
- Rapid pulse.
- Feeling of impending doom.
- Mental changes; confusion; agitation.
- Extreme fatigue and weakness.
- Headache.
- Sore throat.

CAUSES—Some strains of staphylococcal bacteria produce toxins that enter the bloodstream, causing sudden symptoms. Over half of the cases have come from staphylococci in the vagina of women using tampons. Toxic shock syndrome can also arise from wounds or infections in the throat, skin, lungs or bone.

RISK INCREASES WITH
- Continuous or prolonged use of tampons (particularly super absorbent) during menstrual periods.
- Staphylococcal infections.
- Use of an intrauterine contraceptive device (IUD) or diaphragm.
- Previous illness with toxic shock syndrome.
- Postpartum women.
- Postoperative patients, particularly after nasal surgery.

HOW TO PREVENT
- Change tampons frequently, and alternate them at night with sanitary napkins.
- Don't use superabsorbent tampons. Use tampons made of cotton, rather than those made of synthetic fibers.
- Don't use tampons if you have a skin infection, especially near the genitals.
- Wash hands thoroughly before inserting tampons. Staphylococci are commonly found on the hands.
- Get early medical attention for infected wounds.

PROBABLE OUTCOME—Most patients recover with early diagnosis and prompt hospital treatment, but some cases are fatal. Skin of the fingers, palms and soles usually peels during recovery. The disease may recur following treatment.

POSSIBLE COMPLICATIONS
- Severe shock.
- Kidney or liver failure.
- Congestive heart failure.
- Respiratory distress.
- Loss of hair and nails.
- Recurrence of TSS.
- Mortality may be as high as 15% in severe cases.

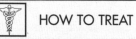 HOW TO TREAT

GENERAL MEASURES
- Diagnostic tests may include laboratory blood studies and mucosal cultures.
- Immediate hospitalization is required to administer intravenous fluids, antibiotics and electrolytes to correct fluid and electrolyte loss and dehydration, and to manage kidney or cardiac problems and provide mechanical breathing support if needed.
- Tampons, diaphragms or other foreign bodies are removed at once. Following removal, the vagina will usually be cleansed with an antiseptic solution to help neutralize the bacteria producing the toxins.

MEDICATION
- Antibiotics, usually intravenous, for infection. Some antibiotics may reduce the effectiveness of oral contraceptives. If you are currently using oral contraceptives for birth control, discuss this with your doctor.
- Intravenous fluids and electrolytes.

ACTIVITY—Resume your normal activities as soon as symptoms improve.

DIET—No special diet after recovery. Intravenous nourishment is usually necessary during hospitalization.

 CALL YOUR DOCTOR IF

- You or a family member has symptoms of toxic shock syndrome. Call immediately! Shock develops rapidly.
- New, unexplained symptoms develop. Drugs used in treatment may produce side effects.

Toxoplasmosis

GENERAL INFORMATION

DEFINITION—A protozoan infection found in humans and many species of mammals and birds. There are several types that occur in humans: congenital toxoplasmosis (passed from infected mother to her unborn child); ocular toxoplasmosis (also called retinochoroiditis, which usually results from congenital toxoplasmosis, but symptoms may not occur until ages 20-40); acute toxoplasmosis in a basically healthy individual; acute toxoplasmosis in an immunocompromised individual (person with AIDS, cancer or on immunosuppressant drugs).

SIGNS & SYMPTOMS
• Usually, no symptoms (70% to 90% of patients).
• Fever.
• Fatigue.
• Swollen lymph glands.
• Muscle aches.
• Sore throat.
• Rash (sometimes).
• Retinitis (inflammation of the retina).

CAUSES—The protozoan, Toxoplasma gondii, usually transmitted by:
• Eating undercooked meats from infected animals.
• Cats who harbor the germ can excrete it in their stools; humans who handle cat litter, or small children who eat soil contaminated with dog or cat feces, can become infected.
• Blood transfusion; organ transplant.
• An infected pregnant woman can transmit it to her unborn child (often with severe effects).

RISK INCREASES WITH
• Immunosuppression due to illness or drugs.
• Contact with cats.
• Improper food preparation.

HOW TO PREVENT
• Avoid eating raw or undercooked meats or eggs, or drinking unpasteurized milk. Use proper techniques for preparation and storage of meat products. Wash hands carefully after handling raw meats.
• Pregnant women at significant risk, or those who are very concerned about toxoplasmosis, can have a laboratory blood test early in pregnancy to determine if they have antibodies to toxoplasmosis. Some patients who suspect early pregnancy infection can request testing again at 16-18 weeks of pregnancy to determine if they have acquired an infection and, if so, may consider a therapeutic abortion.
• Immunocompromised persons and pregnant women should avoid contact with cat feces.
• Protect children's play area, including sand boxes, from cat and dog feces.
• Change cat litter boxes daily; feed indoor cats only canned, dry or cooked meat.

PROBABLE OUTCOME—The majority of infected persons have no symptoms, and those with mild symptoms recover spontaneously with no aftereffects.

POSSIBLE COMPLICATIONS
• For pregnant female—when infection occurs early in pregnancy: miscarriage; stillbirth; various chronic disorders (seizures) and birth defects (blindness, deafness, mental retardation) in the newborn (some may not be apparent for years). An infection later in pregnancy usually has no serious effects.
• For immunocompromised patient—lung and heart damage, brain inflammation, recurrence.
• For nonimmunocompromised patient (basically healthy)—rarely, may develop lung or brain inflammation.
• Ocular toxoplasmosis may cause permanent eye damage, including partial or complete blindness.

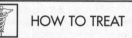

HOW TO TREAT

GENERAL MEASURES
• Diagnosis involves a medical history, physical exam and laboratory studies of blood.
• Treatment is usually unnecessary for a healthy, nonpregnant individual who has no symptoms. For a child under age 5, medications will be prescribed to prevent eye complications.
• For pregnant females, your doctor will discuss the treatment available, the risks involved and the expected outcomes.
• For immunocompromised patients, treatment is with medication.
• Newborns with infection are treated with medications, even if no symptoms are present, since the germs can multiply after birth.
• If drugs are prescribed for you, your doctor will do frequent blood tests to monitor side effects.

MEDICATION
• Pyrimethamine, sulfadiazine or trisulfapyrimidines for 3 to 4 weeks, and folinic acid to reduce the side effects of pyrimethamine are often prescribed.
• Corticosteroids, if necessary, for inflammation.
• Other medications are being evaluated.

ACTIVITY—Level of activity will be determined by severity of symptoms.

DIET—No special diet.

CALL YOUR DOCTOR IF

• You or a family member has symptoms of toxoplasmosis.
• Symptoms worsen or don't improve after diagnosis and treatment.
• New, unexplained symptoms develop. Drugs used in treatment may produce side effects

Urethral Caruncle Removal

GENERAL INFORMATION

DEFINITION—Removal of a urethral caruncle, a small benign tumor that develops at the opening of the female urethra.

REASONS FOR PROCEDURE—Treatment of excessive bleeding or discomfort.

RISK INCREASES WITH
- Adults over 60.
- Obesity; smoking.
- Poor nutrition.
- Recent or chronic illness.
- Alcoholism.
- Use of drugs such as antihypertensives, muscle relaxants, tranquilizers, sleep inducers, insulin, sedatives, beta-adrenergic blockers or cortisone.

DESCRIPTION OF PROCEDURE
- Laboratory blood and urine studies, Pap smear (see Glossary) and pelvic examination are usually performed prior to surgery.
- Surgery is performed in a hospital, outpatient facility or a doctor's office, by a urologist or obstetrician-gynecologist.
- The vagina is held open with a speculum. The caruncle is located, cleansed and anesthetized with local anesthesia.
- The caruncle is then removed with electrocauterization or a scalpel.
- Bleeding is controlled with pressure or electrocauterization.

PROBABLE OUTCOME—Expect complete healing without complications. Allow about 2 weeks for recovery from surgery.

POSSIBLE COMPLICATIONS
- Excessive bleeding.
- Surgical-wound infection.

FOLLOW-UP CARE

GENERAL MEASURES
- Usually, no hospital stay is required.
- Bathe and shower as usual. Wash the vaginal area gently with mild unscented soap and water after urination.
- Use an electric heating pad or a warm compress in the genital area to relieve surgical-wound pain.

MEDICATION
- Prescription pain medication should generally be required for no longer than 4 to 7 days. Use only as much as you need.
- Antibiotics to fight or prevent infection. Antibiotics may reduce the effectiveness of some oral contraceptives. If you are currently using oral contraceptives for birth control, discuss this with your doctor.
- You may use nonprescription drugs, such as acetaminophen, for minor pain. Avoid aspirin.

ACTIVITY
- To help recovery and aid your well-being, resume daily activities, including work, as soon as you are able.
- Avoid vigorous exercise for 2 weeks after surgery.
- Resume driving 3 days after returning home.
- Sexual relations may be resumed when your doctor determines that healing is complete.

DIET—No special diet.

CALL YOUR DOCTOR IF

- Pain, swelling, redness, drainage or bleeding increases in the surgical area.
- Urination is painful or difficult.
- You develop signs of infection: headache, muscle aches, dizziness or a general ill feeling and fever.
- New, unexplained symptoms develop. Drugs used in treatment may produce side effects.

Urethral Caruncle Removal

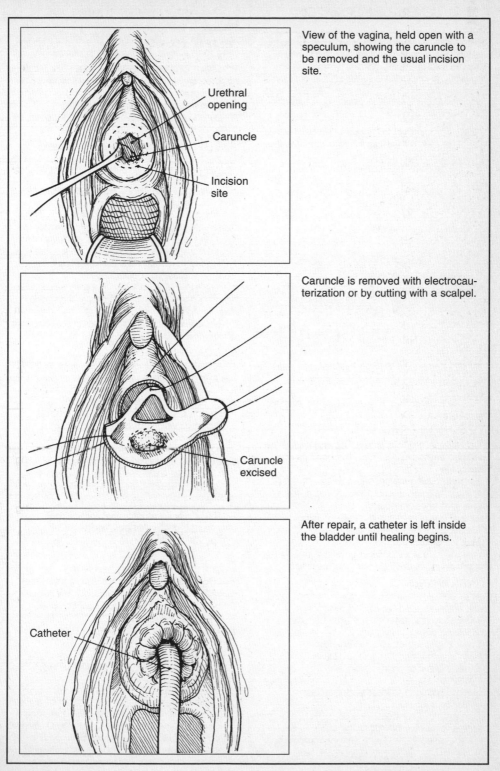

View of the vagina, held open with a speculum, showing the caruncle to be removed and the usual incision site.

Urethral opening

Caruncle

Incision site

Caruncle is removed with electrocauterization or by cutting with a scalpel.

Caruncle excised

After repair, a catheter is left inside the bladder until healing begins.

Catheter

Urethritis

GENERAL INFORMATION

DEFINITION—Inflammation or infection of the urethra (the tube through which urine travels from the bladder to the outside). Urethritis is frequently accompanied by bladder infection or inflammation (cystitis). It can affect all ages and both sexes and is often sexually transmitted.

SIGNS & SYMPTOMS
• No symptoms may be present, but both sexes may be carriers of the causative organisms (i.e., gonococcus, chlamydia).
• Painful or burning urination. The pain can be severe.
• Discharge that may be cloudy, yellow-green mucus, or watery and white.
• Frequent urge to urinate, even when there is not much urine in the bladder.

CAUSES
• The same bacterial infection that causes gonorrhea causes gonococcal urethritis.
• Nonspecific urethritis (also called nongono-coccal urethritis) can be caused by a variety of organisms, including bacteria, yeast and chlamydia.
• Use of a Foley catheter (a tube placed in the bladder to keep the bladder empty, often used during surgery).
• Other causes could be trauma from an injury or surgery, or from a chemical such as an antiseptic.
• Bubble bath or bath oils have been known to cause urethritis.

RISK INCREASES WITH
• Bacterial infection that spreads and enters the urethra from the skin around the genitals and anal area.
• Bruising during sexual intercourse.
• Contact with an infected sexual partner.
• Use of a urinary catheter.
• Use of drugs to which bacteria-causing infection have become resistant.
• Multiple sexual partners.
• Previous kidney stones or genital injury.
• A previous sexually transmitted disease.

HOW TO PREVENT
• After bowel movements, wipe from front to back and wash with soap and water.
• Take showers rather than tub baths; use unscented soap.
• Drink 8 glasses of water every day.
• For causes related to sexual activity:
 Drink a glass of water before sexual intercourse.
 Urinate within 15 minutes after sexual intercourse.
 Use a rubber condom.
 Use a water-soluble lubricant, such as K-Y Lubricating Jelly, during sexual intercourse.
Use varying sexual positions to decrease the chance of trauma to the female urethra.

PROBABLE OUTCOME—Urethritis is usually a low grade infection, seldom producing serious, long-term illness. Recurrence is common.

POSSIBLE COMPLICATIONS
• Chronic urethritis and cystitis, if treatment is inadequate.
• Pelvic inflammatory disease (PID).
• Spread of infection to ureters and kidneys.

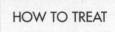

HOW TO TREAT

GENERAL MEASURES
• Diagnostic tests may include laboratory blood and discharge studies and urinalysis.
• Testing (screening) for other sexually transmitted diseases is usually recommended.
• When antibiotics are required, both you and your sexual partner will need to be treated.
• Diagnostic testing may be repeated after treatment to verify a cure.
• To relieve pain, take sitz baths by sitting in a tub of hot water for 15 minutes at least twice a day.
• Keep the area around the genitals clean. Use unscented plain soap.

MEDICATION
• Antibiotics to fight infection. Be sure to finish the prescribed dose, even if symptoms subside. Antibiotics may reduce the effectiveness of some oral contraceptives. If you are currently using oral contraceptives for birth control, discuss this with your doctor.
• In cases of severe pain, medication (phenazopyridine [Pyridium]) may be prescribed that decreases urethral spasm (cause of the pain) until the antibiotic therapy controls the infection. Pyridium produces bright orange (tea) colored urine.

ACTIVITY—No restrictions. Avoid sexual intercourse until you have been free of symptoms for 2 weeks.

DIET
• Drink 8 glasses of water every day.
• Avoid caffeine and alcohol during treatment.
• Drink cranberry juice to acidify urine. Some drugs are more effective with acidic urine.

CALL YOUR DOCTOR IF

• You or a family member has symptoms of urethritis.
• The following occur during treatment:
 Oral temperature of 101°F (38.3°C) or higher.
 Bleeding from the urethra or blood in urine.
 No improvement in 1 week, despite treatment.
• New, unexplained symptoms develop. Drugs used in treatment may produce side effects.

Uterine Bleeding, Dysfunctional (Premenopausal Abnormal Uterine Bleeding)

 GENERAL INFORMATION

DEFINITION—Bleeding that is not related to a woman's normal menstrual pattern and is not associated with tumor, inflammation or pregnancy. Most often occurs in women age 40 years and over, or in adolescents.

SIGNS & SYMPTOMS—Bleeding between menstrual cycles. Blood flow may be irregular, prolonged, sometimes very heavy and may contain clots.

CAUSES—Usually caused by an overgrowth of the endometrium (lining of the uterus) due to estrogen stimulation. With dysfunctional uterine bleeding, ovulation (the development and release of an egg from the ovary) occurs periodically.

RISK INCREASES WITH
• Polycystic ovarian syndrome.
• Obesity.
• Use of synthetic estrogen without added progestin.

HOW TO PREVENT
• Maintain proper weight.
• Follow medical advice regarding any hormone therapy.

PROBABLE OUTCOME—Usually curable with treatment. However, depending on underlying cause, symptoms may recur.

POSSIBLE COMPLICATIONS
• Anemia from excessive blood loss.
• Cancer (rare, but risk is higher if disorder is untreated).

 HOW TO TREAT

GENERAL MEASURES
• Diagnostic tests may include laboratory blood studies, Pap smear, or ultrasound to evaluate the thickness of the uterine lining and exclude other causes for the bleeding. Surgical diagnostic procedures such as endometrial biopsy, laparoscopy or hysteroscopy (see Glossary for these terms) may be performed. Dysfunctional uterine bleeding is the usual diagnosis for patients when these tests show no discernible causes.
• Treatment is directed at stopping the excessive bleeding and correcting anemia if it exists. If bleeding is severe, hospitalization may be necessary to bring it under control.
• Local application of heat may provide some pain relief. Place a heating pad or hot-water bottle on the abdomen or back. Take a warm bath for 10 to 15 minutes as often as needed.

• If hormonal therapy does not control the bleeding, a dilatation and curettage, often referred to as D & C (see Glossary), or a hysteroscopic procedure may be performed for both diagnostic and therapeutic (as a treatment to stop the bleeding) reasons.
• For some patients, when all of the conservative treatment measures have failed, a hysterectomy may be necessary.

MEDICATION
• Hormones to correct a hormone imbalance. For many women, oral contraceptive pills are used for treatment, even in cases when contraception is not required.
• Pain relievers if needed.
• Avoid aspirin, especially if you are anemic; aspirin can cause bleeding to increase.
• Iron supplements may be necessary for anemia.

ACTIVITY
• Stay as active as possible, depending on the underlying condition.
• Ask your doctor about resumption of sexual activities.

DIET—No special diet.

CALL YOUR DOCTOR IF

• You or a family member has abnormal uterine bleeding.
• The following occur during treatment:
   Bleeding becomes excessive (saturating a pad or tampon more often than once an hour).
   Signs of infection develop, such as fever, a general ill feeling, headache, dizziness or muscle aches.
• New, unexplained symptoms develop. Drugs used in treatment may produce side effects.

Uterine Bleeding, Postmenopausal

 GENERAL INFORMATION

DEFINITION—Unexpected vaginal bleeding that begins 6 to 12 or more months after menopause.

SIGNS & SYMPTOMS
• Vaginal bleeding, which may be a light-brown discharge or heavy red bleeding (with or without clots). Mucus may accompany the bleeding. Bleeding episodes vary in length. The type or quality of the bleeding is not as relevant as the fact that it has taken place. Following menopause, women who are being treated with hormonal replacement will likely encounter some bleeding and should consult the doctor about the types of bleeding to be concerned about.
• Pelvic pain (sometimes).

CAUSES
• Hormone therapy that stimulates the endometrium (uterine lining), causing sloughing similar to normal menstruation. Estrogens (female hormones) used irregularly are a common cause of this.
• Cancer of the reproductive system.
• Irritation or infection of the membranes lining the vulva.
• Vaginal or endometrial atrophy (shrinking or wasting away of tissue).
• Injury or trauma to the vagina, associated with reduced estrogen levels.
• Polyps or benign tumors of the cervix.
• Polyps on the inner uterine lining; myomas.
• Disorders of the blood cells, lymphatic system or bone marrow.
• High blood pressure.
• Congestive heart failure.
• Liver disorders.
• Anticoagulant or aspirin-containing drugs.

RISK INCREASES WITH
• Recent vaginal infection.
• Adults over 60, due to fragile blood vessels and thin vaginal or uterine lining.

HOW TO PREVENT—No specific preventive measures.

PROBABLE OUTCOME—Depends on the underlying cause and treatment chosen.

POSSIBLE COMPLICATIONS
• Anemia caused by excessive blood loss.
• If cancer is the cause, it may spread to other body parts.

 HOW TO TREAT

GENERAL MEASURES
• Diagnostic tests may include laboratory blood studies, Pap smear and ultrasound (see Glossary).
• Unexplained postmenopausal bleeding requires further testing. This may include an endometrial biopsy, hysteroscopic examination or dilatation and curettage, referred to as D & C (see Glossary for all of these terms), that may be both diagnostic and a treatment to relieve the bleeding. Sometimes, even after extensive testing, no clear-cut reason for the bleeding is found.
• Specific therapy, such as medications or surgery, is dependent on the cause.
• It may be helpful to take frequent lukewarm baths to relax muscles and relieve discomfort. Sit in a tub of warm water for 10 to 15 minutes as often as necessary. Use heat to relieve pain. Place a heating pad or hot-water bottle on the abdomen or back when resting.
• Surgery (hysterectomy) to remove the uterus may be needed when conservative measures have failed to stop the bleeding.

MEDICATION
• If hormone medications are currently being taken, the dose may need to be adjusted. In other cases, hormones may be prescribed depending on the medical evaluation of the bleeding.
• Medication to treat the underlying disorder, such as antihypertensives for high blood pressure.
• Iron supplements may be necessary for anemia.
• Avoid aspirin, especially if you are anemic; aspirin can cause bleeding to increase.

ACTIVITY
• Resume your normal activities as soon as symptoms improve.
• Sexual relations may be resumed as soon as desired after diagnosis and treatment.

DIET—No special diet.

CALL YOUR DOCTOR IF

• You have postmenopausal vaginal bleeding.
• Bleeding persists for 1 week, despite treatment.
• The bleeding becomes excessive (saturates a pad or tampon more frequently than once each hour).
• Signs of infection develop: fever, a general ill feeling, headache, dizziness and muscle aches.
• New, unexplained symptoms develop. Drugs used in treatment may produce side effects.

Uterine Malignancy (Endometrial Carcinoma)

 GENERAL INFORMATION

DEFINITION—Cancer (malignancy) of the endometrium, which is the lining of the uterus. It usually affects postmenopausal women ages 50 to 60 years and is the most common female pelvic malignancy in the U.S. A second type of uterine cancer, sarcoma, is less common.

SIGNS & SYMPTOMS
Early stages:
- Bleeding or spotting, especially after sexual intercourse. This often occurs after menstrual activity has ceased for 12 months or more. A watery or blood-streaked vaginal discharge may precede bleeding or spotting.
- Uterine cramping or pain.
- Enlarged uterus. It is sometimes a large enough mass to be felt externally.
Later stages:
- Spread to other organs, causing abdominal pain, chest pain and weight loss.

CAUSES—Exact cause unknown. Continuous exposure to estrogen without progesterone is implicated.

RISK INCREASES WITH
- Diabetes mellitus.
- Obesity.
- High blood pressure.
- Use of estrogen without also using progesterone.
- History of breast, ovarian or colon cancer.
- Family history of endometrial cancer.
- History of uterine polyps, menstrual cycles without ovulation or other signs of hormone imbalance, including hirsutism (see Glossary).
- Delayed menopause (after age 55).
- Never having had children.
- Early age of first menstruation.
- Use of tamoxifen for breast cancer.
- Previous pelvic radiation therapy.

HOW TO PREVENT
- Pelvic examinations every 6 to 12 months (cannot prevent cancer, but may aid in early detection, when treatment is more effective). Examinations are especially important for women with risk factors listed above.
- Obtain medical care for any uterine bleeding or spotting after menopause.
- Good general health measures to control diabetes and high blood pressure and maintain ideal body weight.

PROBABLE OUTCOME—With early diagnosis and treatment, 90% of patients survive at least 5 years. Older patients and patients with delayed diagnosis have a poorer prognosis.

POSSIBLE COMPLICATIONS
- Those complications that involve major abdominal surgery or invasive diagnostic testing.
- If bleeding is untreated, severe anemia may occur.
- Spread of cancer to the bladder, rectum and distant organs, which could be fatal.
- Treatment failure or recurrence of the cancer.

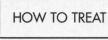 **HOW TO TREAT**

GENERAL MEASURES
- Diagnostic tests may be numerous, first to diagnose the cancer, and then to determine any spread to other body organs (staging). Tests may include laboratory blood tests, Pap smear, liver function tests, chest x-ray, CT scan, mammogram, barium enema, MRI, vaginal ultrasound, endometrial biopsy, dilatation and curettage (D & C). (See Glossary for above terms.)
- Treatment will depend on the extent of the disease and may involve one, or a combination, of the following: surgery, radiation, hormonal therapy and chemotherapy.
- In some cases, other disorders, such as diabetes mellitus, high blood pressure or anemia must be brought under control before the cancer can be treated.
- Surgical treatment usually includes removing the uterus, ovaries and fallopian tubes, along with evaluation of the adjacent pelvic lymph nodes.
- Psychotherapy or counseling for depression may be recommended.
- See the Resource section of this book for additional information.

MEDICATION
- Anticancer drugs, including cortisone drugs.
- Hormone therapy may be prescribed.
- Antibiotic therapy, if needed for infection.

ACTIVITY—Resume your normal activities as soon as symptoms improve after treatment. In most cases, full sexual activity may be resumed after therapy.

DIET—No special diet, but eat a well-balanced diet, even if you lose your appetite from radiation or drug therapy. Vitamin and mineral supplements are helpful.

 CALL YOUR DOCTOR IF

- You or a family member has symptoms of uterine cancer.
- The following occur after surgery:
  Excessive bleeding (soaking a pad or tampon at least once an hour).
  Signs of infection, such as fever, muscle aches and headache.
- New, unexplained symptoms develop. Drugs used in treatment may produce side effects.

Uterine Prolapse

GENERAL INFORMATION

DEFINITION—Weakness of the pelvic supporting structure that allows a uterus to fall or drop from its normal location, causing it to bulge into the vagina. In its most pronounced form, it projects outside the vagina. Associated with prolapse may be urethrocele and cystocele (urethra and/or bladder bulge along the front wall of the vagina) and rectocele (rectal wall bulges into the back wall of the vagina).

SIGNS & SYMPTOMS
- A lump in front or back of the vagina, or a lump that projects outside of the vagina.
- Vague discomfort or pressure in the pelvic region.
- Backache that worsens with lifting.
- Frequent and painful urination.
- Occasional stress incontinence (urine leakage when laughing, sneezing or coughing).
- Difficulty in moving bowels.
- Pain with sexual intercourse.

CAUSES—Prolapse occurs when muscles and ligaments at the base of the abdomen become extremely stretched, usually as a result of childbirth and aging.

RISK INCREASES WITH
- Obesity.
- Repeated childbirth, although one pregnancy and vaginal delivery can weaken the area enough to lead to prolapse eventually.
- Advancing age.
- Conditions that cause increased intra-abdominal pressure such as tumors, chronic coughing, chronic constipation.
- Poor physical fitness.
- Occupations requiring heavy lifting
- Multiple sclerosis; Marfan's syndrome.

HOW TO PREVENT
- Maintain appropriate weight.
- Practice pelvic-strengthening exercises (Kegels) during pregnancy and after childbirth.
- Eat a normal, well-balanced diet.
- Engage in a regular exercise program to maintain good overall muscle strength.
- Avoid constipation.
- Estrogen therapy.

PROBABLE OUTCOME
- Aggressive treatment is not always necessary because prolapse is not a health risk. Exercise can often improve muscle function.
- Severe prolapse can be corrected with surgery.

POSSIBLE COMPLICATIONS
- Ulceration of the cervix.
- Increased risk of infection or injury to pelvic organs.
- Hemorrhoids from straining to overcome constipation.
- Urinary tract obstruction.
- Renal (kidney) failure.

HOW TO TREAT

GENERAL MEASURES
- Diagnostic tests may include pelvic examination, Pap smear, urinalysis, pelvic ultrasound or CT, endometrial biopsy and IVP (see Glossary for these terms).
- Treatment plan will depend on severity of prolapse, age, sexual activity, associated pelvic disorders and desire for future pregnancy.
- Patients with mild symptoms can usually be treated with Kegel exercises (see "Kegel Exercises" in this book), hormone therapy and pessary if needed. Others may need surgery.
- Avoid wearing tight girdles or clothing that may increase intra-abdominal pressure.
- A pessary (a small, often ring-shaped, device that is inserted into the vagina to help maintain the uterus in a normal position) may be prescribed. Pessaries must be removed, cleaned and reinstalled every few months to prevent infection.
- Surgery may be necessary when the prolapse causes significant symptoms. Several surgical methods are available; the choice will depend on a number of variables and the presence of associated conditions.

MEDICATION
- Estrogen therapy can increase blood flow to vaginal tissues and increase tone and strength of supporting tissues.
- Antibiotics will be prescribed if infection develops.

ACTIVITY
- Avoid occupational or physical activities that increase intra-abdominal pressure (e.g., heavy lifting).
- If surgery is necessary, resume your normal activities gradually.

DIET
- A weight loss diet is recommended if you are overweight.
- Eat a diet high in fiber to prevent constipation.

CALL YOUR DOCTOR IF

- You or a family member has symptoms of uterine prolapse.
- Symptoms don't improve in 3 months despite treatment or exercise, or symptoms become intolerable and you wish to consider surgery.
- You are using a pessary and experience unusual vaginal bleeding or discomfort, or have difficulty in urination.

Vaginal Hernias
(Cystocele; Enterocele; Rectocele; Urethrocele)

 GENERAL INFORMATION

DEFINITION—Weakness in the pelvic supporting structure that allows the pelvic organs to descend into the vagina.
• Cystocele is a descent of a portion of the bladder into the vagina.
• Enterocele is a protrusion of the intestine through the back of the vaginal wall.
• Rectocele is a protrusion of the rectum through the vaginal wall.
• Urethrocele is a sagging of the urethra. When associated with a cystocele, it is called a cystourethrocele.

SIGNS & SYMPTOMS
• Sometimes, no symptoms are apparent.
• Stress incontinence (urine leakage that occurs with coughing, sneezing or lifting).
• Incomplete emptying of the bladder.
• Increased urinary frequency.
• Urinary incontinence.
• A sensation of vaginal fullness, pressure or "falling out."
• Pain during sexual intercourse.
• Increased susceptibility to urinary tract infections.
• Constipation caused by a rectocele that interferes with muscle contraction in the rectum.

CAUSE—Weakness in the tissues supporting the pelvis and vaginal walls.

RISK INCREASES WITH
• Multiple pregnancies.
• Prolonged labors.
• Birth of a large baby.
• Lack of estrogen in menopause.
• Obesity.
• Chronic cough, such as in chronic bronchitis.
• Constipation.
• Occupations involving much standing and lifting.
• Large pelvic tumors.
• Congenital malformations.

HOW TO PREVENT
• Pelvic strengthening exercises (Kegel exercises) during and following pregnancy.
• Estrogen therapy after menopause.
• Avoidance or correction of obesity, chronic cough, straining and traumatic deliveries.

PROBABLE OUTCOME
• With small- or moderate-sized hernias, conservative therapy is usually sufficient to relieve symptoms.
• Surgery is an option in severe cases.

POSSIBLE COMPLICATIONS
• Recurrent urinary tract infections.
• Uterine prolapse.
• Chronic constipation. Fecal impaction.

 HOW TO TREAT

GENERAL MEASURES
• Diagnostic tests may include pelvic examination or x-ray, urinalysis, cystoscopy and urethroscopy (see Glossary for these terms).
• Treatment measures will depend on the severity of the symptoms, age of patient and desire for future pregnancies. Treatment steps may include exercises, use of a pessary (see Glossary), medications and surgery.
• Other treatment steps may be recommended for obese patients or those with chronic cough or chronic constipation.
• Kegel exercises (see Glossary) will help to tighten and strengthen the pelvic floor muscles and relieve the symptoms.
• Use of a pessary may provide adequate temporary support. Pessaries must be removed, cleaned and reinstalled every few months to prevent infection.
• Surgery is recommended for severe symptoms and is usually required for final resolution. Surgical methods will depend on the type of defect, any associated conditions, desire for future pregnancies, and age and general health of the patient.
• Rarely, an enterocele may require emergency procedures.

MEDICATION
• Antibiotics if infection is present.
• In postmenopausal women, estrogen replacement therapy may improve the tone and quality of the pelvic support muscles.
• Pain medication if required following surgery.
• Stool-softening laxatives and lubricating rectal suppositories may be necessary for constipation caused by rectocele.

ACTIVITY—Avoid occupations or activities that require heavy lifting or cause intra-abdominal pressure.

DIET
• If overweight, a weight loss diet is recommended.
• Eating a high fiber diet and increasing fluid intake help relieve problems of constipation.

 CALL YOUR DOCTOR IF

• You or a family member has symptoms of a vaginal hernia.
• Symptoms don't improve, or they worsen despite treatment.
• You develop signs of infection, including fever, chills, or body aches.
• You are using a pessary and experience any unusual vaginal bleeding or discomfort, or have difficulty in urination.

Vaginal or Vulvar Cancer

 GENERAL INFORMATION

DEFINITION—Uncontrolled growth of malignant cells in the vagina or on the vulva (vaginal lips). The peak growth occurs in older women in the postmenopausal years. One type (rhabdomyosarcoma) occurs in children.

SIGNS & SYMPTOMS
- Vulvar pruritus (itching).
- Abnormal vaginal bleeding.
- Discomfort or bleeding with intercourse.
- Swollen lymph nodes in the groin area.
- Small or large, firm, ulcerated, painless lesion of the vulva. These growths on the vulva have thick, raised edges and bleed easily.
- Uncomfortable urination, if cancer spreads to the bladder.
- Rectal bleeding, if it spreads to the rectum.

CAUSES
- Intrauterine exposure to DES (diethylstilbestrol, a drug prescribed [up to 1971] to control spotting or bleeding in pregnant women).
- A possible connection may be exposure to human papillomavirus (HPV), the cause of genital warts.

RISK INCREASES WITH
- Family history of cancer of reproductive organs.
- Smoking.
- Multiple sex partners.
- Advanced age.
- Other cancer, especially cervical cancer.

HOW TO PREVENT
- No specific preventive measures. Have a yearly pelvic exam and Pap smear to detect the disease during its early stages when treatment is most effective.
- Become familiar with the appearance of your genitals. (Use a mirror and examine once a month.) Darker spots around the vagina on the labia are generally not associated with vaginal or vulvar cancer but may represent melanoma, a skin cancer. Any dark skin discoloration should be brought to the attention of your doctor for further evaluation.

PROBABLE OUTCOME—Early detection and treatment offer a good chance for normal life expectancy. Symptoms can be relieved or controlled during treatment.

POSSIBLE COMPLICATIONS
- Complications and difficulty in wound healing or lymphedema (see Glossary) following surgery.
- Stress urinary incontinence.
- Fatal spread to other body parts. Common sites of spread are the lymph nodes in the groin, wall of the pelvis, bladder, rectum, bone, lungs or liver.

 HOW TO TREAT

GENERAL MEASURES
- Diagnostic tests may be numerous, first to diagnose the cancer, and then to determine any spread to other body organs. Tests may include laboratory blood studies, Pap smear, chest x-ray, CT scan, mammogram, barium enema, cystoscopy, colposcopy, punch biopsy or sigmoidoscopy (see Glossary for these terms).
- Treatment may include surgery, radiation, or chemotherapy and will depend partly on the location and extent of the disease, as well as the age and physical condition of the patient.
- Surgery may include vulvectomy, vaginectomy, hysterectomy (see Glossary for these terms) and lymph node removal. Laser vaporization is often used for treatment of vulvar cancer.
- Radiation treatment (sometimes). External radiation shrinks the primary tumor. Internal radiation (implants) affects cancer that has spread to adjoining tissues.
- Following treatment, your doctor will usually recommend a pelvic exam and Pap smear (vaginal cancer), or a clinical examination of the groin nodes and vulvar area (vulvar cancer) every 3 to 6 months for 2 years, and then every 6 to 12 months for the next 3 years.
- Annual chest x-rays should be obtained following treatment for either vaginal or vulvar cancer.
- See the Resource section of this book for additional information.

MEDICATION
- Anticancer drugs are usually not prescribed, except when the disease is advanced, or in cases of childhood sarcoma.
- Pain relievers as needed.
- Antibiotics, if urinary tract infection results from use of a urinary catheter during radiation treatment.
- Stool softener or laxative, if needed to prevent constipation.

ACTIVITY
- After surgery, resume your normal activities gradually, allowing 6 weeks for full recovery. Most patients can maintain a fully active lifestyle while receiving radiation therapy.
- Sexual relations may be resumed when healing is complete in 8 to 10 weeks.

DIET—No special diet after treatment.

CALL YOUR DOCTOR IF

- You or a family member has symptoms of cancer of the vagina or vulva.
- You develop signs of infection, including increasing pain, fever and swelling, or excessive vaginal bleeding.

Vaginismus

GENERAL INFORMATION

DEFINITION—Involuntary, painful contraction of the muscles around the vagina and rectum. If vaginismus is severe, the contractions may cause the vagina to close so tightly that sexual intercourse is prevented. It also prevents the insertion of any object into the vagina, such as a tampon, diaphragm or speculum (used for medical examination). Vaginismus can affect females of all ages.

SIGNS & SYMPTOMS
- Pain with vaginal intercourse.
- Inability to use tampons with comfort.
- Reluctance or avoidance of pelvic examination.
- Infertility.

CAUSES
- An unconcious desire to prevent penile penetration because of emotional or psychological factors. These may include fear, anxiety, hostility, anger or a distaste for sex.
- An insensitive sexual partner, insufficient or unskillful foreplay or inadequate vaginal lubrication prior to attempted penetration.
- Anatomic or congenital abnormalities.
- Physical disorders (rare), such as infections, allergic reactions or a rigid, nonperforated hymen.
- Vaginal infection.

RISK INCREASES WITH
- First sexual experience.
- Previous traumatic gynecological examination.
- History of genital or psychic trauma, especially incest or rape.
- Stress.

HOW TO PREVENT—Pelvic examination by a doctor and counseling prior to beginning sexual activity.

PROBABLE OUTCOME—Curable if the underlying cause can be cured or a coping method can be developed through medical treatment and psychological counseling.

POSSIBLE COMPLICATIONS—Psychological trauma caused by guilt, anxiety, loss of self-esteem and feelings of inadequacy, or interpersonal problems resulting from the disorder.

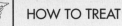 HOW TO TREAT

GENERAL MEASURES
- Diagnostic tests may include pelvic examination to rule out physical disorders (sedation may be necessary for a thorough examination).
- A complete sexual history is important and will include early childhood experiences, family attitudes toward sex, previous and current sexual responses, contraceptive practices, reproductive goals, feelings about your sexual partner and specifics about the pain you experience.
- Treatment will first take care of any medical problems, followed by therapy to eliminate the muscular spasms and psychological problems.
- For muscular spasms, one type of therapy involves dilating the vaginal opening gently and gradually with plastic dilators or your fingers. Office treatments may be necessary up to 3 times a week, and you should practice at home at least twice a day.
- Prior to dilation or attempted intercourse, sit in a tub of warm water for 10 to 15 minutes. Baths often relax muscles and relieve discomfort. Repeat baths as often as is helpful.
- Psychotherapy or counseling is recommended, in addition to dilation therapy, or if dilating treatment is unsuccessful. This may include sensate focus exercises (see Glossary), improving communication with your partner and therapy to resolve any conflicts in your life. In some cases, hypnosis may be recommended.
- Before attempting intercourse, you and your partner should use a lubricant, such as K-Y Lubricating Jelly or Replens.

MEDICATION—Medicine is usually not necessary for vaginismus, but mild sedatives or tranquilizers may be prescribed for short periods of time.

ACTIVITY—No restrictions.

DIET—No special diet.

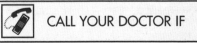 CALL YOUR DOCTOR IF

- You or a family member has symptoms of vaginismus.
- Symptoms don't improve after 3 weeks, despite treatment.
- Symptoms recur after treatment.

Vaginitis, Bacterial (Gardnerella Vaginitis; Nonspecific Vaginitis; Bacterial Vaginosis)

 GENERAL INFORMATION

DEFINITION—Vaginitis means infection or inflammation of the vagina. Nonspecific vaginitis (bacterial vaginosis) implies that any of several infecting germs, including Gardnerella, Escherichia coli, Mycoplasma, streptococci or staphylococci, have caused the infection. These infections are contagious and may be sexually transmitted. Vaginitis can affect all ages, but most often occurs during reproductive years.

SIGNS & SYMPTOMS—Severity of the following symptoms varies among women and from time to time in the same woman.
• Thin, gray-white (sometimes profuse) vaginal discharge that has an unpleasant odor.
• Genital swelling, burning and itching.
• Vaginal discomfort.
• Painful urination.
• Change in vaginal color from pale pink to red.
• Discomfort during sexual intercourse.

CAUSES—The germs normally present in the vagina can multiply and cause infection when the pH and hormone balance of the vagina and surrounding tissue are disturbed. E. coli bacteria normally inhabit the rectum and can cause infection if spread to the vagina. The following conditions increase the likelihood of infections:
• General poor health.
• Allergies to soaps, detergents, bubble bath, feminine deodorant spray or douches.
• Hot weather, nonventilating clothing (especially underwear) or any other condition that increases genital moisture, warmth and darkness. These foster the growth of germs.
• Poor hygiene (sometimes).

RISK INCREASES WITH
• Diabetes mellitus.
• Menopause.
• Illness that has lowered resistance.
• Multiple sexual partners.
• Use of an intrauterine device (IUD).
• HIV infection.

HOW TO PREVENT
• Keep the genital area clean. Use plain unscented soap.
• Use latex condoms during sexual intercourse.
• Take showers rather than tub baths.
• Wear cotton underpants or pantyhose with a cotton crotch.
• Don't sit around in wet clothing, especially a wet bathing suit.
• After urination or bowel movements, cleanse by wiping or washing from front to back (vagina to anus).
• Lose weight if you are obese.
• Avoid vaginal douches, deodorants and bubble baths.
• If you have diabetes, adhere strictly to your treatment program.
• Change tampons or pads frequently.

PROBABLE OUTCOME—Usually curable in 2 weeks with treatment.

POSSIBLE COMPLICATIONS
• Discomfort and decreased pleasure with sexual activity.
• Pelvic inflammatory disease (PID).
• Nonspecific vaginitis in pregnant women has been associated with preterm birth. The disorder should be carefully evaluated and treated when it occurs in pregnancy.

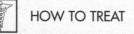 HOW TO TREAT

GENERAL MEASURES
• Diagnostic tests may include laboratory studies of vaginal discharge, Pap smear and pelvic examination.
• Drug therapy will be directed to the specific organism. Your sexual partner may need treatment also. It is best not to do self-treatment for the disorder until the specific cause is determined.
• Don't douche unless prescribed for you.
• If urinating causes burning, urinate through a a toilet-paper roll or plastic cup with the bottom cut out, or pour a cup of warm water over the genital area while you urinate.

MEDICATION
• Antibiotics or antifungals to treat the infection; these are usually vaginal, rather than oral, medications. Metronidazole (Flagyl) is often used for treatment of bacterial vaginosis. Don't drink alcohol or use vinegar when you take metronidazole. Alcohol or vinegar combined with metronidazole causes a violent reaction with nausea, vomiting, weakness and sweating.
• Soothing vaginal creams or lotions for nonspecific forms of vaginitis may be recommended.

ACTIVITY—Avoid overexertion, heat and excessive sweating. Delay sexual relations until after treatment.

DIET—No special diet instructions except those involving alcohol or vinegar (see Medication).

CALL YOUR DOCTOR IF

• You or a family member has symptoms of vaginitis.
• Symptoms persist longer than 1 week or worsen, despite treatment.
• Unusual vaginal bleeding or swelling develops.

Vaginitis, Candidal
(Vaginal Yeast Infection; Monilial Vaginitis)

 GENERAL INFORMATION

DEFINITION—Infection or inflammation of the vagina caused by a yeast-like fungus (usually Candida albicans). The bacteria that causes candidal vaginitis is contagious, and may be sexually transmitted. It is the second most common vaginitis in the U.S. (bacterial vaginitis is the most common).

SIGNS & SYMPTOMS—Severity of the following symptoms varies among women, and from time to time in the same woman.
• White, "curdy" vaginal discharge (resembles lumps of cottage cheese). The odor may be unpleasant, but not foul.
• Swollen, red, tender, itching vaginal lips (labia) and surrounding skin.
• Burning on urination.
• Change in vaginal color from pale pink to red.
• Pain during sexual intercourse (dyspareunia).

CAUSES—The fungus Candida lives in small numbers in a healthy vagina, rectum and mouth. When the vagina's hormone and pH balance is disturbed, the organisms multiply and cause infections. The vaginitis tends to appear before menstrual periods and improves as soon as the period begins.

RISK INCREASES WITH
• Pregnancy.
• Diabetes mellitus.
• Antibiotic treatment.
• Anemia.
• Hypothyroidism.
• HIV infection.
• Oral contraceptives (possibly).
• High carbohydrate intake, especially sugars and alcohol (possibly).
• Hot weather and/or nonventilating clothing, which increase moisture, warmth and darkness, fostering fungal growth.
• Immunosuppression from drugs or disease.

HOW TO PREVENT
• Keep the genital area clean. Use plain unscented soap.
• Take showers rather than tub baths.
• Avoid tight-fitting clothes; wear cotton underpants or pantyhose with a cotton crotch.
• Don't sit around in wet clothing, especially a wet bathing suit.
• Avoid douches, vaginal deodorants, bubble baths and colored or perfumed toilet paper.
• Limit your intake of sweets and alcohol.
• After urination or bowel movements, cleanse by wiping or washing from front to back (vagina to anus).
• Lose weight if you are obese.
• If you have diabetes, adhere strictly to your treatment program.

• Avoid use of antibiotics unless prescribed by the doctor.

PROBABLE OUTCOME—Usually curable after 1 to 2 weeks of treatment (sometimes less). Recurrences are common.

POSSIBLE COMPLICATIONS
• Secondary bacterial infections of the vagina and other pelvic organs.
• In some cases, the vaginitis becomes chronic.

 HOW TO TREAT

GENERAL MEASURES
• Diagnostic tests may include laboratory studies of vaginal discharge, Pap smear and pelvic examination.
• Treatment is usually with a vaginal cream or suppository. Your doctor may prescribe an oral antifungal medication in addition to, or in place of, vaginal medications. Treatment for your sexual partner may be recommended also. It is best not to do self-treatment for the disorder until the specific cause is determined.
• Don't douche unless prescribed for you.
• If urinating causes burning, urinate through a tubular device, such as a toilet-paper roll or plastic cup with the bottom cut out, or pour a cup of warm water over the genital area while you urinate.

MEDICATION—Antifungal drugs may be prescribed, either in oral form (rare) or in vaginal creams or suppositories (usually). Keep creams or suppositories in the refrigerator. After treatment, you may keep a refill of the medication so you can begin treatment quickly if the infection recurs. Follow the directions carefully. Nonprescription treatments (Gyne-Lotrimin, Mycelex, etc.) are effective.

ACTIVITY—Avoid overexertion, heat and excessive sweating. Delay sexual relations until symptoms cease.

DIET—Increase consumption of yogurt, buttermilk or sour cream. Reduce alcohol and sugars.

 CALL YOUR DOCTOR IF

• You or a family member has symptoms of vaginitis.
• Despite treatment, symptoms worsen or persist longer than 1 week.
• Unusual vaginal bleeding or swelling develops.
• After treatment, symptoms recur.
• New, unexplained symptoms develop. Drugs used in treatment may produce side effects.

Vaginitis, Postmenopausal (Atrophic Vaginitis)

 GENERAL INFORMATION

DEFINITION—Infection or inflammation of the vagina caused by lowered estrogen levels in the body that upset the vagina's normal hormone and pH balance. The estrogen deficiency causes a thinning and atrophy (shrinking) of the female genital tissues, which makes the vaginal tissues more prone to injury and infection. Postmenopausal vaginitis is not contagious.

SIGNS & SYMPTOMS—Severity of the following symptoms varies greatly among women, and from time to time in the same woman.
• Vaginal discharge that is usually thin, whitish and sometimes tinged with blood. It may have a strong odor.
• Vaginal dryness; decreased vaginal secretions.
• Genital pain and itching.
• Discomfort during sexual intercourse.
• Change in vaginal color from pale pink to red.

CAUSES—Germs that inhabit the vagina cause infection when the normal physiology of the vagina is disturbed. After menopause, the estrogen level that helped maintain a normal vaginal environment decreases, leaving the vagina more vulnerable to infection. The following conditions increase the likelihood of atrophic vaginitis.
• General poor health.
• Hot weather, nonventilating clothing, especially underwear, or any other condition that increases genital moisture, warmth and darkness. These foster the growth of germs.
• Radiation of the pelvis.
• Premature ovarian failure; oophorectomy (removal of the ovaries) which causes surgical menopause.

RISK INCREASES WITH
• Diabetes mellitus.
• Illness that has lowered resistance.
• More frequent sexual intercourse.
• HIV infection.

HOW TO PREVENT
• Keep the genital area clean. Use plain unscented soap.
• Take showers rather than tub baths.
• Wear cotton panties or pantyhose with a cotton crotch; avoid tight-fitting slacks or jeans.
• Don't sit around in wet clothing, especially a wet bathing suit.
• After urination or bowel movements, cleanse by wiping or washing from front to back.
• Lose weight if you are obese.
• Avoid douches, vaginal deodorants and bubble baths.
• If you have diabetes, adhere strictly to your treatment program.

• Seek medical advice about replacement estrogen.

PROBABLE OUTCOME—Usually curable in 10 days with treatment.

POSSIBLE COMPLICATIONS
• Side effects associated with estrogen replacement therapy.
• Secondary bacterial infection in any pelvic organ.

 HOW TO TREAT

GENERAL MEASURES
• Diagnostic tests may include laboratory studies of vaginal discharge, Pap smear, pelvic examination and biopsy (to rule out cancer).
• Treatment will usually be with estrogen replacement therapy (ERT), which will alleviate the symptoms as well as reverse the thinning of the genital tissues which can cause vaginal dryness and susceptibility to infections. In addition, a vaginal cream which contains estrogen may be prescribed. Progesterone may also be prescribed to offset the effects of estrogen on the uterus.
• Don't douche unless prescribed for you.
• If urinating causes burning, urinate through a toilet-paper roll or plastic cup with the bottom cut out, or pour a cup of warm water over the genital area while you urinate.
• Cool baths may help to relieve discomfort.

MEDICATION
• Topical or oral estrogen or both may be prescribed. If you use a cream or suppository, use a small sanitary pad to protect clothing. Keep creams or suppositories in the refrigerator. After treatment, you may want to keep a refill of the medication so you can begin treatment quickly if the infection recurs. Follow the prescription directions carefully.
• Other creams, ointments or suppositories to suppress the organisms causing the infection may be prescribed.

ACTIVITY—Avoid overexertion, heat and excessive sweating. Delay sexual relations until you are well.

DIET—No special diet.

 CALL YOUR DOCTOR IF

• You or a family member has symptoms of vaginitis.
• Symptoms persist longer than 1 week or worsen, despite treatment.
• Unusual vaginal bleeding or swelling develops.
• Symptoms recur after treatment.
• New, unexplained symptoms develop. Drugs used in treatment may produce side effects.

Vaginitis, Trichomonal (Trichomoniasis)

GENERAL INFORMATION

DEFINITION—Infection or inflammation of the vagina caused by a parasite that lives in the lower genitourinary tract. It is very contagious between sexual partners. The disorder involves the vagina, urethra and bladder in women. In men, it affects the prostate gland and urethra.

SIGNS & SYMPTOMS
- Often, no symptoms.
- Foul-smelling, frothy vaginal discharge that is usually most noticeable several days after a menstrual period.
- Vaginal itching and pain.
- Pelvic pain.
- Redness of the vaginal lips (labia) and vagina.
- Painful urination, if urine touches inflamed tissue.
- The severity of discomfort varies greatly from woman to woman, and from time to time in the same woman. Infected men may have no symptoms.

CAUSES—Infection from a tiny parasite, Trichomonas vaginalis. The parasite passes from person to person during sexual intercourse. It is possible, but rare, for Trichomonas to be passed through nonsexual contact, as the organism can survive for several hours in a moist environment. It may live in its host for years without producing symptoms. Then, perhaps from altered resistance, it will suddenly multiply rapidly and cause distressing symptoms. Since it thrives in both the male and female, both sexual partners must receive treatment.

RISK INCREASES WITH—Multiple sexual partners.

HOW TO PREVENT—Use rubber condoms during sexual intercourse.

PROBABLE OUTCOME—Curable with treatment.

POSSIBLE COMPLICATIONS—Secondary bacterial infections or recurrent infection.

HOW TO TREAT

GENERAL MEASURES
- Diagnostic tests may include laboratory studies of vaginal discharge, Pap smear and pelvic examination.
- Testing (screening) for other sexually transmitted diseases may be recommended.
- Both sexual partners require simultaneous treatment.
- Don't douche unless prescribed for you.
- Wear cotton underpants or pantyhose with a cotton crotch.
- Take showers instead of tub baths.
- If urinating causes burning, urinate through a tubular device, such as a toilet-paper roll or plastic cup with the bottom cut out, or pour a cup of warm water over the genital area while you urinate.
- Don't sit around in wet clothing, especially in a wet bathing suit.

MEDICATION—Metronidazole (Flagyl) is usually prescribed for you and your sexual partner or partners. Follow directions carefully. Don't drink alcohol or use vinegar when you take metronidazole. Alcohol or vinegar and metronidazole interact to cause a violent reaction with nausea, vomiting, sweating, weakness and other symptoms.

ACTIVITY
- Avoid overexertion, heat and excessive sweating.
- Delay sexual relations until you are well and both you and your partner (or partners) have been treated. Reinfection is likely if all partners are not successfully treated.
- Allow about 10 days for recovery.

DIET—No special diet instructions except those involving alcohol and vinegar (see Medication).

CALL YOUR DOCTOR IF

- You or a family member has symptoms of trichomonal vaginitis.
- Symptoms persist longer than 1 week or worsen, despite treatment.
- Unusual vaginal bleeding or swelling develops.
- After treatment, symptoms recur.
- New, unexplained symptoms develop. Drugs used in treatment may produce side effects.

Vulvovaginitis before Puberty

GENERAL INFORMATION

DEFINITION—Infection or inflammation of the vagina or vulva before a young girl reaches puberty. Affects female infants and children.

SIGNS & SYMPTOMS
• Redness, pain and itching around the genital area.
• Vaginal discharge, which may or may not have an offensive odor.
• Pain with urination.
• Bleeding from the affected area (sometimes).

CAUSES
• Infections caused by bacteria, parasites (including pinworms), yeast-like fungi or viruses.
• Allergies to synthetic fabrics, soap or other items in contact with the genitals.
• Scratches, abrasions or genital injury from insertion of foreign bodies in the vagina by the child or a playmate.
• Genital injury from sexual abuse.
• Irritation from sources such as bubble bath or bath additives.

RISK INCREASES WITH
• Poor hygiene.
• Trauma or abuse.
• Diabetes mellitus.
• Infection elsewhere in the body (e.g., otitis media or pharyngitis).
• Infrequent bathing or unsanitary living conditions.

HOW TO PREVENT
• Teach the child to wipe from the vagina toward the anus after bowel movements.
• Don't let the child sit around in wet clothing, especially a wet bathing suit.
• Don't use dyed or perfumed toilet tissue, scented soap or bubble baths.
• Provide the child with cotton underpants or nylon underpants with a cotton crotch, and have the child avoid wearing tight-fitting pants which may irritate the vagina.
• Teach your child to resist and report any attempted sexual contact by anyone.

PROBABLE OUTCOME—Usually curable in 10 days with treatment.

POSSIBLE COMPLICATIONS—Adhesions (fibrous tissue within the body that joins normally unconnected parts; they are usually from scar tissue formed after inflammation).

HOW TO TREAT

GENERAL MEASURES
• Diagnostic tests may include laboratory blood studies, examination of the vagina and culture of the vaginal discharge.
• Removal of any foreign object in the vagina.
• Drug therapy will be directed to the specific organism which is causing the infection.
• Discontinuance of the source of any irritation or allergy, such as soap or bubble bath.
• If urinating causes burning, the child may urinate while bathing or urinate through a toilet-paper roll or plastic cup with the bottom cut out, or pour a cup of warm water over the genital area while urinating. This prevents urine from stinging inflamed skin.

MEDICATION
• Medication appropriate for the infection, including antibiotics, antifungal or antiparasitic drugs. If metronidazole is prescribed, have the child avoid drinking alcohol or using vinegar while taking this medication. Alcohol or vinegar and metronidazole interact to cause a violent reaction with nausea, vomiting, dizziness, sweating and other symptoms.
• Topical ointments to relieve pain and itching.

ACTIVITY—No restrictions.

DIET—No special diet, except to avoid alcohol and vinegar if taking metronidazole (see Medication).

CALL YOUR DOCTOR IF

• Your child has symptoms of vulvovaginitis.
• You suspect your child has been sexually abused.
• Symptoms don't improve in 7 to 10 days or symptoms worsen, despite treatment.
• Unusual vaginal bleeding or swelling develops.
• New, unexplained symptoms develop. Drugs used in treatment may produce side effects.

Warts, Genital
(Condyloma Acuminata; Human Papillomavirus [HPV]; Venereal Warts)

 GENERAL INFORMATION

DEFINITION—Warts in the genital area (including the urethra, genitals and rectum). These are more contagious than other warts. They are a sexually transmitted disease and can affect both sexes. Incubation period may be several months' duration, so someone can have the infection and show no signs or symptoms.

SIGNS & SYMPTOMS—Genital warts have the following characteristics:
• Warts appear on moist surfaces, especially the penis, vulva, labia, cervix and anus.
• Warts may be small, flat, flesh-colored bumps, or tiny, cauliflower-like bumps.
• Each wart measures 1 mm to 2 mm in diameter, but clusters may be quite large.
• They may produce no symptoms or cause itching, burning, tenderness or pain.
• Genital warts in children may be a sign of sexual abuse.

CAUSES—Genital warts (condyloma acuminata) are caused by a subtype of the same virus that causes other warts, the human papillomavirus (HPV). More than 60 distinct types of HPV have been identified. They spread easily on the skin of the infected person and are transmitted via sexual activity to other people. They have an incubation period of 1 to 6 months but can take years to develop.

RISK INCREASES WITH
• Presence or history of other sexually transmitted disease.
• Multiple sexual partners; not using condoms.
• Crowded or unsanitary living conditions; poor hygiene.
• Smoking.
• Immunosuppression.

HOW TO PREVENT
• Maintain a mutually monogamous sexual relationship.
• Using condoms may help prevent transmission; however, condoms can't always cover all affected skin (e.g., scrotum).

PROBABLE OUTCOME
• These small warts usually cause no symptoms. If untreated, some will disappear spontaneously. However, because the virus may be sexually transmitted, it is important to obtain medical treatment. The warts may grow rapidly during pregnancy, but often resolve postpartum.
• Recurrence is common.

POSSIBLE COMPLICATIONS
• Cervical dysplasia (atypical, precancerous cells).
• In pregnancy, the warts can cause the skin of the vagina to tear more easily and make it more difficult to repair if an episiotomy procedure is performed. In addition, there is a small risk that the newborn can acquire the infection whether the birth is vaginal or by cesarean section.
• Some types of HPV have been associated with an increased risk of genital cancer. For this reason, women who have had genital warts should have Pap smears at least once a year.

 HOW TO TREAT

GENERAL MEASURES
• Genital warts can often be diagnosed with a physical examination. Vinegar placed on the skin turns the warts white. Sexual partners should also be screened and treated.
• Other diagnostic tests may include microscopic examination, Pap smear or tissue biopsy.
• Treatment will be determined by size and location of warts. Even though the warts can be removed, the viral infection can't be cured, and the warts often return. Pregnant women with genital warts require special treatment.
• Small warts may be treated with topical medication.
• Cryotherapy (see Glossary) may be used to remove some warts.
• Some larger warts require laser treatment, electrocoagulation or surgical excision.
• Don't treat these warts with nonprescription drugs used for wart removal on the hands. They can make the genital area very sore.
• Obtain annual pelvic examinations and Pap smears.

MEDICATION
• A topical medication may be prescribed; apply to small areas at a time. Use petroleum jelly on surrounding healthy tissue first, and then apply the cream carefully to avoid damaging healthy tissue. Using too much may cause irritation or absorption of the drug. Wash off after 4 hours. Keep the medication out of eyes.
• Alpha interferon injections into each wart with a very small needle may be recommended.

ACTIVITY—No restrictions, except to avoid sexual relations until treatment is completed.

DIET—No special diet.

 CALL YOUR DOCTOR IF

• You or a family member has symptoms of genital warts.
• You develop signs of infection, including red, swollen, painful or tender skin; fever; chills; headache or muscle aches.

Contraception

Cervical Cap

 GENERAL INFORMATION

DEFINITION
• The goal of contraception (or birth control) is to prevent an unplanned pregnancy. The majority of methods of contraception enable sexually active couples to temporarily avoid pregnancy. Permanent birth control is accomplished through sterilization. Be sure you know and understand the different types of birth control available to you, the risks and benefits of each and any side effects, so that you can make an informed choice.
• The cervical cap is a small cup-like device (thimble shaped) made of soft rubber (or rigid plastic) about 1 1/2 inches long. The cap is inserted into the vagina where it fits tightly over the cervix and blocks only the entrance into the cervix. Suction holds it in place. A cervical cap is considered a barrier method of birth control because it provides a mechanical barrier to sperm transport. It is used with a spermicide that helps the suction and inactivates any sperm that might get by the cap.

ADVANTAGES
• Generally effective for contraception (82%-94%). Proper and consistent usage increases the effectiveness.
• Easily transported.
• May be used only when needed.
• May be used during light menstruation to temporarily contain the menstrual flow.
• May offer some protection against sexually transmitted diseases.
• Should not have any effect on a woman's future ability to become pregnant.
• Does not involve the use of hormones, as in some other forms of birth control that can have side effects.
• May be left in place 1 to 2 days (however, a foul discharge may develop after the first day).
• Low cost and long wear.

DISADVANTAGES
• Not 100% effective for birth control or prevention of sexually transmitted diseases.
• Must be prescribed and fitted by a health-care provider.
• May be difficult to fit properly. The existing sizes may not fit all women, especially those who have had several children.
• Requires high degree of motivation and fair degree of manual dexterity to position the cap correctly over the cervix.
• Must be used simultaneously with a spermicide; some women find that spermicides irritate the vagina.
• Must be left in place for at least 6 hours following intercourse.
• May develop undetectable flaws.
• Disagreeable to some couples to use spermicidal jellies and creams during oral sex.
• May become dislodged during intercourse.
• May contribute to urinary tract infections.
• Has been associated with mildly abnormal Pap smears in some women.

 GENERAL MEASURES

INSTRUCTIONS FOR USE
• Make sure that you are carefully fitted by a competent medical person. The cap comes in 4 sizes.
• Repeat fittings after childbirth, miscarriage, abortion, any surgical operation involving the female genitals, or weight gain or loss of 12 or more pounds.
• Practice inserting the cervical cap before attempting to use it with your partner.
• The cap should be inserted up to 2 hours before intercourse.
• Leave the cap in place at least 6 hours after intercourse to ensure that the spermicide has had enough time to kill all the sperm. You may leave it in for up to 2 days if you choose. Do not leave it in place beyond the initial time period if you are menstruating.
To insert:
• Before insertion, fill cap 1/3 full with a spermicide, preferably a jelly.
• Never use a petroleum lubricant.
• Squat or recline to position the cap. Insert the cap fully into the vagina and press the rim around the cervix until the dome covers it entirely.
To remove:
• Wait at least 6 hours after intercourse. You must exert pressure with a fingertip to break the seal, then hook your finger over the rim of the cap and pull it down out of the vagina. Take care to avoid injuring the rubber with fingernails.
• Wash the cap with mild unscented soap and water.
• Hold up to the light after each removal to check for holes. If any defects are found, call your doctor for advice.
• Store in a dry place in its container.
Note: Follow the special written instructions that come with the cervical cap if they differ from those discussed in this chart.

MEDICATIONS—No restrictions.

 CALL YOUR DOCTOR IF

• You are interested in a cervical cap for contraception.
• You are using a cervical cap that is uncomfortable or seems to be dislodged by intercourse.
• You find defects in a cervical cap you are using.

Contraception Methods Compared
(continued on next page)

 GENERAL INFORMATION

DEFINITION

Choosing a method of birth control is a highly personal decision, based on individual preferences, medical history, lifestyle and other factors. Each method carries with it a number of risks and benefits of which the user should be aware.

Each method of birth control has a failure rate (an inability to prevent pregnancy over a one-year period); sometimes the failure rate is due to the method and sometimes it is due to human error. Each method has possible side effects, some minor and some serious. Some methods require lifestyle modifications, such as remembering to use the method with each and every sexual intercourse. Some cannot be used by individuals with certain medical problems. (The following information is adapted in part from the *FDA Consumer*, the magazine of the U.S. Food & Drug Administration.)

SPERMICIDES USED ALONE

Spermicides, which come in many forms (foams, jellies, gels and suppositories) work by forming a physical and chemical barrier to sperm. They should be inserted into the vagina within an hour before intercourse. If intercourse is repeated, more spermicide should be inserted. The active ingredient in most spermicides is the chemical nonoxynol-9. The failure rate for spermicides in preventing pregnancy when used alone is from 20% to 30%. Spermicides are available without a prescription. Discontinue use if you experience burning or irritation with these products.

BARRIER METHODS

There are five barrier methods of contraception: male condoms, female condoms, sponge, diaphragm and cervical cap. Each of these methods works by keeping the sperm and egg apart. Usually, these methods have only minor side effects. One possible side effect is an allergic reaction to either the material of the barrier or the spermicides that are used with them.

Male Condom:
• A male condom is a sheath that covers the penis during sex. Condoms are made of either latex rubber or natural skin (also called "lamb-skin" but actually made from sheep intestines). Only latex condoms have been shown to be highly effective in helping to prevent sexually transmitted diseases (STDs). Latex provides a good barrier to even small viruses such as HIV and hepatitis B. Each condom can be used only once. Condoms have a birth control failure rate of about 15%.
• Some condoms have spermicide added. This may give some additional contraceptive protection. Vaginal spermicides may also be added before sexual intercourse.
• Some condoms have lubricants added. These do not improve birth control or STD protection. Non–oil-based lubricants can also be used with condoms. However, oil-based lubricants such as petroleum jelly (Vaseline) should not be used because they weaken the latex. Condoms are available without a prescription.

Female Condom:
• The Reality Female Condom consists of a lubricated polyurethane sheath with a flexible polyurethane ring on each end. One ring is inserted into the vagina much like a diaphragm, while the other remains outside, partially covering the labia. The female condom may offer some protection against STDs, but for highly effective protection, male latex condoms must be used. The estimated failure rate for the Reality Female Condom is from 21% to 26%.

Sponge:
• In 1995, the only company in the U.S. manufacturing the sponge discontinued its production. It may become available again at some future date. The sponge is made of white polyurethane foam. It is shaped like a small doughnut and contains the spermicide nonoxynol-9. Like the diaphragm, it is inserted into the vagina to cover the cervix during and after intercourse. It does not require fitting by a health professional and is available without prescription. It is to be used only once and then discarded. The failure rate is between 18% and 28%. An extremely rare side effect is toxic shock syndrome (TSS), a potentially fatal infection caused by a strain of Staphylococcus aureus, and more commonly associated with tampon use.

Diaphragm:
• The diaphragm is a flexible rubber disk with a rigid rim. Diaphragms range in size from 2 to 4 inches in diameter and are designed to cover the cervix during and after intercourse so that sperm cannot reach the uterus. Spermicidal jelly or cream must be placed inside the diaphragm for it to be effective.
• The diaphragm must be fitted by a health professional and the correct size prescribed to ensure a snug seal with the vaginal wall. If intercourse is repeated, additional spermicide should be added with the diaphragm still in place. The diaphragm should be left in place for at least six hours after intercourse. The diaphragm used with spermicide has a failure rate between 6% to 18%.
• In addition to possible allergic reactions or irritation, there have been some reports of bladder infections with this method. As with the contraceptive sponge, toxic shock syndrome (TSS) is an extremely rare side effect.

Contraception Methods Compared (cont.)

Cervical Cap:
The cervical cap is a dome-shaped rubber cap in various sizes that fits snugly over the cervix. Like the diaphragm, it is used with a spermicide and must be fitted by a health professional. It is more difficult to insert than the diaphragm but may be left in place for up to 48 hours. In addition to the allergic reactions that can occur with any barrier method, users have reported an unpleasant odor and/or discharge. There also appears to be an increased incidence of irregular Pap tests in the first six months of using the cap, and toxic shock syndrome (TSS) is an extremely rare side effect. The cap has a failure rate of about 18%.

HORMONAL CONTRACEPTION
Hormonal contraception involves ways of delivering forms of two female reproductive hormones, estrogen and progestogen, that help regulate ovulation (release of an egg), the condition of the uterine lining and other parts of the menstrual cycle. Unlike barrier methods, hormones interact with the body and have the potential for serious side effects, though these are rare. When properly used, hormonal methods are also extremely effective. Hormonal methods are available only by prescription.

Birth Control Pills:
• There are two types of birth control pills: combination pills, which contain both estrogen and a progestin (a natural or synthetic progesterone), and "mini-pills," which contain only progestin. The combination pill prevents ovulation, while the mini-pill reduces cervical mucus and causes it to thicken. This prevents sperm from reaching the egg. Also, progestins stop the uterine lining from thickening. This prevents the fertilized egg from implanting in the uterus. The failure rate for the mini-pill is 1% to 3%; for the combination pill, 1% to 2%.
• Combination oral contraceptives offer significant protection against ovarian and endometrial cancers, iron-deficiency anemia, pelvic inflammatory disease and fibrocystic breast disease. Women who take combination pills have a lower risk of ovarian cysts.
• Smokers and women with certain medical conditions should not take the pill. These conditions include a history of blood clots; heart attacks, strokes or angina; cancer of the breast, vagina, cervix or uterus; any undiagnosed, abnormal vaginal bleeding; liver tumors; jaundice due to pregnancy or use of birth control pills.
• Women with the following conditions should discuss with a health professional whether the benefits of the pill outweigh its risks: high blood pressure; heart, kidney or gallbladder disease; a family history of heart attack or stroke; severe headaches or depression; elevated cholesterol or triglycerides; epilepsy or diabetes.

• Serious side effects of the pill include blood clots that can lead to stroke, heart attack, pulmonary embolism or death. A clot may, on rare occasions, occur in the blood vessel of the eye, causing impaired vision or even blindness. The pills may also cause high blood pressure that returns to normal after oral contraceptives are stopped. Minor side effects, which usually subside after a few months' use, include fluid retention, nausea, headaches, breast swelling, weight gain, irregular bleeding and depression. Sometimes taking a pill with a lower dose of hormones can reduce these side effects.
• The effectiveness of birth control pills may be reduced by a few other medications, including some antibiotics, barbiturates and antifungal medications. On the other hand, birth control pills may prolong the effects of theophylline and caffeine. They also may prolong the effects of benzodiazepines such as Valium, Librium and Xanax. Women should always tell their health professionals when they are taking birth control pills.

Norplant:
• In a minor surgical procedure, six matchstick-sized capsules containing progestin are placed just underneath the skin of the upper arm. The implant is effective within 24 hours and provides progestin for up to five years or until it is removed. Both the insertion and the removal must be performed by a qualified professional.
• Because contraception is automatic and does not depend on the user, the failure rate is less than 1% for women who weigh less than 200 pounds. Women who weigh more have a higher pregnancy rate after the first two years.
• Women who cannot take birth control pills for medical reasons should not consider Norplant a contraceptive option. The potential side effects of the implant include irregular menstrual bleeding, headaches, nervousness, depression, nausea, dizziness, skin rash, acne, enlargement of the ovaries or fallopian tubes, change of appetite, breast tenderness, weight gain and excessive growth of body and facial hair. These side effects may subside after the first year.

Depo-Provera:
• Depo-Provera is an injectable form of a progestin. It has a failure rate of 1%. Each injection provides contraceptive protection for 14 weeks. It is injected every three months into a muscle in the buttocks or arm by a trained professional.
• The side effects are similar to those for Norplant listed above. In addition, there may be irregular bleeding and spotting during the first months, followed by episodes of amenorrhea (no menstrual period). About 50% of the women who use Depo-Provera for one year or longer report amenorrhea.

Contraception Methods Compared
(continued on next page)

OTHER TEMPORARY CONTRACEPTIVE METHODS

Intrauterine Device (IUD):
- IUDs are small, plastic, flexible devices that are inserted into the uterus through the cervix by a trained clinician. Only two IUDs are presently marketed in the United States: ParaGard T380A, a T-shaped device partially covered by copper and effective for ten years, and Progestasert, which is also T-shaped but contains a progestin released over a one-year period. After that time, the IUD should be replaced. Both IUDs have a 4% to 5% failure rate.
- It is not known exactly how IUDs work. At one time it was thought that the IUD affected the uterus so that it would be inhospitable to implantation. New evidence, however, suggests that uterine and tubal fluids are altered, particularly in the case of copper-bearing IUDs, inhibiting the transport of sperm through the cervical mucus and uterus.
- The risk of pelvic inflammatory disease (PID) with IUD use is highest in those with multiple sex partners or with a history of previous PID. Therefore, the IUD is recommended primarily for women in mutually monogamous relationships.
- In addition to PID, other complications include perforation of the uterus, septic abortion or tubal pregnancy. Women may also experience some short-term side effects such as cramping and dizziness at the time of insertion; bleeding, cramps and backache that may continue for a few days after the insertion; spotting between periods and longer and heavier menstruation during the first few periods after insertion.

Periodic Abstinence—Periodic abstinence entails not having sexual intercourse during the woman's fertile period. Sometimes this method is called natural family planning or "rhythm." Using periodic abstinence is dependent on the ability to identify the approximately 10 days in each menstrual cycle that a woman is fertile. Methods include:
- The basal body temperature method is based on the knowledge that just before ovulation a woman's basal body temperature drops several tenths of a degree and after ovulation it returns to normal. The method requires that the woman take her temperature each morning before she gets out of bed.
- The cervical mucus method depends on a woman recognizing the changes in cervical mucus that indicate ovulation is occurring or has occurred. There are now electronic thermometers with memories and electrical resistance meters that can more accurately pinpoint a woman's fertile period.
- Maintaining a calendar record of menstrual cycles is an additional step women can take to help determine ovulation.
- The periodic abstinence method has a failure rate of 14% to 47%. It has none of the side effects of artificial methods of contraception.

SURGICAL STERILIZATION
- Surgical sterilization must be considered permanent. Tubal ligation seals a woman's fallopian tubes so that an egg cannot travel to the uterus. Vasectomy involves closing off a man's vas deferens so that sperm will not be carried to the penis.
- Vasectomy is considered safer than female sterilization. It is a minor surgical procedure, most often performed in a doctor's office under local anesthesia. The procedure usually takes less than 30 minutes. Minor post-surgical complications may occur.
- Tubal ligation is an operating-room procedure performed under general or regional anesthesia. The fallopian tubes can be reached by a number of surgical techniques and, depending on the technique, the operation is sometimes an outpatient procedure or requires only a one-night stay. Following vaginal delivery, patients often choose to have a tubal ligation performed as a minilaparotomy or laparoscopy; both of these methods are replacing the traditional laparotomy (see Glossary for these terms).
- Major complications, which are rare in female sterilization, include infection, hemorrhage and problems associated with the use of general or regional anesthesia. It is estimated that major complications occur in 1.7% of the cases, while the overall complication rate has been reported to be between 0.1% and 15.3%.
- The failure rate of laparoscopy and minilaparotomy procedures, as well as vasectomy, is less than 1%. Although there has been some success in reopening the fallopian tubes or the vas deferens, the success rate is low, and sterilization should be considered irreversible.

 CALL YOUR DOCTOR IF

You want additional information on contraception.

Contraception Methods Compared (cont.)

A guide to information on various birth control methods. Effectiveness estimates are based on a number of different studies. This chart summarizes the contraception methods previously mentioned.

Type	Estimated Effectiveness	Risks	STD Protection	Convenience	Availability
Male condom	88-98%	Rarely, irritation and allergic reactions	Latex condoms help protect against sexually transmitted diseases, including herpes and AIDS	Applied immediately before intercourse —	Nonprescription
Female condom	74-79%	Rarely, irritation and allergic reactions	May give some protection against sexually transmitted diseases, including herpes and AIDS; not as effective as male latex condom	Applied immediately before intercourse; used only once and discarded	Nonprescription
Spermicides used alone	70-80%	Rarely, irritation and allergic reactions	Unknown	Applied no more than 1 hour before intercourse	Nonprescription
Sponge (manufacture discontinued in 1995 in U.S.)	72-82%	Rarely, irritation and allergic reactions; difficulty in removal; vary rarely, toxic shock syndrome	None	Can be inserted hours before intercourse and left in place up to 24 hours; used only once and discarded	Nonprescription
Diaphragm with spermicide	82-94%	Rarely, irritation and allergic reactions; bladder infection; very rarely, toxic shock syndrome	None	Inserted before intercourse; can be left in place 24 hours; additional spermicide must be inserted if intercourse is repeated	Prescription
Cervical cap with spermicide	At least 82%	Abnormal Pap test; genital infections; very rarely, toxic shock syndrome	None	Can remain in place for 48 hours; not necessary to reapply spermicide if intercourse repeated; may be difficult to insert	Prescription

Contraception Methods Compared (cont.)

Type	Estimated Effectiveness	Risks	STD Protection	Convenience	Availability
Oral contraceptives (combination pill or mini-pill)	97-99%	Blood clots, heart attacks and strokes, gallbladder disease, liver tumors, water retention, hypertension, mood swings, dizziness and nausea, not for smokers	None	Pill must be taken on daily schedule, regardless of the frequency of intercourse	Prescription
Implant (Norplant)	99%	Menstrual cycle irregularity, headaches, nervousness, depression, nausea, dizziness, change of appetite, breast tenderness, weight gain, enlargement of ovaries and/or fallopian tubes, excessive growth of body and facial hair, may subside after 1st year	None	Effective 24 hours after implantation for approximately 5 years; can be removed by physician at any time; minor outpatient surgical procedure	Prescription
Injection (Depo-Provera)	99%	Amenorrhea, weight gain and other side effects similar to those with Norplant	None	One injection every 3 months	Prescription
Intrauterine device (IUD)	95-96%	Cramps; bleeding; pelvic inflammatory disease; infertility; rarely, perforation of the uterus	None	After insertion, stays in place until physician removes it	Prescription
Periodic abstinence (natural family planning)	Variable, perhaps 53-86%	None	None	Requires frequent monitoring of body functions and periods of abstinence	Instructions from physician or clinic
Surgical sterilization	Over 99%	Pain, infection and, for female tubal ligation, possible surgical complications	None	Vasectomy is a one-time procedure usually performed in a doctor's office; tubal ligation is a one-time procedure performed in an operating room	Surgery

Diaphragm

GENERAL INFORMATION

DEFINITION
• The goal of contraception (or birth control) is to prevent an unplanned pregnancy. The majority of methods of contraception enable sexually active couples to temporarily avoid pregnancy. Permanent birth control is accomplished through sterilization. Be sure you know and understand the different types of birth control available to you, the risks and benefits of each and any side effects, so that you can make an informed choice.
• The diaphragm is made of soft rubber in the shape of a shallow cup or dome, with a flexible metal spring rim. It is considered a barrier method of birth control because it provides a mechanical barrier to sperm transport. A diaphragm is inserted into the vagina and fits over the cervix behind the pubic bone. It must be used with a spermicidal cream or jelly to inactivate any sperm that may happen to move around the rim.

ADVANTAGES
• Generally effective for birth control (82%-94%). Proper and consistent usage increases the effectiveness.
• Easily transported.
• May be used only when needed.
• Does not involve the use of hormones that can have side effects.
• May be left in place up to 24 hours following intercourse.
• Low cost and long wearing (should last about 2 years with proper care).
• Offers some protection against sexually transmitted diseases (STDs).
• Should not have any effect on a woman's future ability to become pregnant.

DISADVANTAGES
• Not 100% effective for birth control or prevention of sexually transmitted diseases.
• Must be prescribed and fitted by a health-care provider.
• Putting in the diaphragm may be awkward at first. It does become quicker and easier with time.
• Must be used simultaneously with a spermicide. The discharge from the cream or jelly can be a nuisance.
• May develop undetectable flaws.
• Disagreeable to some couples to use spermicidal jellies and creams during oral sex.
• May become dislodged during intercourse.
• May contribute to urinary tract infections.

GENERAL MEASURES

INSTRUCTIONS FOR USE
• Make sure that you are carefully fitted for the diaphragm by a competent health-care provider. The diaphragm comes in various sizes to accommodate the majority of women.
• Repeat the fitting every 2 years or after childbirth, miscarriage, abortion, any surgical operation involving the female genitals, or weight gain or loss of 12 or more pounds.
• Practice inserting the diaphragm before attempting to use it with your partner.
• The diaphragm can be inserted up to 6 hours before intercourse.
• Leave the diaphragm in place at least 6 hours after intercourse, to ensure that the spermicide has had enough time to kill all of the sperm. You may leave it in for up to 24 hours if you choose.
To insert:
• Before insertion, place 1 teaspoonful to 1 tablespoonful of spermicide cream or jelly into the shallow cup.
• Never use a petroleum lubricant.
• Crouch, squat, lie down or stand with one foot propped on a chair. Squeeze the diaphragm, with the dome side down, into a long narrow shape with one hand while holding the lips of the vagina open with the other.
• Slide the diaphragm deeply into the vagina until the lower part of the rim passes the cervix.
• Push the front rim under the pubic bone, making sure the cervix is encircled. Feel your cervix through the diaphragm (it feels firm, similar in shape to the tip of your nose) to confirm that the diaphragm is positioned correctly.
• Don't douche while the diaphragm is in place.
To remove:
• Wait at least 6 hours after intercourse. (Do not leave it in place past this initial time period if you are menstruating.)
• Choose a comfortable position. Slip a finger or two under the lower rim and carefully force the diaphragm out by pulling on the rim. Avoid puncturing the diaphragm with a fingernail.
• Wash the diaphragm with mild unscented soap and water. Dust it with corn starch if desired; never use a talcum powder.
• Hold the diaphragm up to the light after each removal to check for holes. If you find any defects, call your doctor for advice.
• Store in a dry place in its container.
Note: Follow the special written instructions that come with the diaphragm if they differ from those discussed in this chart.

MEDICATIONS—No restrictions.

CALL YOUR DOCTOR IF

• You are interested in a diaphragm for contraception.
• You find defects in a diaphragm you are using, or have trouble using your diaphragm.

Female Condom

GENERAL INFORMATION

DEFINITION
• The goal of contraception (or birth control) is to prevent an unplanned pregnancy. The majority of methods of contraception enable sexually active couples to temporarily avoid pregnancy. Permanent birth control is accomplished through sterilization. Be sure you know and understand the different types of birth control available to you, the risks and benefits of each and any side effects, so that you can make an informed choice.
• The female condom (or vaginal pouch) is a disposable nonprescription birth control device. The recommended type is a sheath made of thin polyurethane material with 2 flexible rings, one at each end. One ring fits into the depth of the vagina and the other sits outside the vagina after the insertion. When it is in place, the pouch covers the vaginal wall and creates a covered passageway for the penis. The female condom is intended for one-time use only.

ADVANTAGES
• Generally effective for birth control (74%-79%). Proper and consistent usage increases the effectiveness.
• Easily transported.
• May be used only when needed.
• One size fits all women.
• Can be inserted long before intercourse (whereas a male condom needs to be used right at the time of intercourse).
• Does not require a visit to a doctor's office for fitting.
• Allows female to be in control of birth control method.
• Does not involve the use of hormones, as in some other forms of birth control, that can have side effects.
• It comes prelubricated and does not require precise placement over the cervix.
• The polyurethane is stronger than latex used in male condoms and is less likely to tear.
• Offers some protection against sexually transmitted diseases (STDs).
• Should not have any effect on a woman's future ability to have children.

DISADVANTAGES
• Not 100% effective for birth control or prevention of sexually transmitted diseases.
• Some women, as well as some men, are bothered by the feel of the device during intercourse or find the outside ring to be bothersome.
• Must be removed after a single act of intercourse; may not be used more than once.
• Inserting the condom is a little cumbersome and may take some practice.
• More costly than male condoms.

GENERAL MEASURES

INSTRUCTIONS FOR USE
• Practice inserting the condom before attempting to use one with a partner.
• Don't use after the expiration date.
• Don't use a male condom at the same time as a female condom; the female condom may not stay in place or be as effective.
To insert:
• Squeeze the inner ring and insert the pouch into the vagina just past the pubic bone using the index finger (similar to tampon insertion).
• The inner ring should cover the cervix. The outer ring plus about 1 inch of the condom stays outside the vagina.
• Using your finger, check to be sure the sheath is not twisted and that it will be easy for the penis to enter into the vagina. Also check to make sure that the inner ring covers the cervix, that the polyurethane sheath covers the walls of the vagina and that the outer ring is just outside the vaginal lips (labia).
• A lubricant may be added if desired.
• Do not leave it in place beyond the initial time period if you are menstruating.
To remove:
• After your partner ejaculates, squeeze and twist the outer ring to keep sperm inside the condom.
• Pull gently to remove.
• Wrap condom in tissue and throw in waste basket; it should not be flushed down the toilet.
• Use a new female condom for each act of intercourse.
Note: Follow the special written instructions that come with the product if they differ from those discussed in this chart.

MEDICATIONS—No restrictions.

CALL YOUR DOCTOR IF

You have questions about using a female condom for contraception.

Hormone Implants (Norplant)

GENERAL INFORMATION

DEFINITION
• The goal of contraception (or birth control) is to prevent an unplanned pregnancy. The majority of methods of contraception enable sexually active couples to temporarily avoid pregnancy. Permanent birth control is accomplished through sterilization. Be sure you know and understand the different types of birth control available to you, the risks and benefits of each and any side effects, so that you can make an informed choice.
• Hormone implants consist of 6 small capsules (the size of matchsticks) containing a progestin hormone. They are surgically inserted just under the skin of the upper arm. The implants provide birth control for 5 years by slowly releasing the hormones in the capsules into the body. Hormones work by blocking ovulation and by thickening the cervical mucus to make sperm penetration more difficult; they also change the endometrium (lining of the uterus) to make it unsuitable for implantation of a fertile egg.

ADVANTAGES
• Very effective for contraceptive use (over 99%); one of the most effective temporary forms of birth control available.
• The hormone used in the implants, progestin, provides a birth control option for women who cannot take estrogen hormones.
• The implants require no daily routine.
• Spontaneous sexual intercourse.
• Although they cannot be discontinued as easily as discontinuing a daily pill (oral contraceptives), they can be removed at any time by a trained health-care provider.
• They are effective for up to 5 years. There is no significant delay in restoration of fertility following removal.

DISADVANTAGES
• They require a minor surgical procedure with a local anesthetic for insertion. Some minor skin side effects may occur at the implantation site.
• Some women experience problems when the implants are removed, including a longer surgical time, pain and scarring.
• Side effects from the implants include menstrual irregularities, headaches, depression and weight gain. The side effects tend to diminish with time.
• They should not be used in women who have a blood clotting disorder, heart problems, undiagnosed vaginal bleeding, liver problems or breast cancer.
• Up-front costs are high since there is a one-time payment, but the overall costs for a 5-year period are comparable to oral contraceptives.
• High failure rate in women over 200 lbs.

• Will not protect against sexually transmitted diseases (STDs). A form of barrier protection (e.g., a latex condom) will need to be used.

GENERAL MEASURES

INSTRUCTIONS FOR USE
• The implants are usually inserted during the first 7 days of a woman's menstrual cycle, and then are effective within 24 hours after insertion. However, they can be inserted anytime if pregnancy has been ruled out; another form of birth control (nonhormonal) should then be used for the remainder of the cycle.
• A patient information booklet will be provided for you to read prior to implant insertion. Be sure any questions or concerns you have are answered or explained.
To insert:
• The procedure will be done in a health-care provider's office. It should take about 15 minutes.
• A local anesthetic is injected into the upper arm (may cause some stinging).
• A small incision is made and, one by one, the 6 capsules are placed under the skin in a fan-shape position.
• A protective bandage is placed over the incision which can be removed in a few days.
• There may be some discoloration, bruising or swelling in the incision area for a few days.
To remove:
• Again, the procedure will be done in a health-care provider's office and should take less than 30 minutes.
• The capsules are located by being palpated (felt); a local anesthetic is then injected.
• An incision is made and the capsules are withdrawn one by one.
• The site should be kept clean, dry and bandaged for 3 to 4 days.

MEDICATIONS
• Carbamazepine, rifampin and phenytoin all reduce the effectiveness of the hormone implants and may increase the risk of pregnancy.
• Advise anyone who prescribes a medicine for you, or before any anesthetic is used, that you have the hormone implants.

CALL YOUR DOCTOR IF

• You are interested in hormone implants for contraception.
• After implantation, unexpected side effects occur, such as severe abdominal pain.
• You have pus, bleeding or severe pain at the insertion site.
• Heavy vaginal bleeding develops.
• You have had the hormone implants for about 5 years and they need to be replaced.

Hormone Injection
(Depo-Provera)

 GENERAL INFORMATION

DEFINITION

• The goal of contraception (or birth control) is to prevent an unplanned pregnancy. The majority of methods of contraception enable sexually active couples to temporarily avoid pregnancy. Permanent birth control is accomplished through sterilization. Be sure you know and understand the different types of birth control available to you, the risks and benefits of each and any side effects, so that you can make an informed choice.

• The most widely used injectable form of birth control Is Depo-Provera (depo-medroxyproges-terone acetate). The drug, which is sometimes abbreviated DMPA, contains a long-acting, synthetic form of the hormone progesterone. Depo-Provera suppresses ovulation, makes the mucus of the cervix less likely to be penetrated by viable sperm and induces changes in the uterine lining that make it more difficult for a fertilized egg to implant. Depo-Provera is given by an injection every 90 days.

ADVANTAGES

• Very effective for birth control (over 99%); one of the most effective forms available.

• Quickly and easily administered by a health-care provider.

• The hormone used, progestin, provides a birth control option for women who cannot take estrogen hormones that are used in oral contraceptives.

• The injections require no daily routine.

• Freedom from concern of pregnancy allows enjoyment of spontaneous sexual intercourse.

• Future fertility does not appear to be affected, but it may take as long as 12 months for ovulation to occur once the injections are discontinued.

• May provide some protection against endometrial cancer.

• Does not interfere with breast-feeding, much like progesterone-only pills, when used postpartum.

DISADVANTAGES

• Presence of other medical problems may affect the use of these injections. These include allergies, liver disorder, cancer or a history of cancer, diabetes mellitus, epilepsy, unexplained vaginal bleeding, other bleeding problems or stroke.

• Side effects or adverse reactions can include irregular uterine bleeding, cessation of menstrual periods (amenorrhea), headaches, fluid retention and bloating, weight gain, bleeding disorders, skin reactions to the injections.

• The injections may lead to depression, fatigue, nervousness and loss of sexual desire (rarely).

• Bone mineral density may be reduced; bone density usually returns to normal once a woman's use of Depo-Provera has been discontinued.

• Requires injections every 3 months in a health-care provider's office.

• Cannot be reversed as easily as discontinuing use of a daily birth control pill. Following discontinuation of Depo-Provera, ovulation may not occur for as long as 12 months; women desiring future conception should take this into consideration before beginning use of DMPA.

• Long-term effects are still being studied.

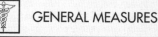 GENERAL MEASURES

INSTRUCTIONS FOR USE

• The injections will be prescribed for you after the health-care provider has studied your medical history and the results of a physical examination.

• The first injection is often given during the first 5 days of the menstrual period so that pregnancy has been ruled out.

• The injections are injected into a muscle once every 3 months (usually in a large muscle such as the buttocks muscle). The contraceptive levels of hormone persist for up to 4 months (allowing a 2- to 4-week margin of safety).

• Follow-up medical examinations are recommended at least once a year or more frequently.

MEDICATIONS

There may be some interaction with other medications. Advise any health-care provider treating you or prescribing for you that you have these hormone injections.

 CALL YOUR DOCTOR IF

• You are interested in hormone injections as a method of temporary contraception.
After the injections:

• You suspect you are pregnant.

• Unexpected vaginal bleeding occurs or other changes in your menstrual cycle develop.

• You develop pain or swelling in the calf or any unusual leg pain.

• There are changes in your blood pressure.

• Other unexplained symptoms develop.

Intrauterine Device (IUD)

 GENERAL INFORMATION

DEFINITION
• The goal of contraception (or birth control) is to prevent an unplanned pregnancy. The majority of methods of contraception enable sexually active couples to temporarily avoid pregnancy. Permanent birth control is accomplished through sterilization. Be sure you know and understand the different types of birth control available to you, the risks and benefits of each and any side effects, so that you can make an informed choice.
• An intrauterine device (IUD) is a tiny object (usually made of plastic) that is inserted into the uterus to prevent pregnancy. One or more plastic strings attached to the IUD will extend out through the cervical canal. These strings enable periodic checking for position and aid IUD removal. IUDs are visible on x-ray should one become "lost." The IUD interferes with the transportation of both sperm and egg with the end result being that fertilization does not take place. One type of IUD, containing a hormone (progesterone), needs to be changed every year. A second type, containing copper, is effective for 10 years.

ADVANTAGES
• IUDs are 95%-96% effective for birth control.
• The device is easily fitted and tolerated by most women.
• Enjoyment of spontaneous sexual intercourse; freedom from concern once IUD is in place.
• The IUD requires no daily routine.
• Although they cannot be discontinued as easily as discontinuing a daily pill (oral contraceptives), they can be removed at any time by a trained health-care provider.
• With the progesterone-containing IUD, there will probably be less bleeding during menstrual cycles.
• Fertility for a woman after removal of the IUD should probably be the same as it was before using the IUD.

DISADVANTAGES
• Cramping and bleeding may occur the first few days after insertion.
• Spontaneous expulsion of the IUD. Occurs more frequently within the first year. It is noticed in most instances, but some women may not be aware of the device being expelled.
• Occasional bleeding between menstrual periods; changes in amount of menstrual flow; increased pain with periods.
• IUDs offer no protection against sexually transmitted diseases. A form of barrier protection (e.g., condoms) will need to be used.
• In rare situations, IUDs will perforate the uterus and travel into the abdomen. "Lost" IUDs require special examinations.

• IUDs can increase the risk for pelvic infections, such as pelvic inflammatory disease (PID), which can impair future fertility.
• If pregnancy occurs with an IUD in place, there is a 50% chance of miscarriage. The IUD should be removed if pregnancy occurs.
• IUDs may increase the risk of ectopic pregnancy.
• Not recommended for women who have a diagnosed gynecological problem or are pregnant. Women who have certain chronic disorders or STDs, who have not yet had a child or who have multiple sexual partners are also not good IUD candidates.

GENERAL MEASURES

INSTRUCTIONS FOR USE
• You will have a full medical examination, including a pelvic exam, Pap smear testing, breast exam, pregnancy test and tests for STDs before insertion of an IUD.
• The device will be inserted by a trained health-care provider.
• The timing for the insertion can vary; it may be done during a menstrual period, between periods or 6 weeks after childbirth or abortion.
To insert:
• The IUD is straightened out in a plastic tube (like a straw) and the tube is inserted through the vagina and cervix into the uterus. The IUD is pushed through the tube and it springs back into shape in the uterus.
• The tube is removed and the IUD stays in the uterus with its string dangling into the vagina. You will be instructed on how to check for the string.
• There may be pain during the insertion and sometimes cramping for the rest of the day.
To remove:
Consult your doctor.

MEDICATIONS—Ask your health-care provider about the need for pain medication during and after the insertion procedure.

CALL YOUR DOCTOR IF

• You are interested in an intrauterine device (IUD) for contraception.
• Following insertion of an IUD, unexpected side effects develop, including excessive or irregular vaginal bleeding, abdominal cramps, vaginal discharge, or you develop signs of infection (fever, chills, muscle aches).
• You cannot find the string of the IUD when you search for it.
• The IUD has been in place for the recommended length of time.

Male Condom

GENERAL INFORMATION

DEFINITION
• The goal of contraception (or birth control) is to prevent an unplanned pregnancy. The majority of methods of contraception enable sexually active couples to temporarily avoid pregnancy. Permanent birth control is accomplished through sterilization. Be sure you know and understand the different types of birth control available to you, the risks and benefits of each and any side effects, so that you can make an informed choice.
• The condom is a contraceptive device that looks like a skinny balloon and is usually made of thin latex rubber or polyurethane. The male wears this sheath over the erect penis during intercourse to prevent the sperm from being deposited in the vagina. The condom may also be effective in preventing spread of some sexually transmitted diseases (STDs). The male condom is also called a prophylactic or rubber. It is the only form of temporary birth control a man can use. Some condoms are made of animal intestine, but these are not effective for preventing STDs.

ADVANTAGES
• Generally effective for contraceptive use (88%-98%). Proper and consistent usage increases the effectiveness.
• The condom is readily available, inexpensive and easy to use. Women can buy and carry condoms.
• No medical appointment or prescription is required to purchase condoms.
• In addition to birth control, it gives good protection against some STDs, including HIV.
• Some condoms contain a spermicide which offers further protection in case a condom breaks during intercourse. In addition, using a small amount of spermicide (nonoxynol-9) with the condom increases protection.
• There are no systemic side effects from condom use.
• Since the condom catches the semen, a woman has less leaking (discharge) following intercourse.
• Condoms have no effect on a couple's future ability to have children.

DISADVANTAGES
• Since the condom needs to be used right at the time of sexual intercourse, it may decrease the spontaneity of sex for some couples.
• Condoms may lessen the male's sensation since the penis does not touch the vaginal walls directly.
• The friction caused by using a condom may irritate a woman's vagina unless a lubricant is used.
• Condoms can deteriorate if exposed to heat. Do not store them for very long in a pocket or wallet. If not exposed to heat, latex condoms have a shelf life of about 5 years.
• Allergic reaction to latex (rare).

GENERAL MEASURES

INSTRUCTIONS FOR USE
• When opening a condom, handle the package gently. Don't use teeth, sharp fingernails, scissors, or other sharp instruments as these may damage the condom. And make sure you can see what you're doing!
• After you open the package, inspect the condom. If the material sticks to itself or is gummy, the condom is no good. Check the condom top for obvious damage such as tears, holes or brittleness; don't unroll the condom to check it because this could damage it.
• Use a new condom for every act of intercourse and oral sex.
• Put the condom on after the penis is erect and before any contact is made between the penis and any part of the partner's body.
• If using a spermicide, put some inside the condom tip.
• If the condom does not have a reservoir tip, pinch the tip enough to leave a half-inch space for semen to collect. Make sure to eliminate any air in the tip to help keep the condom from breaking.
• Holding the condom by the rim (and pinching the half-inch tip, if necessary), place the condom on top of the penis. Then, continuing to hold it by the rim, unroll it all the way to the base of the penis. If you are using a water-based lubricant, such as K-Y Jelly, you may put more on the outside of the condom.
• Never use lubricants which contain oils, fats or grease, such as a petroleum-based jelly (Vaseline), baby oil or lotions or hand or body creams. These can seriously weaken latex, causing the condom to break easily.
• If you feel the condom break, stop immediately, withdraw and put on a new condom.
• After ejaculation, and before the penis gets soft, grip the rim of the condom and carefully withdraw the penis from the vagina.
• To remove the condom, gently pull it off the penis, being careful the semen doesn't spill out.
• Wrap the used condom in a tissue and throw it in the trash. Because condoms may cause problems in sewers, don't flush them down the toilet. Afterwards, wash your hands with soap and water.

MEDICATIONS—No restrictions.

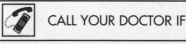

CALL YOUR DOCTOR IF

You are interested in using condoms for contraception and want additional information.

Morning-After Pill

GENERAL INFORMATION

DEFINITION
• The goal of contraception (or birth control) is to prevent an unplanned pregnancy. The majority of methods of contraception enable sexually active couples to temporarily avoid pregnancy. Permanent birth control is accomplished through sterilization. Be sure you know and understand the different types of birth control available to you, the risks and benefits of each and any side effects, so that you can make an informed choice.
• The morning-after pill (or postcoital pill) consists of a series of very high doses of estrogens (generally diethylstilbestrol [DES]), progesterones or combination pills. They may be effective in preventing pregnancy if initiated within 72 hours of sexual intercourse. This method of birth control works by altering the ability of a fertilized egg to implant and grow. It is usually not recommended as a routine birth control method; rather, it is reserved for special circumstances.
• The drug mifepristone (also known as RU-486), which has been used in Europe for over a decade, is also effective in terminating pregnancy. However, while it has recently been approved by the Food and Drug Administration (FDA) for use in the United States, political controversy over its use remains, and difficulty continues in finding a U.S. company to manufacture and distribute the drug. Until such time as a U.S. manufacturer has been established, RU-486 will remain largely unobtainable in the U.S.

ADVANTAGES
• Generally effective for birth control (97%-99%), but effectiveness varies depending on the time of the woman's menstrual cycle; if taken at mid-cycle, the failure rate is higher.
• It is an immediate form of birth control should unexpected intercourse occur, such as rape.
• It is a backup birth control option for couples experiencing failure of other methods: expulsion of an intrauterine device (IUD), condom breakage or diaphragm displacement.
• Should have no effect on a woman's future ability to become pregnant.

DISADVANTAGES
• Not 100% effective for birth control.
• Must be prescribed by a health-care provider.
• Side effects occur including nausea, vomiting, headache, breast tenderness, bloated feeling and swelling of hands and feet. The side effects may be less with the combination pill and more severe with the use of the high-dose estrogen alone.
• If these drugs are inadvertently consumed during an early pregnancy, there may be significant effects on the developing embryo. Pregnancy termination may have to be considered. If pregnancy occurs despite proper use of the medication at the time of conception, developmental effect is unlikely.
• Will not protect against sexually transmitted diseases.
• The long-term effects of even one-time use of diethylstilbestrol have not been studied.

GENERAL MEASURES

INSTRUCTIONS FOR USE
• You should be examined by a doctor before taking a morning-after pill.
• The pills may be taken beginning within 24 hours and not later than 72 hours after unprotected intercourse. Generally, the high-dose estrogen is taken once daily for 5 days; the combination pill method consists of taking 2 birth control pills (such as Ovral) containing a synthetic estrogen (often ethinyl estriadol) combined with a progestin (often levonorgestrel), and then taking 2 more of these tablets 12 hours later.
• A follow-up examination in 3 to 4 weeks is recommended to assess the effectiveness of the treatment. Another form of birth control, if needed, should be discussed with your doctor.

MEDICATIONS—Don't take any other medications during the time of treatment with the morning-after pill without medical approval.

CALL YOUR DOCTOR IF

• You have had unprotected intercourse and want information about birth control options available to you.
• Following treatment with the morning-after pill, you experience unexpected side effects.
• You suspect you are pregnant after undergoing treatment.

Oral Contraceptives

GENERAL INFORMATION

DEFINITION
• The goal of contraception (or birth control) is to prevent an unplanned pregnancy. The majority of methods of contraception enable sexually active couples to temporarily avoid pregnancy. Permanent birth control is accomplished through sterilization. Be sure you know and understand the different types of birth control available to you, the risks and benefits of each and any side effects, so that you can make an informed choice.
• Oral contraceptives prevent ovulation and, therefore, make pregnancy unlikely or impossible. There are two types of contraceptive pills: combination and daily progestogen (sometimes called the mini-pill). The combination type, combining both estrogen and a synthetic progestogen, are the most popular and the most effective.

ADVANTAGES
• Effective, with lowest failure rate of any nonpermanent method—less than 0.1 pregnancy per 100 women per year, if all pills are taken as prescribed.
• Freedom from fear of pregnancy.
• Spontaneity of sexual experiences.
• Regular and less painful menstrual periods.
• Decrease in the amount of menstrual bleeding in most women.
• Decreased risk of fibrocystic breasts.
• Less likelihood of anemia or arthritis.
• Decrease in incidence of pelvic inflammatory disease.
• Decrease in incidence of cancer of the lining of the uterus and ovarian cancer.

DISADVANTAGES
• There are many conditions that might prevent you from taking the pill. Your doctor will take a thorough medical history and perform a physical examination prior to prescribing oral contraceptives. If any of the conditions are present that preclude prescribing the pill, or if you are a smoker, another form of birth control will be recommended.
• There may be side effects from the pill. Many of these occur rarely and will frequently decrease with the passage of time. Most patients experience no side effects at all. Side effects may include enlargement of fibroid tumors; breast fullness or tenderness; fluid retention; missed periods; acne; mild headache; high blood pressure; thrombophlebitis; weight gain; nausea; vomiting; diarrhea; stroke (rare); depression or easy mood shifts; change in sex drive; decrease in levels of some vitamins and minerals; increase in incidence of gallstones; increased likelihood of vaginal yeast infection; elevation of triglycerides and cholesterol; depigmentation of areas of the skin.

• Will not protect against sexually transmitted diseases (STDs). A form of barrier protection will need to be used.

GENERAL MEASURES

INSTRUCTIONS—Note: For most types of pills, you will need to use a second contraceptive method during your first cycle of pills. Otherwise, you will be inadequately protected against pregnancy.
Combination pills:
• Count the first sign of your menstrual cycle as day 1.
• On day 5, begin taking 1 pill each day. Pick a time that suits you and stick to it as your routine.
• Continue taking the pills for 21 days.
• Stop taking the pills for 7 days.
• Begin taking pills again for the next cycle after these 7 days, no matter when menstrual bleeding begins or ends.
• If you forget a combination pill, take it as soon as you remember. Take the next pill at the regular time (with very low dose pills, another form of contraception should be used for the remainder of the cycle).
• If you forget 2 days in a row, take 2 pills as soon as you remember and 2 pills the next day. Also, for the remainder of this cycle, use an additional form of contraception.
• If you forget for 3 or more days, stop taking any pills, wait 7 days, then start on a brand new packet. Use another form of contraception for a month.
Note: Some packets come with 28 pills. Follow instructions on the package.
Mini-pills:
• Start on day 5 as explained above, but continue to take a pill every day without interruption.
• If you forget a mini-pill, take 2 as soon as you remember, but use an additional contraception method for a month.

MEDICATIONS—Do not use any medicines, even nonprescription, before discussing them with your doctor.

CALL YOUR DOCTOR IF

You experience any of the following symptoms:
• Changes in your menstruation.
• Pain during, or bleeding after, intercourse.
• A sensation of pressure on your bladder or rectum.
• Severe chest pain or shortness of breath.
• Increased blood pressure.
• Abdominal pain, fever, jaundice, nausea.
• You see flashing lights or blurred images, or your ability to see decreases.
• Swelling or unusual pain in your legs.

RU-486
(Mifepristone; Abortion Pill, RU-486)

 GENERAL INFORMATION

DEFINITION
• RU-486 is a drug that has been used in Europe for some years as a nonsurgical way to terminate a pregnancy. The generic drug name is mifepristone, but it is more commonly known as RU-486. RU-486 has been approved by the FDA for use in the U.S., however, as of this writing, political controversy over its use remains and difficulty continues in finding a U.S. company to manufacture and distribute the drug. Until such time as a U.S. manufacturer has been established, RU-486 will remain largely unobtainable to women in the U.S. The following information and instructions are based on the assumption that you have had counseling and competent guidance in making your decision to seek this procedure for termination of the pregnancy.
• RU-486 also has potential as a menstrual inducer, to be taken several days before a woman's period is due. It is also being studied as a treatment for other disorders such as endometriosis, breast cancer and Cushing's syndrome.

REASONS FOR PROCEDURE
• Personal concerns about the social or economic aspects of an unplanned pregnancy.
• Continuing with the pregnancy may pose a threat to the life of the mother.
• Mother or father has a genetic condition that the fetus is at significant risk of acquiring, or the fetus has been tested and is known to have the condition (such as cystic fibrosis).
• Pregnancy resulted from a rape.
• Fetus is affected with a major disorder such as a chromosomal abnormality or birth defect.
• Fear that the fetus has been harmed by medications or other conditions.

RISK INCREASES WITH—Women who are hypersensitive to the drugs used.

DESCRIPTION OF PROCEDURE
• For the first step, the RU-486 drug is taken in a tablet form. Its action is to prevent implantation of a fertilized egg in the uterus or to bring on menses even if implantation has taken place.
• Two days later, a second drug is given in the doctor's office. This drug (a prostaglandin) will cause contractions of the uterus and enhance effectiveness of RU-486. A 4-hour time period is spent in the doctor's office for medical observation. After returning home, the fertilized egg is expelled. This stage can be somewhat painful, protracted and messy. Other negative effects may include abdominal cramps, dizziness, vomiting and diarrhea.

PROBABLE OUTCOME
• Termination of the pregnancy. This method is 96% to 99% effective when given before the 6th week of pregnancy.
• Recovery is rapid.
• 12 days after the procedure, a follow-up visit to the doctor is necessary to verify the abortion is complete.

POSSIBLE COMPLICATIONS
• In a few situations, women who do not completely abort will need to undergo a surgical procedure to complete the abortion.
• Excessive bleeding that may require a blood transfusion (rare).

 FOLLOW-UP CARE

GENERAL MEASURES
• Following the procedure, rest quietly at home for the remainder of the day.
• To reduce pain, place a heating pad or hot-water bottle on the abdomen or back. Hot baths can promote muscle relaxation and relieve discomfort. Repeat the baths as necessary.
• You will probably experience intermittent bleeding for the next 10 to 14 days, which may be light or moderately heavy and may increase with activity. Use external sanitary pads for bleeding.
• If contraception is desired, it can often be initiated shortly after the procedure. If you wish to take birth control pills, begin taking them either on the night following the procedure or the next day. If you prefer an IUD, diaphragm or cervical cap, the fitting can be made during your next doctor's appointment.
• Your next menstrual period should begin 4 to 6 weeks after the procedure. If you take birth control pills, your first period will begin after you complete the first cycle of pills.

MEDICATION—You may use nonprescription drugs, such as acetaminophen, for minor pain.

ACTIVITY
• Normal activities may be resumed almost immediately.
• You should have no sexual relations for 1 week following the procedure.

DIET—No special diet.

 CALL YOUR DOCTOR IF

• You experience increased frequency, amount or duration of bleeding (heavier than the heaviest day of your period).
• You develop signs of infection: fever, chills, or muscle aches.
• New, unexplained symptoms develop. Drugs used in treatment may produce side effects.

Spermicides

GENERAL INFORMATION

DEFINITION
• The goal of contraception (or birth control) is to prevent an unplanned pregnancy. The majority of methods of contraception enable sexually active couples to temporarily avoid pregnancy. Permanent birth control is accomplished through sterilization. Be sure you know and understand the different types of birth control available to you, the risks and benefits of each and any side effects, so that you can make an informed choice.
• The vaginal spermicide (in various forms) is a chemical compound that contains one ingredient that kills sperm and another that provides a harmless base to carry the spermicidal agent. The base material is heavy and offers added protection by blocking the opening into the cervix. The choice between a foam, jelly, cream, tablet or suppository will generally depend on personal preference. Most studies reveal that the tablets and suppositories are not as effective as other forms of chemical barriers. Foams are probably the most effective since they spread more evenly to coat the vagina and cervix.

ADVANTAGES
• The effectiveness for birth control ranges from 70% to 80%.
• Do not involve the hormones used in some other forms of birth control that can have side effects.
• Inexpensive; readily available; easy to use.
• Do not require a prescription.
• Provide some degree of lubrication that is helpful for some couples during sexual intercourse.
• Do not interfere with sensation during sex (as a condom sometimes does).
• There is nothing to remove later.
• Can be used as a supplement to other methods of birth control (male and female condoms; diaphragms).
• Easily transported.
• May be used when needed.
• Do not interfere with a woman's future ability to become pregnant, should pregnancy be desired at a later date.
• Offer some protection against sexually transmitted diseases (STDs).

DISADVANTAGES
• Not 100% effective for birth control.
• Some of the products may not fully dissolve in the vagina and can cause friction during sexual intercourse.
• The product must be applied before intercourse and left in the vaginal tract for at least 6 hours afterward (you cannot bathe or shower).
• Some people have minor allergic reactions or irritation to the products; switching brands may help.
• Tend to be messy following intercourse; cause increased leakage (discharge) for most women.

GENERAL MEASURES

INSTRUCTIONS FOR USE
• If an aerosol foam product is used, shake the can vigorously before use to ensure an even distribution of the spermicidal chemical.
• Fill the applicator with the product to be used. Current products use either nonoxynol-9 or octoxynol-3 as the spermicidal agent.
• Gently insert the applicator as far up into the vagina as you can make it go. This will be easier to do if you lie on your back.
• Depress the plunger or squeeze the tube to deliver the product into the vagina.
• Do not apply the product sooner than 1 hour before intercourse. You need not wait longer than 2 or 3 minutes after the application (except for suppositories, which take 10 minutes to melt) before starting intercourse.
• Wait at least 6 hours after intercourse before showering or bathing. If douching is desired, wait at least 8 hours following intercourse.
• For proper use, always follow the directions that come with each particular product; manufacturer's directions may vary from these instructions.

MEDICATIONS—No restrictions.

CALL YOUR DOCTOR IF

You are interested in using a spermicide for contraception and need additional information.

Tubal Ligation

GENERAL INFORMATION

DEFINITION—A method of sterilization that involves blocking the fallopian tubes in such a way that the ovum (egg) is inaccessible for fertilization. Sterilization is considered a permanent form of birth control. In some cases it can be surgically reversed, generally at a considerable cost and with increased risks for subsequent pregnancies (e.g., ectopic pregnancy). It is important to receive personal counseling before deciding to undergo this procedure.

REASONS FOR PROCEDURE—Prevention of unwanted pregnancy.

RISK INCREASES WITH
- Obesity; smoking; poor nutrition.
- Recent or chronic illness.
- Use of drugs such as antihypertensives, muscle relaxants, tranquilizers, sleeping pills, insulin, sedatives, beta-adrenergic blockers or cortisone.

DESCRIPTION OF PROCEDURE
- The procedure may be performed in a hospital or outpatient surgical facility.
- A local anesthetic, a spinal anesthetic, or a general anesthetic may be administered.
- One of several techniques is used to expose the fallopian tubes for surgery.
 Laparoscopy (the most common procedure) involves the use of a telescopic instrument with fiberoptic light and generally requires a pencil-size incision just below the umbilicus (belly button). A second tiny incision may also be made just above the pubic hairline.
 Minilaparotomy involves a vaginal approach and an incision at or just above the pubic hairline. This procedure is often favored in women having the tubal ligation immediately following delivery.
 Laparotomy, which requires a standard surgical incision through the abdomen, is a more complicated method and is usually reserved for cases when other methods have failed, or when there is scarring from previous surgery.
 Posterior colpotomy (rare) is an approach through an incision in the rear of the vagina.
- When the surgery is performed with a laparoscope, the surgeon will first pump either carbon dioxide or nitrous oxide gas into the abdominal cavity in order to elevate the uterus against the abdominal wall. This allows for better visualization of the fallopian tubes and reduces the risk of accidentally damaging other internal organs.
- Once the fallopian tubes are exposed, a small section of each tube is cut free and removed. The severed ends are tied (ligated) or blocked completely by coagulation using an electric current. In some cases, the tubes are clamped off using a clip or band.

- The skin is closed with sutures or clips, which can usually be removed about 1 week after surgery. Often, the sutures are absorbable and don't need to be removed.

PROBABLE OUTCOME
- Expect complete healing, without complications, and sterility for life. Your menstrual periods will continue as usual. Allow about 2 weeks for recovery from surgery.
- You may experience slight abdominal pain and distention (bloating) for a few days after surgery. If gas was used during surgery, you may also have some shoulder pain.

POSSIBLE COMPLICATIONS
- Inadvertent injury to surrounding structures.
- Infection or excessive bleeding.
- Failure of the sterilization procedure (less than 1%). This may result in an ectopic pregnancy.
- Heavier, more painful periods or ovarian cysts following surgery (possibly).

FOLLOW-UP CARE

GENERAL MEASURES
- With most procedures, you will be allowed to return home the same day.
- Use an electric heating pad, a heat lamp or a warm compress to relieve surgical-wound pain.
- Bathe and shower as usual. You may wash the incision gently with mild unscented soap.
- Use another method of birth control until the next menstrual period in case ovulation has occured prior to surgery.

MEDICATION
- Prescription pain medication should generally be required for only 2 to 7 days following the procedure.
- You may use nonprescription drugs, such as acetaminophen, for minor pain.
- Stool softener laxative, for constipation.
- Antibiotics to fight infection.

ACTIVITY
- Return to daily activities and work after one week. Avoid vigorous exercise for 2 weeks.
- Resume driving 3 days after returning home.
- Sexual relations may be resumed when your doctor has determined that healing is complete.

DIET—No restrictions.

CALL YOUR DOCTOR IF

- Pain, swelling, redness, drainage or bleeding increases in the surgical area.
- You develop signs of infection: headache, muscle aches, dizziness, fever or chills.
- You experience nausea, vomiting, constipation or abdominal swelling.
- New, unexplained symptoms develop. Drugs used in treatment may produce side effects.

Tubal Ligation

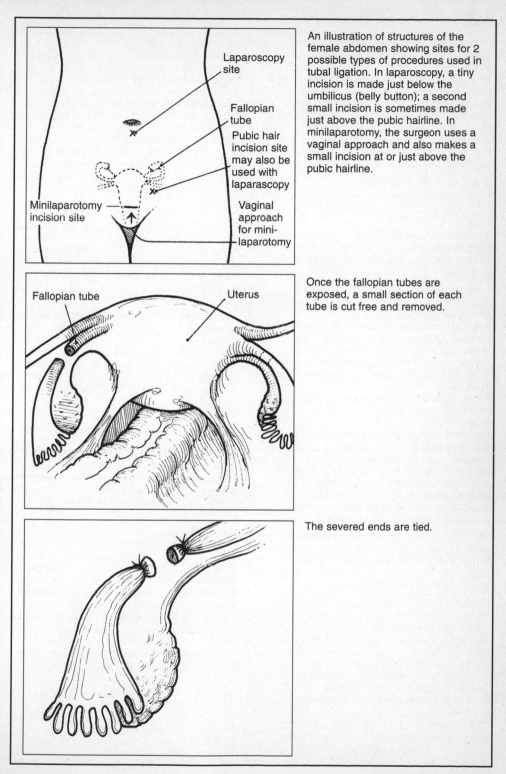

An illustration of structures of the female abdomen showing sites for 2 possible types of procedures used in tubal ligation. In laparoscopy, a tiny incision is made just below the umbilicus (belly button); a second small incision is sometimes made just above the pubic hairline. In minilaparotomy, the surgeon uses a vaginal approach and also makes a small incision at or just above the pubic hairline.

Laparoscopy site

Fallopian tube

Pubic hair incision site may also be used with laparascopy

Vaginal approach for mini-laparotomy

Minilaparotomy incision site

Once the fallopian tubes are exposed, a small section of each tube is cut free and removed.

Fallopian tube

Uterus

The severed ends are tied.

Vasectomy

GENERAL INFORMATION

DEFINITION— A method of sterilization that involves cutting and tying the vas deferens (sperm channels inside the scrotum). The surgery stops the flow of sperm and provides a safe, effective form of birth control without affecting sexual desire or ability. Sterilization is considered a permanent form of birth control. In some cases it can be surgically reversed. Personal counseling prior to the procedure is important to be sure you and your partner understand all aspects of a vasectomy.

REASONS FOR PROCEDURE
• Voluntary sterilization.
• Recurrent epididymitis when caused by chronic prostate infection.

RISK INCREASES WITH
• Emotional instability.
• Recent illness, especially one with fever.

DESCRIPTION OF PROCEDURE
• The procedure may be performed in the doctor's office, outpatient surgical facility or hospital.
• A local anesthetic by injection is administered.
• Incisions are made on both sides of the scrotum. The vas deferens is identified, tied in two places and cut between the ties.
• The divided vas deferens is returned to the scrotum.
• The edges of incised skin are reconstructed with fine sutures, which usually fall out in about 7 days.
• Another method utilized for vasectomy is called no-scalpel technique. It requires 2 specialized instruments and avoids the usual surgical incision. It requires no sutures to close the surgical site and may result in fewer complications. Some men may not be appropriate candidates for this procedure because of differences in scrotal anatomy.

PROBABLE OUTCOME—
Your partner should expect sterility without complications. He may have up to 30 ejaculations before sperm completely disappear from semen. Allow 2 to 3 days for full recovery from surgery.

POSSIBLE COMPLICATIONS
• Collection of blood in the scrotum.
• Surgical-wound infection.
• Sperm granuloma (benign lump in the surgical area).
• Small possibility of reestablishing fertility.
• Pregnancy may still occur in about 1% of cases (often as a result of unprotected intercourse too soon after the procedure).

FOLLOW-UP CARE

GENERAL MEASURES
• He should have someone drive him home. He should wear an athletic support for 24 hours (or longer) and rest in bed for 24 hours.
• He should apply ice bags to both sides of the scrotum (outside the athletic support) for 20 minutes per hour for the first 6 to 8 hours.
• Hard blunt ridges should form along the incisions. While healing, the ridges will recede gradually. Keep the incision area clean and dry.
• Your partner should use an electric heating pad, a heat lamp or a warm compress to relieve incisional pain (beginning 24 hours after surgery).
• He can shower as usual (avoid hot baths for 24 to 48 hours following surgery). He may wash the incision gently with mild unscented soap.
• Use another form of birth control until his sterility is confirmed by the doctor. He will be asked to bring a semen sample to the doctor's office for testing.

MEDICATION
• Prescription pain medication should generally be required for only 2 to 7 days following the procedure.
• He may use nonprescription drugs, such as acetaminophen, for minor pain. Avoid aspirin because of increased bleeding risk.
• Antibiotics, if needed to fight infection.

ACTIVITY
• Your partner should return to daily activities and work as soon as possible (usually 2 to 3 days after surgery).
• He should avoid strenuous activity for 5 to 7 days. Don't swim until the incision is healed.
• Sexual relations may be resumed 1 week after surgery. Use birth control measures until laboratory studies confirm sterility (about 12 weeks).

DIET—No special diet.

 ## CALL YOUR DOCTOR IF

• Pain, swelling, redness, drainage or bleeding increases in the surgical area.
• Signs of infection develop: headache, muscle aches, dizziness or a general ill feeling and fever.
• New, unexplained symptoms develop. Drugs used in treatment may produce side effects.

Vasectomy

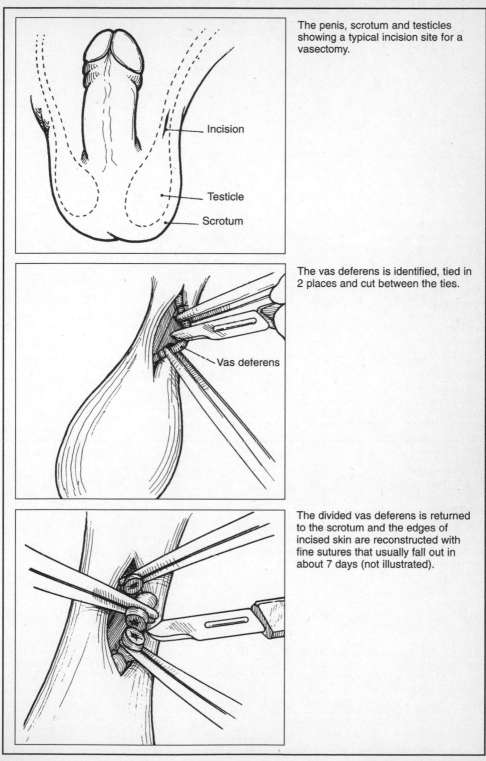

The penis, scrotum and testicles showing a typical incision site for a vasectomy.

Incision

Testicle

Scrotum

The vas deferens is identified, tied in 2 places and cut between the ties.

Vas deferens

The divided vas deferens is returned to the scrotum and the edges of incised skin are reconstructed with fine sutures that usually fall out in about 7 days (not illustrated).

Pregnancy

Abortion, Dilatation and Extraction (D & E)

GENERAL INFORMATION

DEFINITION—A D & E is a technique of emptying the uterus of a pregnancy. It can be used to terminate a pregnancy or to remove a fetus that has died in utero. This method of abortion is recommended only if your pregnancy test was positive and your last menstrual period was 12 to 20 weeks ago. This information and instruction is based on the assumption that you have had counseling and competent guidance in making your decision to seek this procedure for termination of the pregnancy.

REASONS FOR PROCEDURE
• A fetus is no longer alive and emptying the uterus via several methods is being considered.
• Personal concerns about the social or economic aspects of an unplanned pregnancy.
• Continuing with the pregnancy may pose a threat to the life of the mother.
• Mother has a genetic condition that the fetus is at significant risk of acquiring, or the fetus has been tested and is known to have the condition (such as cystic fibrosis).
• Pregnancy resulted from a rape or incest.
• Fetus is affected with a major disorder such as chromosomal abnormality or birth defect.
• Fear that the fetus has been harmed by medications or other conditions.

RISK INCREASES WITH
• Obesity.
• Smoking.
• Poor nutrition.
• Recent or chronic illness.
• Use of drugs such as antihypertensives, muscle relaxants, tranquilizers, sleep inducers, insulin, sedatives, narcotics, beta-adrenergic blockers or cortisone.

DESCRIPTION OF PROCEDURE
• In most instances, the D & E is an outpatient, operative procedure carried out under a sedative and local anesthetic. Sometimes, a general anesthesia is used.
• The cervix is dilated to make it ready for the procedure. Sometimes, laminaria (rods of sterile seaweed) are inserted into the cervix 2 to 24 hours before the abortion to help slowly soften and dilate the cervix. Other times, a series of increasingly larger rods are used for dilatation.
• Surgical instruments are then used to remove the fetal tissue and placentae. A curettage (scraping of the uterus) may follow.

PROBABLE OUTCOME
• Emptying of the pregnant uterus.
• Recovery is rapid, with the patient usually returning home within hours.

POSSIBLE COMPLICATIONS
• Complications such as lacerations or tearing of the cervix, perforation of the uterus, and heavy bleeding do occur, but they are rare.

• In some cases, a repeat procedure may be required (uncommon).

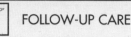

FOLLOW-UP CARE

GENERAL MEASURES
• Following the procedure, rest quietly at home for the remainder of the day.
• If you have pain, place a heating pad or hot-water bottle on the abdomen or back. Hot baths frequently promote muscle relaxation and relieve discomfort. Repeat the baths as often as they provide comfort.
• You will probably experience intermittent bleeding for the next 10 to 14 days, which may be light or moderately heavy; bleeding may decrease with rest and increase with standing, walking or other activity. Use external sanitary pads for bleeding.
• Contraception can often be initiated shortly after the procedure. If you wish to take birth control pills, begin taking them either on the night you return from surgery or the next day. If you prefer an IUD, diaphragm or cervical cap, the fitting can often be made during your next doctor's appointment.
• Your next menstrual period should begin 4 to 6 weeks after the procedure. If you take birth control pills, your first period will begin after you complete the first cycle of pills.

MEDICATION
• Prescription pain medication should generally be required for only 2 to 7 days following the procedure.
• You may use nonprescription drugs, such as acetaminophen, for minor pain. Avoid aspirin.
• Antibiotics to reduce the risk of infection.
• Drugs such as methylergonovine (Methergine) or oxytocin (Pitocin), to help your uterus contract, will usually be prescribed.

ACTIVITY
• Normal activities may be resumed almost immediately.
• You should have no sexual relations, should not use tampons, and should not douche for at least 2 weeks following the operation.

DIET—No special diet.

CALL YOUR DOCTOR IF

• You experience increased frequency, amount, or duration of bleeding (heavier than the heaviest day of your period).
• You develop fever, with a temperature of over 100° F orally.
• You experience prolonged abdominal pain or pressure on the bladder or rectum.
• New, unexplained symptoms develop. Drugs used in treatment may produce side effects.

Abortion, Dilatation and Extraction (D & E)

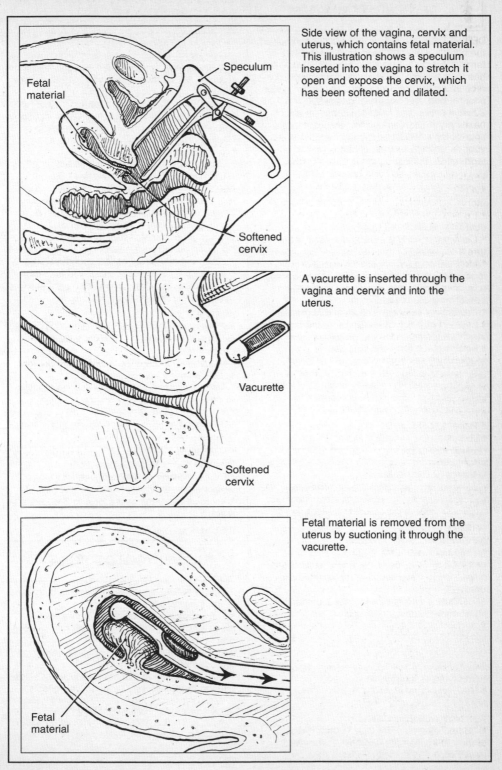

Fetal material

Speculum

Softened cervix

Side view of the vagina, cervix and uterus, which contains fetal material. This illustration shows a speculum inserted into the vagina to stretch it open and expose the cervix, which has been softened and dilated.

Vacurette

Softened cervix

A vacurette is inserted through the vagina and cervix and into the uterus.

Fetal material is removed from the uterus by suctioning it through the vacurette.

Fetal material

Abortion, Hysterotomy

GENERAL INFORMATION

DEFINITION—The hysterotomy is a technique of emptying the uterus of a pregnancy. It can be used to terminate a pregnancy or to remove a fetus that has died in utero. In this method, a surgical procedure similar to a cesarean section is performed. It is reserved for special circumstances (i.e., failure to complete a midtrimester abortion due to cervical stenosis or other complications) and usually is not the primary abortion method chosen. This information and instruction is based on the assumption that you have had, or will have, counseling and competent guidance in making your decision to seek this procedure for termination of the pregnancy.

REASONS FOR PROCEDURE
• A fetus is no longer alive and emptying the uterus via several methods is being considered.
• Personal concerns about the social or economic aspects of an unplanned pregnancy.
• Continuing with the pregnancy may pose a threat to the life of the mother.
• Mother has a genetic condition that the fetus is at significant risk of acquiring, or the fetus has been tested and is known to have the condition (such as cystic fibrosis).
• Pregnancy resulted from a rape or incest.
• Fetus is affected with a major disorder such as chromosomal abnormality or birth defect.
• Fear that the fetus has been harmed by medications or other conditions.

RISK INCREASES WITH
• Obesity.
• Smoking.
• Poor nutrition.
• Recent or chronic illness.
• Use of drugs such as antihypertensives, muscle relaxants, tranquilizers, sleep inducers, insulin, sedatives, narcotics, beta-adrenergic blockers or cortisone.

DESCRIPTION OF PROCEDURE
• A general anesthesia is used.
• An incision is made in the abdomen and then in the uterus. Fetal tissue and placentae are removed.
• The uterine wall is sewed back together and the abdominal opening closed.

PROBABLE OUTCOME
• Emptying of the pregnant uterus.
• Expect complete healing without complications. Allow yourself several weeks for recovery from surgery.

POSSIBLE COMPLICATIONS
• Excessive bleeding.
• Surgical-wound infection.
• Depending on the the type of uterine scar, there is often an increased risk of uterine rupture in a future pregnancy.

FOLLOW-UP CARE

GENERAL MEASURES
• Use sanitary pads for bleeding, which may last for several days. If bleeding continues more than 14 days after surgery, you may then use tampons.
• If you have pain, place a heating pad or hot-water bottle on the abdomen or back. Hot baths frequently aid muscle relaxation and relieve discomfort. Repeat baths as often as they provide comfort.
• Contraception can often be initiated shortly after the procedure. If you wish to take birth control pills, begin taking them either on the night you return from surgery or the next day; a backup form of contraception should be used for the first month. If you prefer an IUD, diaphragm or cervical cap, the fitting can often be made during your next doctor's appointment.
• Your next menstrual period should begin 4 to 6 weeks after the procedure. If you take birth control pills, your first period will begin after you complete the first cycle of pills.

MEDICATION
• Prescription pain medication should generally be required for only 2 to 7 days following the procedure.
• Stool softener laxative, if needed to prevent constipation.
• Antibiotics are sometimes prescribed to fight or prevent infection.
• You may use nonprescription drugs, such as acetaminophen, for minor pain. Avoid aspirin.

ACTIVITY
• Have someone drive you home from surgery. Resume normal activities slowly.
• Do not douche or use tampons for at least 2 weeks after surgery.
• Avoid sexual intercourse for 4 to 6 weeks after surgery.

DIET—No special diet.

CALL YOUR DOCTOR IF

• Pain, swelling, redness or drainage increases in the surgical area.
• You develop signs of infection: headache, muscle aches, dizziness or a general ill feeling and fever.
• You experience nausea, vomiting, constipation or abdominal swelling.
• New, unexplained symptoms develop. Drugs used in treatment may produce side effects.

Abortion, Hysterotomy

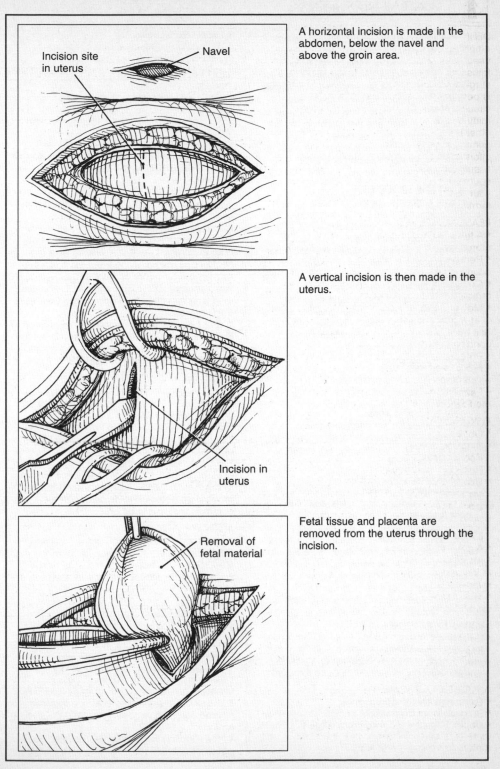

Incision site in uterus

Navel

A horizontal incision is made in the abdomen, below the navel and above the groin area.

Incision in uterus

A vertical incision is then made in the uterus.

Removal of fetal material

Fetal tissue and placenta are removed from the uterus through the incision.

Abortion, Intra-amniotic Instillation

GENERAL INFORMATION

DEFINITION—Intra-amniotic instillation is a technique of electively terminating a pregnancy. This method involves amniocentesis (see Glossary) and injection of various fluids into the amniotic sac to initiate labor. It is recommended only if your pregnancy test was positive and your last menstrual period was 16 to 24 weeks ago. This information and instruction is based on the assumption that you have had counseling and competent guidance in making your decision to seek this procedure for termination of the pregnancy.

REASONS FOR PROCEDURE
• Personal concerns about the social or economic aspects of an unplanned pregnancy.
• Continuing with the pregnancy may pose a threat to the life of the mother.
• Mother has a genetic condition that the fetus is at significant risk of acquiring, or the fetus has been tested and is known to have the condition (such as cystic fibrosis).
• Pregnancy resulted from a rape or incest.
• Fetus is affected with a major disorder such as chromosomal abnormality or birth defect.
• Fear that the fetus has been harmed by medications or other conditions.

RISK INCREASES WITH
• Obesity.
• Smoking.
• Poor nutrition.
• Recent or chronic illness.
• Use of drugs such as antihypertensives, muscle relaxants, tranquilizers, sleep inducers, insulin, sedatives, narcotics, beta-adrenergic blockers or cortisone.

DESCRIPTION OF PROCEDURE
• The procedure is performed in a hospital.
• The cervix is usually dilated ahead of the procedure using sterile seaweed (laminaria).
• Under local anesthesia, the doctor will carefully insert a hollow needle into the uterus through the abdomen. The needle's penetration of the uterus will cause some pain, but it should not last long and should hurt no worse than an injection in any other part of the body.
• Amniotic fluid is withdrawn and a solution is introduced into the cavity, either in a single dose or as 2 doses 6 hours apart.
• Contractions begin 12 to 24 hours later and the dead fetus and placenta are delivered. A synthetic hormone may be given to continue contractions until all tissue has been expelled.

PROBABLE OUTCOME
• Termination of the pregnancy.
• Complete healing without complications. Allow about 1 week for recovery from surgery.

POSSIBLE COMPLICATIONS
• Retained placenta (usually can be removed with the use of surgical instruments).
• Excessive bleeding.
• Perforation or infection of the uterus.
• Cervical laceration (tearing).
• Failure of the procedure to expel all the tissue.

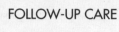

FOLLOW-UP CARE

GENERAL MEASURES
• Use sanitary pads for bleeding, which may last for several days. If bleeding continues more than 14 days after surgery, you may then use tampons.
• If you have pain, place a heating pad or hot-water bottle on the abdomen or back. Hot baths often aid muscle relaxation and relieve discomfort. Repeat baths as often as needed.
• Contraception can often be initiated shortly after the procedure. If you wish to take birth control pills, begin taking them either on the night you return from surgery or the next day. If you prefer an IUD, diaphragm or cervical cap, the fitting can often be made during your next doctor's visit.
• Your next menstrual period should begin 4 to 6 weeks after the procedure. If you take birth control pills, your first period will begin after you complete the first cycle of pills.

MEDICATION
• Prescription pain medication should generally be required for only 2 to 7 days following the procedure.
• Stool softener laxative to prevent constipation.
• Antibiotics are sometimes prescribed to fight or prevent infection.
• You may use nonprescription drugs, such as acetaminophen, for minor pain. Avoid aspirin.
• Drugs such as methylergonovine (Methergine) or oxytocin (Pitocin), to help your uterus contract, will usually be prescribed.

ACTIVITY
• Have someone drive you home from surgery. Rest quietly there for the remainder of the day. Resume normal activities slowly the next day.
• Abstain from sexual relations for 2 weeks after surgery.

DIET—No special diet.

CALL YOUR DOCTOR IF

• Unexplained vaginal bleeding develops.
• You experience nausea, vomiting, constipation, diarrhea or abdominal swelling.
• You develop signs of infection: headache, muscle aches, dizziness or a general ill feeling and fever.
• New, unexplained symptoms develop. Drugs used in treatment may produce side effects.

Abortion, Intra-amniotic Instillation

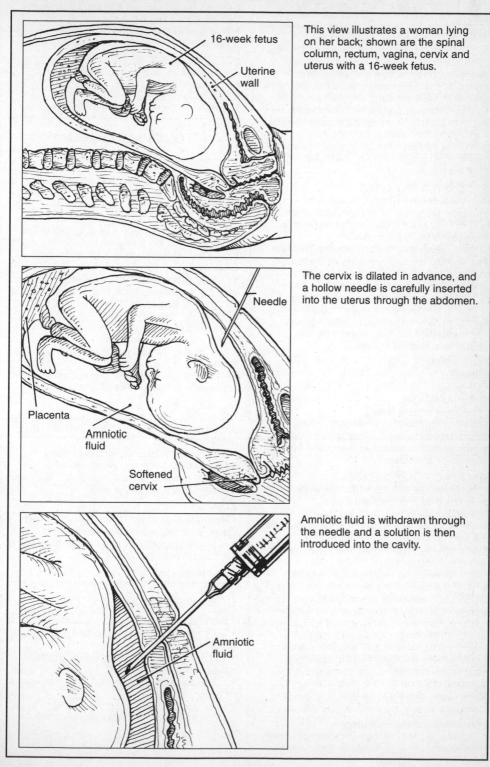

16-week fetus

Uterine wall

This view illustrates a woman lying on her back; shown are the spinal column, rectum, vagina, cervix and uterus with a 16-week fetus.

Needle

Placenta

Amniotic fluid

Softened cervix

The cervix is dilated in advance, and a hollow needle is carefully inserted into the uterus through the abdomen.

Amniotic fluid

Amniotic fluid is withdrawn through the needle and a solution is then introduced into the cavity.

Abortion, Menstrual Extraction

GENERAL INFORMATION

DEFINITION—Menstrual extraction is a technique of electively terminating a pregnancy. This procedure is done in the early weeks of pregnancy, no more than 2 weeks after a missed period. Pregnancy may or may not have been diagnosed, as some women do not wish to know if they are pregnant. This information and instruction is based on the assumption that you have had, or will have, counseling and competent guidance in making your decision to seek this procedure for termination of the pregnancy.

REASONS FOR PROCEDURE
• Personal concerns about the social or economic aspects of an unplanned pregnancy.
• Continuing with the pregnancy may pose a threat to the life of the mother.
• Mother has a genetic condition that the fetus is at significant risk of acquiring, or the fetus has been tested and is known to have the condition (such as cystic fibrosis).
• Pregnancy resulted from a rape or incest.
• Fetus is affected with a major disorder such as chromosomal abnormality or birth defect.
• Fear that the fetus has been harmed by medications or other conditions.

RISK INCREASES WITH
• Obesity.
• Smoking.
• Poor nutrition.
• Recent or chronic illness.
• Use of drugs such as antihypertensives, muscle relaxants, tranquilizers, sleep inducers, insulin, sedatives, narcotics, beta-adrenergic blockers or cortisone.

DESCRIPTION OF PROCEDURE
• The procedure may be performed in the doctor's office or an outpatient clinic.
• There is usually no need for an anesthetic, however a local anesthesia may be injected into the area around the cervix if necessary.
• When the cervix is dilated, there may be some feelings of pressure.
• A thin plastic tube (a cannula) is inserted through the canal of the cervix into the cavity of the uterus. The tube is connected to a suction apparatus such as a syringe or other suction machine. Gentle suction is applied for just a few minutes while the doctor sweeps the tube around inside the uterus. These maneuvers gently remove the implanted fertilized egg.
• During the procedure, you may experience cramping discomfort of the uterus, some nausea, and sweating or a feeling of faintness.

PROBABLE OUTCOME
• Termination of the pregnancy.
• Expect complete healing without complications. Allow about 1 week for recovery from surgery.

• There is no evidence of problems with later pregnancies for women who have had uncomplicated first-trimester suction abortions.
• Your next menstrual period should begin 4 to 6 weeks after the procedure.

POSSIBLE COMPLICATIONS
• Rarely, the procedure is unsuccessful in terminating the pregnancy.
• Excessive bleeding.
• Perforation or infection of the uterus.

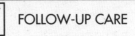

FOLLOW-UP CARE

GENERAL MEASURES
• Use sanitary pads for bleeding, which may last for several days. If bleeding continues more than 14 days after surgery, you may then use tampons.
• If you have pain, place a heating pad or hot-water bottle on the abdomen or back. Hot baths frequently aid muscle relaxation and relieve discomfort.
• Contraception can often be initiated shortly after the procedure. If you wish to take birth control pills, begin taking them within 24 hours after the procedure. The fitting for an IUD, diaphragm or a cervical cap can often be made during your next doctor's visit.
• Your next menstrual period should begin 4 to 6 weeks after the procedure. If you take birth control pills, your first period will begin after you complete the first cycle of pills.

MEDICATION
• Prescription pain medication should generally be required for only 2 to 7 days following the procedure.
• Stool softener laxative for constipation.
• Antibiotics to fight or prevent infection.
• You may use nonprescription drugs, such as acetaminophen, for minor pain.

ACTIVITY
• Rest quietly at home for the rest of the day. Resume normal activities slowly the next day.
• Avoid sexual relations and the use of tampons for 2 weeks after surgery.

DIET—No special diet.

CALL YOUR DOCTOR IF

• Pain, swelling, redness or drainage increases in the genital area.
• You develop signs of infection: headache, muscle aches, or a general ill feeling and fever.
• You experience nausea, vomiting, constipation or abdominal swelling.
• New, unexplained symptoms develop. Drugs used in treatment may produce side effects.

Abortion, Menstrual Extraction

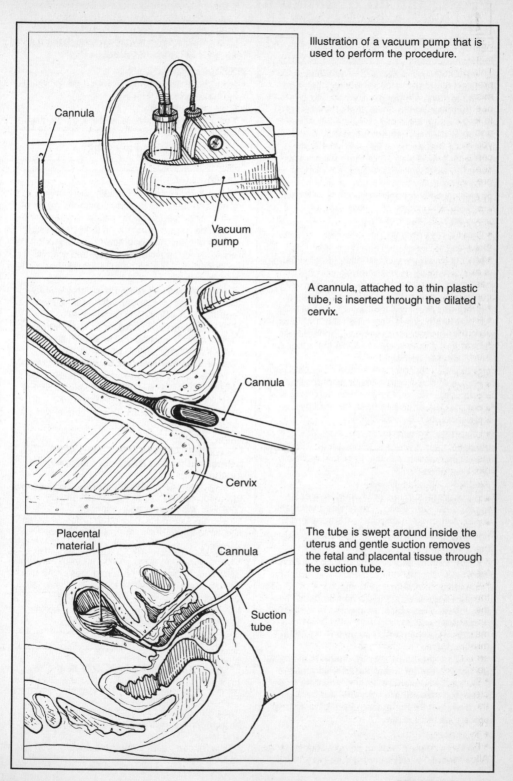

Illustration of a vacuum pump that is used to perform the procedure.

Cannula

Vacuum pump

A cannula, attached to a thin plastic tube, is inserted through the dilated cervix.

Cannula

Cervix

The tube is swept around inside the uterus and gentle suction removes the fetal and placental tissue through the suction tube.

Placental material

Cannula

Suction tube

Abortion, Prostaglandin Induced (Prostaglandin Instillation)

 GENERAL INFORMATION

DEFINITION—This procedure is a technique of emptying the uterus of a pregnancy. It can be used to terminate a pregnancy or to remove a fetus that has died in utero. In this method of abortion, drugs are used to initiate labor; this method is usually recommended only if your pregnancy test was positive and your last menstrual period was 16 or more weeks ago. This information and instruction is based on the assumption that you have had, or will have, counseling and competent guidance in making your decision to seek this procedure for termination of the pregnancy.

REASONS FOR PROCEDURE
• A fetus is no longer alive and emptying the uterus via several methods is being considered.
• Personal concerns about the social or economic aspects of an unplanned pregnancy.
• Continuing with the pregnancy may pose a threat to the life of the mother.
• Mother has a genetic condition that the fetus is at significant risk of acquiring, or the fetus has been tested and is known to have the condition (such as cystic fibrosis).
• Pregnancy resulted from a rape or incest.
• Fetus is affected with a major disorder such as chromosomal abnormality or birth defect.
• Fear that the fetus has been harmed by medications or other conditions.

RISK INCREASES WITH
• Obesity.
• Smoking.
• Poor nutrition.
• Recent or chronic illness.
• Use of drugs such as antihypertensives, muscle relaxants, tranquilizers, sleep inducers, insulin, sedatives, narcotics, beta-adrenergic blockers or cortisone.

DESCRIPTION OF PROCEDURE
• Prostaglandins stimulate uterine contractions. Either vaginal prostaglandin E2 in the form of a suppository or intramuscular injections of 15(S)-15-methyl prostaglandin F2a can be used. The prostaglandin may also be injected directly into the amniotic sac.
• The drugs are repeated every few hours until abortion occurs.
• If needed, there are several methods available that help soften (or ripen) the cervix to make it ready for the procedure. Often, laminaria (rods of sterile seaweed) are placed in the cervix a few hours before the procedure begins, to help facilitate cervical dilation.

PROBABLE OUTCOME
• Complete healing without complications. Allow about 1 week for recovery from surgery.

• Side effects from the drugs can include nausea, vomiting, diarrhea, facial flushing and shortness of breath (bronchospasm).

POSSIBLE COMPLICATIONS
• Retained placentae (usually can be removed with the use of surgical instruments).
• Excessive bleeding.
• Failure of the procedure to expel all the tissue.

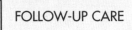 FOLLOW-UP CARE

GENERAL MEASURES
• Use sanitary pads for bleeding, which may last for several days. If bleeding continues 10 to 14 days after surgery, you may then use tampons.
• If you have pain, place a heating pad or hot-water bottle on the abdomen or back. Hot baths frequently aid muscle relaxation and relieve discomfort. Repeat baths as often as they provide comfort.
• Contraception can often be initiated shortly after the procedure. If you wish to take birth control pills, begin taking them either on the night you return from surgery or the next day; a backup form of contraception should be used for the first month. If you prefer an IUD, diaphragm or cervical cap, the fitting can often be made during your next doctor's appointment.
• Your next menstrual period should begin 4 to 6 weeks after the procedure. If you take birth control pills, your first period will begin after you complete the first cycle of pills.

MEDICATION
• Prescription pain medication should generally be required for only 2 to 7 days following the procedure.
• Drugs such as methylergonovine (Methergine) or oxytocin (Pitocin), to help your uterus contract, will usually be prescribed.
• You may use nonprescription drugs, such as acetaminophen, for minor pain. Avoid aspirin.

ACTIVITY
• Have someone drive you home from surgery. Rest quietly there for the remainder of the day. Resume normal activities slowly the next day, if you feel able.
• Avoid sexual relations and do not douche or use tampons for 2 weeks after surgery.

DIET—No special diet.

 CALL YOUR DOCTOR IF

• Excessive vaginal bleeding develops.
• You develop signs of infection: headache, muscle aches, dizziness or a general ill feeling and fever.
• New, unexplained symptoms develop. Drugs used in treatment may produce side effects.

Abortion, Prostaglandin Induced
(Prostaglandin Instillation)

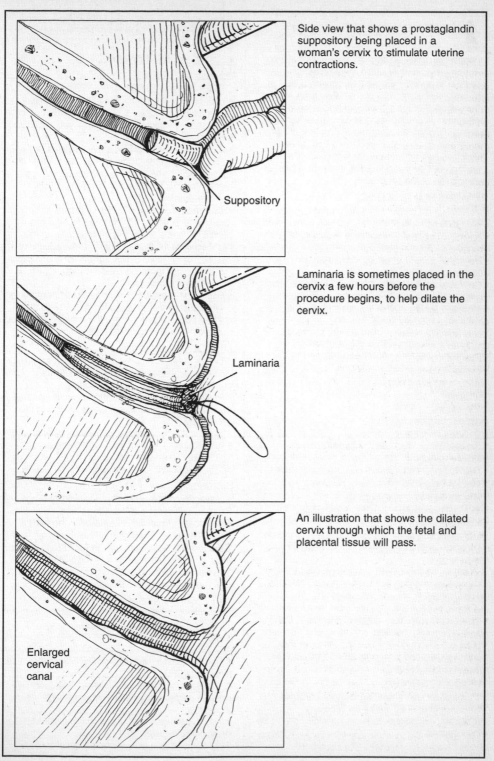

Side view that shows a prostaglandin suppository being placed in a woman's cervix to stimulate uterine contractions.

Suppository

Laminaria is sometimes placed in the cervix a few hours before the procedure begins, to help dilate the cervix.

Laminaria

An illustration that shows the dilated cervix through which the fetal and placental tissue will pass.

Enlarged cervical canal

Abortion, Suction Curettage

GENERAL INFORMATION

DEFINITION—Suction curettage is a technique of emptying the uterus of a pregnancy. It can be used to terminate a pregnancy or to remove a fetus that has died in utero. It involves the removal of a fetus and accompanying tissue of the pregnancy from the uterus with instrumental evacuation through the vagina and is usually performed in pregnancies of 12 weeks duration or less. This information and instruction is based on the assumption that you have had, or will have, counseling and competent guidance in making your decision to seek this procedure for termination of the pregnancy.

REASONS FOR PROCEDURE
• A fetus is no longer alive and emptying the uterus via several methods is being considered.
• Concerns about the social or economic aspects of an unplanned pregnancy.
• Continuing with the pregnancy may pose a threat to the life of the mother.
• Mother has a genetic condition that the fetus is at significant risk of acquiring, or the fetus has been tested and is known to have the condition (such as cystic fibrosis).
• Pregnancy resulted from a rape or incest.
• Fetus is affected with a major disorder.
• Fear that the fetus has been harmed by medications or other conditions.

RISK INCREASES WITH
• Obesity.
• Smoking.
• Poor nutrition.
• Recent or chronic illness.
• Use of drugs such as antihypertensives, muscle relaxants, tranquilizers, sleep inducers, insulin, sedatives, narcotics, beta-adrenergic blockers or cortisone.

DESCRIPTION OF PROCEDURE
• A local anesthetic is used, sometimes accompanied by a tranquilizer.
• The opening of the cervix is dilated by the use of instruments or laminaria (rods of sterile seaweed).
• A small, hollow plastic tube is passed through the vagina and cervix into the uterus. The tube is connected to a suction apparatus.
• Gentle suction through the tube removes the uterine contents. You may feel cramps in the lower abdomen, nausea, sweating and faintness.
• The tube is removed and the lining of the uterus is scraped with a curette to be sure all the placental tissue is removed.

PROBABLE OUTCOME
• Expect complete healing without complications. Allow about 1 week for recovery.
• The procedure should have no effect on future pregnancies.

POSSIBLE COMPLICATIONS
• Excessive bleeding.
• Perforation or infection of the uterus.
• Potential psychological problems.

FOLLOW-UP CARE

GENERAL MEASURES
• Use sanitary pads for bleeding, which may last for several days. If bleeding continues for more than 14 days after surgery, you may use tampons.
• If you have pain, place a heating pad or hot-water bottle on the abdomen or back. Hot baths frequently aid muscle relaxation and relieve discomfort. Repeat baths as often as they provide comfort.
• Contraception can often be initiated shortly after the procedure. If you wish to take birth control pills, begin taking them either on the night you return from surgery or the next day. If you prefer an IUD, diaphragm or cervical cap, the fitting can often be made during your next doctor's appointment.
• Your next menstrual period should begin 4 to 6 weeks after the procedure. If you take birth control pills, your first period will begin after you complete the first cycle of pills.

MEDICATION
• Drugs such as methylergonovine (Methergine) or oxytocin (Pitocin), to help your uterus contract, will usually be prescribed.
• Prescription pain medication should generally be required for only 2 to 7 days following the procedure.
• Stool softener laxative to prevent constipation.
• Antibiotics to fight or prevent infection.
• You may use nonprescription drugs, such as acetaminophen, for minor pain. Avoid aspirin.

ACTIVITY
• Have someone drive you home from surgery. Rest quietly for the remainder of the day.
• Resume normal activities slowly the next day, if you feel able. Light or moderate vaginal bleeding will occur on and off for 10 to 14 days after surgery. Bed rest will reduce bleeding.
• Avoid sexual relations and do not douche or use tampons for 2 weeks after surgery.

DIET—No special diet.

CALL YOUR DOCTOR IF

• Pain, swelling, redness or drainage increases in the surgical area.
• You develop signs of infection: headache, muscle aches, dizziness or a general ill feeling and fever.
• You experience nausea, vomiting, constipation or abdominal swelling.
• New, unexplained symptoms develop. Drugs used in treatment may produce side effects.

Abortion, Suction Curettage

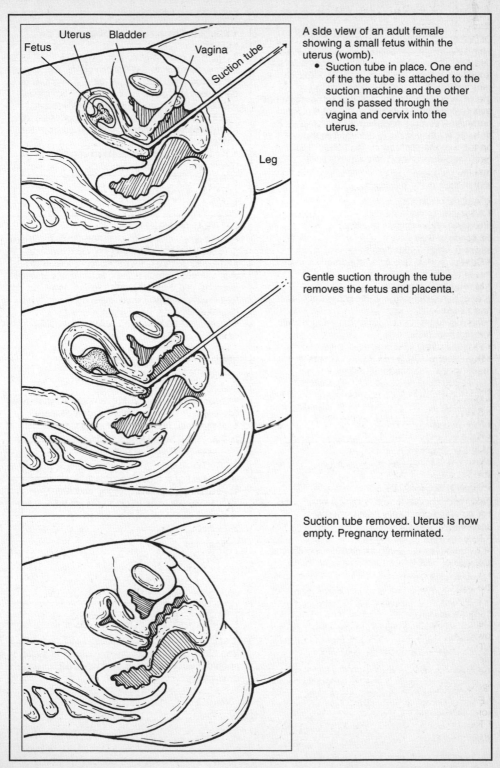

A side view of an adult female showing a small fetus within the uterus (womb).

- Suction tube in place. One end of the the tube is attached to the suction machine and the other end is passed through the vagina and cervix into the uterus.

Gentle suction through the tube removes the fetus and placenta.

Suction tube removed. Uterus is now empty. Pregnancy terminated.

Labels: Fetus, Uterus, Bladder, Vagina, Suction tube, Leg

Abruptio Placentae
(Placental Abruption)

 GENERAL INFORMATION

DEFINITION—Separation of the placenta (also called the after-birth) from the wall of the uterus, generally occurring in the latter half of pregnancy. The placenta carries all nourishment and oxygen to the unborn child. If the placenta partially separates prematurely, the child's life may be endangered. Treatment depends on the severity of the separation, the condition of the fetus and the duration of the pregnancy.

SIGNS & SYMPTOMS
Small separation of the placenta:
• Vaginal bleeding.
• Mild pain or discomfort.
• Unborn child remains healthy.
Large separation:
• Heavy vaginal bleeding.
• Severe pain in the lower abdomen or back.
• Uterine contractions.
• Hard, tender abdomen.
• Shock (rapid heartbeat, rapid breathing and dizziness).
• Fetal distress; heartbeat of the unborn child may be inaudible.
• Coagulopathy (disseminated intravascular coagulopathy [DIC])—certain elements of the placenta are released into the mother's circulation causing blood clotting defects. Symptoms can include nosebleed, blood in the urine, oozing from puncture sites, bleeding into the skin, round red spots on the skin.

CAUSES—Unknown.

RISK INCREASES WITH
• High blood pressure (hypertension).
• Smoking.
• Women over age 35.
• Women who have had several pregnancies.
• A previous pregnancy with placental separation.
• A direct blow to the uterus.
• Chronic disease, such as diabetes mellitus.
• Abuse of illicit drugs (particularly cocaine).

HOW TO PREVENT
• If pregnant, don't engage in activity more vigorous than what you were accustomed to before pregnancy.
• Avoid risk factors (listed above) when possible.
• Since the cause is unknown, there is no assured way to prevent the problem.

PROBABLE OUTCOME—When the separation is less severe and with immediate medical care, the outlook for mother and fetus is good.

POSSIBLE COMPLICATIONS
• Shock or life-threatening bleeding in the mother.
• Death of unborn child and/or mother.
• Brain damage to the unborn child.
• If preterm placental separation is slight and early delivery of unborn child is not deemed necessary, intrauterine growth retardation (IUGR) (see Glossary) may occur, possibly due to decreased blood and nourishment from the placenta.
• 10% to 17% of patients have abruptio placentae in a future pregnancy.

 HOW TO TREAT

GENERAL MEASURES
• Abruptio placentae is an emergency, but there is usually time to obtain advice by telephone and arrange safe transportation to the hospital. Panic is not helpful. If the placental separation is slight, you may be able to return home for bed rest and close observation after examination.
• Hospitalization required (except for mild cases).
• Surgery to deliver the unborn child by cesarean section or vaginal delivery (sometimes).

MEDICATION
• Oxytocin (Pitocin), a drug to induce labor, may be used if immediate delivery is necessary.
• Intravenous fluids may be necessary.
• Blood transfusion may be necessary to replace the amount of blood lost.

ACTIVITY—If you are able to remain at home, rest in bed until bleeding and other symptoms cease. Do not resume normal activities until specific instructions to do so are given to you.

DIET
• If you are resting at home, continue with your regular diet.
• If hospitalized, a liquid-only diet may be prescribed until it is determined that surgery is not likely. Solid food may cause risk if emergency surgery becomes necessary.

 CALL YOUR DOCTOR IF

You have bleeding (anything more than slight spotting) during pregnancy. This is an emergency!

Alpha-Fetoprotein Assessment (Triple Screen; Human Chorionic Gonadotropin Test; Unconjugated Estriol Test)

 GENERAL INFORMATION

DEFINITION—A relatively common screening of a blood sample taken from the mother usually during the 15th to 20th week of pregnancy. Many women find this prenatal testing useful; 40% of pregnant women have the test each year. The primary measurement on the triple screen is for maternal serum alpha-fetoprotein (MSAFP or AFP), a protein produced by the liver cells of every fetus, which is present in both the amniotic fluid and the mother's blood. Testing for human chorionic gonadotropin (hCG) and unconjugated estriol (uE3) is combined with the AFP test to help improve the results.

REASONS FOR PROCEDURE—To help rule out possible fetal abnormalities. The triple test is for screening purposes only and further testing is always necessary for accurate diagnosis of any problem.

RISK INCREASES WITH—No expected risks with the blood test itself. Testing results may be inaccurate if there is an uncertain or imprecise estimate of the gestational age of the pregancy. In cases when the due date is at all uncertain, an ultrasound to confirm the fetal size should be obtained first.

DESCRIPTION OF PROCEDURE—Blood is usually drawn by needle from the upper arm (sometimes from the finger, heel or earlobe). The sample is then sent to a laboratory for testing. Results are available in a few days.

PROBABLE OUTCOME
• The majority of time (over 95%), the test results fall within the normal range.
• About 3% to 5% of women tested will have AFP levels outside the normal range the first time and 3% of these women will still have abnormal levels on a repeat blood test. These women will be offered genetic counseling, which may lead to further testing such as amniocentesis, ultrasound or other prenatal tests to help verify if a problem exists.
• Higher concentrations of AFP levels may indicate:
  A neural tube defect such as spina bifida (failure of the spinal column to close completely).
  Other rarer abnormalities.
  Threatened abortion.
  Twins (or triplets) are expected.
  Abruptio placentae.
  The pregnancy is inaccurately dated.
  The fetus is no longer alive.

• AFP levels can be abnormally low, which may indicate:
  The pregnancy is inaccurately dated.
  Trisomy-21 (Down syndrome).

POSSIBLE COMPLICATIONS
• Some discoloration, soreness or swelling may develop at the puncture site.
• False-positive results of the test which can cause anxiety and worry for the parents-to-be.

 FOLLOW-UP CARE

GENERAL MEASURES
• Use warm compresses if blood collects under the puncture site or if the area becomes tender, red or painful.
• Before you take any action on the basis of the results of your MSAFP screen or any other prenatal testing, be sure that any results that show a possible abnormality have been evaluated by an experienced physician who specializes in genetics, or by a genetic counselor. If you continue to have any doubts after consulting with a genetics specialist, obtain a second medical opinion.

MEDICATION—Medicine is usually not necessary.

ACTIVITY—No restrictions.

DIET—No special diet.

 CALL YOUR DOCTOR IF

• Following the test, you have any unusual pain or reaction at the puncture site.
• You need further information about the testing or test results.

Amniocentesis

GENERAL INFORMATION

DEFINITION—Removal of fluid from the amniotic sac during pregnancy.

REASONS FOR PROCEDURE—Laboratory examination of amniotic fluid helps diagnose abnormalities of the unborn child. Although genetic amniocentesis may be done as early as the 11th week of pregnancy, or as late as the third trimester, the best time is usually between the 14th and 20th weeks of pregnancy. There is ample fluid for the testing, time to treat certain problems before the baby is born and enough time exists if the parents decide not to continue with the pregnancy. Amniocentesis may also be performed in the third trimester to assess fetal lung development. Amniocentesis is often done for one or more of the following reasons:
- Maternal age is over 35 years.
- Patient had abnormal results from blood screening test, such as maternal serum alpha-fetoprotein (MSAFP or AFP) test.
- Metabolic disease risk (because of previous experience or family history).
- Neural tube defect risk (because of previous experience or family history).
- Either parent has a chromosome abnormality.
- Mother has previously had a child with a chromosome abnormality, such as Down syndrome.
- Mother carries a sex-linked abnormality, and the sex of the unborn child must be determined.
- Mother produces antibodies, most commonly to the fetal blood cells, that can cause the unborn child to be anemic. The amniotic fluid is tested for a chemical (bilirubin) that serves as a marker for fetal anemia.
- Unborn child's maturity or other conditions must be determined late in pregnancy.
- To evaluate pregnancy for infection.
- To evaluate fetal lung maturity.
- To remove excess amniotic fluid, most commonly in twins when one baby has too much amniotic fluid and the other has too little.

RISK INCREASES WITH
- Obesity.
- Previous abdominal surgery.
- Previous infection in pelvic organs.

DESCRIPTION OF PROCEDURE
- A local anesthetic may be injected into the abdomen.
- A hollow needle is inserted through the abdominal wall into the uterus. The needle will cause temporary pain but should not hurt more than any injection. Some women report mild to moderate cramping, or a feeling of pressure, during the procedure.
- Amniocentesis is usually performed using continuous ultrasound to allow constant view of the needle's path.
- A small amount of amniotic fluid is suctioned through the needle, and the needle is then removed. Your body will make more fluid to replace the amount that is removed.

PROBABLE OUTCOME—Results of the laboratory test of the amniotic fluid take 10–14 days. More than 95% of amniocentesis tests indicate no abnormalities. Some couples who may have high risk factors have the procedure done to reduce their anxiety during pregnancy. However, normal amniocentesis results cannot guarantee a child without defects. At present there are not tests for all abnormalities.

POSSIBLE COMPLICATIONS
- Miscarriage triggered by procedure (rare).
- Damage to the baby (uncommon), such as slight dimpling of the skin where the baby was poked during the procedure and, very rarely, death. With standard amniocentesis at 14 to 20 weeks, the rate of miscarriage or fetal death as a result of the procedure is less than 1%.
- Excessive bleeding (rare).
- Surgical-wound infection (uncommon).

FOLLOW-UP CARE

GENERAL MEASURES
- Arrange to have someone drive you home following the procedure.
- Bathe and shower as usual. You may wash the injection site gently with mild unscented soap.
- You may experience some mild lower abdominal cramping.
- Before you take any action on the basis of the results of your amniocentesis or any other prenatal testing, be sure that any results that show a possible abnormality have been evaluated by an experienced physician who specializes in genetics, or by a genetic counselor. If you continue to have any doubts after consulting with a genetics specialist, obtain a second medical opinion.

MEDICATION—Usually not necessary.

ACTIVITY—Rest for 4 to 6 hours following the procedure. There are usually no further restrictions on your normal activities unless the doctor advises you differently.

DIET—No special diet.

CALL YOUR DOCTOR IF

- You experience a loss of fluid from the vagina.
- You experience nausea and vomiting.
- You experience significant cramping or pain in the lower abdomen or shoulder.
- You bleed from the vagina or puncture site.
- You develop signs of infection: headache, muscle aches, dizziness or a general ill feeling and fever.

Amniocentesis

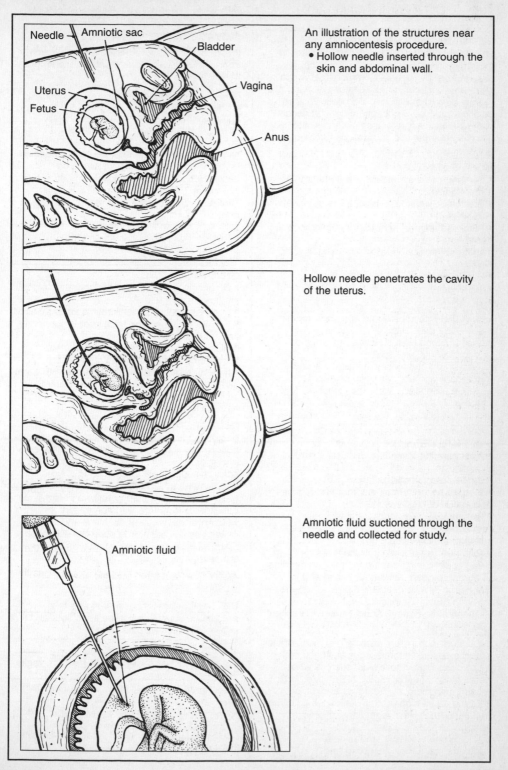

Needle — Amniotic sac
Bladder

Uterus
Fetus
Vagina

Anus

An illustration of the structures near any amniocentesis procedure.
- Hollow needle inserted through the skin and abdominal wall.

Hollow needle penetrates the cavity of the uterus.

Amniotic fluid suctioned through the needle and collected for study.

Amniotic fluid

Anemia during Pregnancy

 GENERAL INFORMATION

DEFINITION—An inadequate level of hemoglobin during pregnancy. Hemoglobin is the protein inside red blood cells that carries oxygen to body tissues. Common anemias in pregnancy include iron-deficiency anemia (75% to 85% of cases) and folic-acid deficiency. In addition, glucose-6-phosphate dehydrogenase (G6PD) deficiency, thalassemia and sickle cell anemia have genetic implications and should receive special evaluation.

SIGNS & SYMPTOMS
• Sometimes no symptoms are apparent.
• Breathlessness.
• Tiredness, weakness, paleness or fainting.
Infrequent:
• Palpitations or an abnormal awareness of the heartbeat.
• Inflamed, sore tongue.
• Nausea.
• Headache.
• Jaundice.

CAUSES
• Poor diet with inadequate iron consumption.
• Folic-acid deficiency.
• Loss of blood from bleeding hemorrhoids or gastrointestinal bleeding.
• Even if iron and folic-acid intake are sufficient, a pregnant woman may become anemic because pregnancy alters the digestive process. The unborn child consumes some of the iron or folic acid normally available to the mother's body.

RISK INCREASES WITH
• Poor nutrition, especially multiple vitamin deficiencies.
• Excess alcohol consumption.
• Medical history of any disorder that reduces absorption of nutrients.
• Pregnancies with multiple fetuses (e.g., twins, triplets, etc.).
• Use of anticonvulsant drugs.
• Previous use of oral contraceptives.
• G6PD deficiency is more common in persons of Mediterranean, African American and Sephardic Jewish descent. Sickle cell anemia is found in African Americans and in persons of Italian, Middle Eastern and East Indian descent.

HOW TO PREVENT
• Eat foods rich in iron, such as liver, beef, whole-grain breads and cereals, eggs and dried fruit.
• Eat foods high in folic acid, such as wheat germ, beans, peanut butter, oatmeal, collards mushrooms, broccoli, beef liver and asparagus.
• Eating foods high in vitamin C, such as citrus fruits and fresh, raw vegetables, makes iron absorption more efficient.
• Take prenatal vitamin and mineral supplements, if they are prescribed.

• Screening for several anemias (e.g., G6PD deficiency and sickle cell disease in high-risk women) should be considered prior to any attempt to become pregnant.

PROBABLE OUTCOME—Usually curable with iron and folic-acid supplements by mouth or by injection.

POSSIBLE COMPLICATIONS
• Premature labor.
• Intrauterine growth retardation (IUGR).
• Dangerous anemia from normal blood loss during labor, requiring blood transfusions.
• Low-birthweight and fetal neural tube defects (such as spina bifida) are known to be associated with maternal folic-acid deficiency.
• Increased risk of spontaneous abortion.
• Increased susceptibility to maternal infection after childbirth.

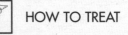 HOW TO TREAT

GENERAL MEASURES
• Diagnosis is determined by laboratory blood studies.
• For most anemias, supplements are prescribed.
• For G6PD deficiency, treatment is supportive and educational.
• Sickle cell anemia in pregnant women requires careful medical management.
• If the tongue is red and sore, rinse with warm salt water 3 or 4 times a day. Use 1 teaspoon salt to 8 ounces warm water.
• Brush teeth with a soft toothbrush.

MEDICATION—Iron, folic acid and other supplements may be prescribed. For better absorption, take iron supplements 1 hour before eating or between meals. If you are taking a calcium supplement in addition to an iron supplement, take them at different times of day (e.g., one in the morning and one at night), as calcium can interfere with iron absorption. Iron will turn bowel movements black and often causes constipation. Iron sometimes may be taken with meals if it has caused an upset stomach.

ACTIVITY—Rest often until the anemia disappears.

DIET—Eat a well-balanced diet and take prescribed supplements. Increase fiber and fluid intake to prevent constipation.

 CALL YOUR DOCTOR IF

• You have symptoms of anemia during pregnancy.
• The following occurs during treatment:
  Diarrhea, nausea, abdominal pain or constipation.
  Any unusual bleeding, even slight.

Baby's First Weeks, What You Need

GENERAL INFORMATION

DESCRIPTION—The following list suggests the very basic supplies needed to care for your baby. If your budget allows, you can add extra items. Buy ahead of time as much as you need to feel prepared and to care for the baby without feeling hassled. Purchase other items as you need them. Items do not need to be new—just safe and clean. Watch for garage sales, other special sales, or exchange items with family or friends.

CLOTHING—Adjust the number needed depending on your laundry facilities. Avoid buying large quantities of newborn sizes that your baby will quickly outgrow.
• Diapers, washable—3-4 dozen. (Even if you are using disposable diapers, cloth diapers work nicely as burp cloths, and 1-2 dozen are helpful to have.)
• Diapers, disposable—12 per day.
• Diaper pins—8-12 (if using cloth diapers).
• Diaper wipes—1 box. (Use soft, cotton washcloths and water, or cotton balls and water, for diaper changes for the first few weeks.)
• Pairs of booties or socks—4-6.
• Shirts (tie-front or snap)—6-8.
• Sleepers, kimonos, nightgowns—4-6.
• One-piece rompers (above the knees; snap at the crotch; for spring or summer baby)—4-6.
• One-piece stretchies (long pants; with or without feet)—4-6 (fall or winter baby); 2-3 (spring or summer baby).
• Bibs, washable (to protect clothes from spit-up)—4-6.
• Sweaters—2.
• Waterproof pants (if using cloth diapers)—3-4.
• Caps (knitted for winter; brimmed for summer)—1.
• Blanket sleepers (winter)—2-3.
• Bunting or hooded jacket (winter)—1.

BEDDING
• Receiving blankets—4-5.
• Quilted mattress pads (optional)—2.
• Flannel waterproof pads—3-4.
• Fitted sheets—3-4.
• Bumper pad—1.
• Lightweight blankets—1-2.

BATHING
• Hooded towels—2-3.
• Wash cloths—8-12.
• Mild soap—1 bar or bottle.
• No-tears baby shampoo—1 bottle.
• Oil or lotion—1 bottle.
• Baby bathtub (optional)—1.

BREAST-FEEDING SUPPLIES
• Support/nursing bra—3-6.
• Bra pads—5-6 washable; 2-3 dozen disposable.
• Breast pump (if working or often away from home)—1.

FORMULA EQUIPMENT/SUPPLIES
• 4-oz bottles, nipples and caps (even if breast-feeding)—4.
• 8-oz bottles, nipples and caps—4-8.
• Extra nipples and caps—2-4.
• Disposable bottle inserts (if using this type)—1 box of each size (4 oz and 8 oz).
• Formula (as prescribed) in ready-to-feed, powdered or liquid concentrate form—1-week supply, then purchase as needed.
• Boiled, sterile water for mixing with powdered or liquid formula concentrate—1 gallon.
• Can opener—1.

EQUIPMENT
• Crib/bassinet/cradle (one that meets current federal safety standards)—1.
• Mattress—1.
• Changing table (optional)—1.
• Diaper pail with cover—1.
• Fever thermometer—1.
• Diaper bag for supplies—1.
• Infant carrier/car seat (may want to consider loaner or rental programs)—1.
• Stroller (optional)—1.
• Intercom/baby monitor (optional)—1.
• Baby swing (optional)—1.
• Rocking chair (optional)—1.
• Portable crib or playpen (optional)—1.
• Soft carrier or backpack (optional)—1.

OTHER
• Rubbing alcohol/cotton balls for cord care—1 bottle/1 package.
• Petroleum jelly (such as Vaseline) for lubricating rectal thermometer and circumcision care (if applicable)—1.
• Sterile gauze pads (if baby is a boy and will be circumcised)—1 package.
• Ointment for diaper rash (such as A&D or Desitin)—1 tube.

CALL YOUR DOCTOR IF

You have questions about what you need or don't need for your baby's first few weeks.

Birth Method Choices

GENERAL INFORMATION

DEFINITION—The options in childbirth include selecting a practitioner, the type of medical practice the practitioner works in, the delivery facility and type of anesthetic. Expectant parents should explore their choices and select those that match their preferences and requirements. There are limitations in many cases due to complications of a pregnancy, lack of options in smaller communities, economic constraints, prepaid health plans or insurance restrictions, and laws in some states that control who can perform deliveries in hospital facilities.

PRACTITIONERS
• Physician—medical doctor (MD) or osteopath (DO). The practitioner may be a family doctor or an obstetrician/gynecologist. If your pregnancy appears to be routine, either practitioner may be selected. If the pregnancy is considered high-risk, you will likely need an obstetrician or a maternal-fetal medicine specialist.
• Midwife—certified nurse-midwife (CNM), or independent midwife who may be trained and certified without becoming a nurse first (CM). Midwives are trained to handle low-risk pregnancies and to attend uncomplicated births.

TYPES OF PRACTICES
• Solo medical practice—there is only one physician in the practice (or office). When that physician is away or unavailable, a covering physician will take care of the patients.
• Partnership or group medical practice—two or more physicians work in the practice (or office). They may be of the same specialty (family practice or obstetrics/gynecology) or a combination of two or more specialties, such as often found in an HMO (health maintenance organization).
• Other medical practice—may combine the services of a certified midwife and a physician, or a certified midwife as primary caregiver with a physician on call as needed.

BIRTHING LOCATIONS
• Hospital—most often it is a full-care facility that is equipped to handle all aspects of child-birth and any possible emergencies.
• Birthing center or maternity center—may be a stand-alone facility or located in a hospital. The focus is on a home-like environment with family/friends sharing the birth. Often, one room is used for labor, delivery and recovery.
• Home delivery—is sometimes the first choice for a few women with a normal pregnancy and expecting a normal delivery. A qualified physician or certified midwife will attend the birth. Arrangements are made in advance for emergency transfer to a hospital if it becomes necessary.

PAIN RELIEF AND ANESTHETICS
• General anesthesia—produces unconsciousness with an inhalant that is administered by an anesthesiologist in an operating delivery room. General anesthesia is most often used in surgical births and sometimes used when complications occur. It is not routinely used for normal vaginal deliveries.
• Regional nerve block—an injected anesthesia that numbs a portion of the body. With surgical deliveries, the numbed area may be from the waist down, while with vaginal deliveries, the numbed area may be smaller. The most commonly used blocks are epidural, spinal and pedundal (see Glossary for these terms). The mother is awake and alert during delivery.
• Pain medication—is sometimes administered intravenously or intramuscularly once labor is well established. Most frequently used is meperidine (Demerol); the amount of pain relief with Demerol varies among women. The drug can slow labor if given too early. Newer pain drugs, such as nalbuphine (Nubain) or butorphanol (Stadol) take less time to recover from and have less effect on the fetus.
• Hypnosis—is an acceptable method for helping to control pain. It varies in effectiveness from just making a woman more relaxed and comfortable to eliminating any feelings of pain. Hypnosis training needs to begin weeks to months prior to delivery time.
• Other pain-relief methods—for women who do not want to use drugs for various reasons, additional options include acupuncture, TENS (see Glossary), massage and heat.

BIRTHING POSITION
• Lithotomy—use of a delivery table with the woman's feet in stirrups.
• Birthing bed—a special bed designed for comfort during the labor period and then converted into a bed suitable for delivery. The back can be raised so the mother is in a squatting position and the foot of the bed is removed. After delivery, it is converted back to a regular bed for recovery.
• Birthing chair—a chair that supports a woman in a sitting position during delivery. The idea is to allow gravity to help with the birth.
• Additional options—LeBoyer births, underwater births and others are rarely used but are available in some areas.

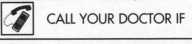

CALL YOUR DOCTOR IF

You have questions or concerns about the options available for childbirth.

Breast-Feeding
(continued on next page)

 GENERAL INFORMATION

DEFINITION
• New parents want to give their babies the very best. When it comes to nutrition, the best first food for babies is breast milk. More than two decades of research have established that breast milk is perfectly suited to nourish infants and protect them from illness. Breast-fed infants have lower rates of hospital admissions, ear infections, diarrhea, rashes, allergies and other medical problems than bottle-fed babies.
• Babies should be breast-fed for 6 to 12 months. The only acceptable alternative to breast milk is infant formula. Solid foods can be introduced when the baby is 4 to 6 months old, but a baby should drink breast milk or formula, not cow's milk, for a full year. There aren't any rules about when to stop breast-feeding. As long as the baby is eating age-appropriate solid foods, a mother may nurse for 2 years if she wishes. A baby needs breast milk for the first year of life, and then as long as desired after that.

BENEFITS TO INFANTS
• The primary benefit of breast milk is nutritional. Human milk contains just the right amount of fatty acids, lactose, water and amino acids for human digestion, brain development and growth. Cow's milk contains a different type of protein than breast milk. This is good for calves, but human infants can have difficulty digesting it. Bottle-fed infants tend to be fatter than breast-fed infants, but not necessarily healthier.
• Because human milk transfers to the infant the mother's antibodies to disease, breast-fed babies have fewer illnesses. About 80% of the cells in breast milk are macrophages, cells that kill bacteria, fungi and viruses. Breast-fed babies are protected, in varying degrees, from a number of illnesses, including pneumonia, botulism, bronchitis, staphylococcal infections, influenza, ear infections and German measles. Furthermore, mothers produce antibodies to whatever disease is present in their environment, making their milk custom-designed to fight the diseases their babies are exposed to as well.
• A breast-fed baby's digestive tract contains large amounts of Lactobacillus bifidus, beneficial bacteria that prevent the growth of harmful organisms. Human milk straight from the breast is always sterile, never contaminated by polluted water or dirty bottles that can lead to diarrhea in the infant.
• Human milk contains at least 100 ingredients not found in formula. No babies are allergic to their mother's milk, although they may have a reaction to something the mother eats. If she eliminates it from her diet, the problem resolves itself.
• Sucking at the breast promotes good jaw development as well. It's harder work to get milk out of a breast than a bottle, and the exercise strengthens the jaws and encourages the growth of straight, healthy teeth. The baby at the breast can control the flow of milk by sucking and stopping. With a bottle, the baby must constantly suck or react to the pressure of the nipple placed in the mouth.
• Nursing may have psychological benefits for the infant as well, creating an early bond between mother and child. At birth, infants see only 12 to 15 inches, the distance between a nursing baby and its mother's face. Studies have found that infants as young as 1 week prefer the smell of their own mother's milk.
• Many psychologists believe the nursing baby enjoys a sense of security from the warmth and presence of the mother, especially when there's skin-to-skin contact during feeding. Parents of bottle-fed babies may be tempted to prop bottles in the baby's mouth, with no human contact during feeding. But a nursing mother must cuddle her infant closely many times during the day. Nursing becomes more than a way to feed a baby; it's a source of warmth and comfort.

BENEFITS TO MOTHER
• Breast-feeding is good for new mothers as well as for their babies. There are no bottles to sterilize and no formula to buy, measure and mix. It may be easier for a nursing mother to lose the pounds of pregnancy as well, since nursing uses up extra calories. Lactation stimulates the uterus to contract back to its original size.
• A nursing mother is forced to get needed rest. She must sit down, put her feet up and relax every few hours to nurse. Nursing at night is easy as well. No one has to stumble to the refrigerator for a bottle and warm it while the baby cries. If she's lying down, a mother can doze while she nurses.
• Nursing is also nature's contraceptive; if the infant receives primarily breast milk during the first six months of life, nursing will provide the mother with contraceptive protection which is comparable to that of the birth control pill. Frequent nursing suppresses ovulation, making it less likely for a nursing mother to menstruate, ovulate or get pregnant. Mothers who are uncertain of their breast-feeding plans, or who want extra contraceptive protection, can safely use other methods to complement the contraception provided by nursing. Hormone injections and implants are safe during nursing, as are all barrier methods of birth control. The labeling on birth control pills says that, if possible, another form of contraception should

Breast-Feeding (cont.)

be used until the baby is weaned. If birth control pills are selected, pills with progesterone only are preferable, because they have no recognized effect on milk production or quality.

• Breast-feeding is also economical. Even though a nursing mother works up a big appetite and consumes extra calories, the extra food for her is less expensive than buying formula for the baby. Nursing saves money while providing the best nourishment.

WHEN YOU SHOULD NOT BREAST-FEED

• There are very few medical reasons why a mother shouldn't breast-feed. Most common illnesses, such as colds, flu, skin infections or diarrhea, cannot be passed through breast milk. In fact, if a mother has an illness, her breast milk will contain antibodies to it that will help protect her baby from those same illnesses.

• A few viruses can pass through breast milk, however. HIV, the virus that causes AIDS, is one of them. Women who are HIV positive should not breast-feed.

• A few other illnesses—such as herpes, hepatitis and beta-streptococcus infections—can also be transmitted through breast milk. But that doesn't always mean a mother with those diseases should not breast-feed. Each case must be evaluated on an individual basis.

• Breast cancer is not passed through breast milk. Women who have had breast cancer can usually breast-feed from the unaffected breast. There is some concern that the hormones produced during pregnancy and lactation may trigger a recurrence of cancer, but so far this has not been proven. Studies have shown, however, that breast-feeding a child reduces a woman's chance of developing breast cancer later.

• Silicone breast implants usually do not interfere with a woman's ability to nurse, but if the implants leak, there is some concern that the silicone may harm the baby. If a woman with implants wants to breast-feed, she should first discuss the potential benefits and risks with her child's doctor.

POSSIBLE PROBLEMS

• For all its health benefits, breast-feeding does require some training and improves with experience. In the early weeks, it can be painful. A woman's nipples may become sore or cracked. She may experience engorgement more than a bottle-feeding mother, when the breasts become so full of milk they're hard and painful. Some nursing women also develop clogged milk ducts, which can lead to mastitis, a painful infection of the breast. Mastitis requires prompt medical care.

• Nursing can affect a woman's entire lifestyle. A nursing mother with baby-in-tow must wear clothes that enable her to nurse anywhere, or she'll have to find a private place to undress. Increasingly, clothing manufacturers are producing very fashionable and attractive clothing that affords easy access to the breast. She should eat a balanced diet and she might need to avoid foods that irritate the baby. She also shouldn't smoke, which can cause vomiting, diarrhea, restlessness and respiratory problems for the baby, as well as decreased milk production.

• Women who plan to go back to work soon after birth will have to plan carefully if they want to breast-feed. If her job allows, a new mother can pump the breast milk several times during the day and refrigerate or freeze it for the baby to take in a bottle later. Some women alternate nursing at night and on weekends with daytime bottles of formula.

• The immediate demands of nursing are potentially greater than those imposed by bottle-feeding. However, if you consider the additional childhood illnesses, risk of colic or poor tolerance to formula, breast-feeding may actually be both easier and more time-efficient. Instead of feeling it's a chore, nursing mothers often cite this close relationship as one of the greatest joys of nursing. Besides, nursing mothers can get away between feedings if they need a break.

• Finally, some women just don't feel comfortable with the idea of nursing. They don't want to handle their breasts, or they want to think of them as sexual, not functional. They may be concerned about modesty and the possibility of having to nurse in public. They may want a break from child care to let someone else feed the baby, especially in the wee hours of the morning.

• If a woman is unsure whether she wants to nurse, she can try it for a few weeks and switch if she doesn't like it. It's very difficult to switch to breast-feeding after bottle-feeding is begun.

• If she plans to breast-feed, a new mother should learn as much as possible about it before the baby is born. Doctors, childbirth instructors, nurses and midwives can all offer information about nursing. But perhaps the best ongoing support for a nursing mother is someone who has successfully nursed a baby.

• La Leche League, a national support organization for nursing mothers, has chapters in many cities that meet regularly to discuss breast-feeding problems and offer support. Most La Leche League chapters allow women to come to a few meetings without charge. League leaders offer advice by phone as well. To find a convenient La Leche League chapter, call 1-800-LA-LECHE.

Breast-Feeding (cont.)

MEDICATIONS
- Most medicines have not been tested in nursing mothers.
- A nursing mother should advise any health-care professional who prescribes a medication for her that she is breast-feeding.
- Read the instructions on nonprescription drugs to see if they are safe for breast-feeding. Ask your pharmacist or doctor if you are unsure.
- Avoid all drugs of abuse if breast-feeding.
- Some drugs can be taken by a nursing mother if she stops breast-feeding for a few days or weeks. To maintain milk supply, she can pump her breasts and discard the milk; baby can be fed formula temporarily.

BREAST-FEEDING INSTRUCTIONS—It's helpful for a woman who wants to breast-feed to learn as much about it as possible before delivery. The following tips can help foster successful nursing:
- Get an early start: Nursing should begin shortly after delivery, if possible, when an infant is awake and the sucking instinct is strong. Even though the mother won't be producing milk yet, her breasts contain colostrum, a thin fluid that contains antibodies to disease.
- Proper positioning: The baby's mouth should be wide open, with the nipple as far back into his or her mouth as possible. This minimizes soreness for the mother. A nurse, midwife or other knowledgeable person can help her find a comfortable nursing position.
- Nurse on demand: Newborns need to nurse frequently, at least every two hours, and not on any strict schedule. This will stimulate the mother's breasts to produce plenty of milk. Later, the baby can settle into a more predictable routine. But because breast milk is more easily digested than formula, breast-fed babies often eat more frequently than bottle-fed babies.
- No supplements: Nursing babies don't need sugar water or formula supplements. These may interfere with their appetite for nursing, which can lead to a diminished milk supply. The more the baby nurses, the more milk the mother will produce.
- Delay artificial nipples: It's best to wait a week or two before introducing a pacifier, so that the baby doesn't get confused. Artificial nipples require a different sucking action than real ones. Sucking at a bottle could also confuse some babies in the early days. They, too, are learning how to breast-feed.

- Air dry: In the early postpartum period or until her nipples toughen, the mother should air dry them after each nursing to prevent them from cracking, which can lead to infection. If her nipples do crack, the mother can coat them with breast milk or other natural moisturizers to help them heal. Vitamin E oil and lanolin are commonly used, although some babies may have allergic reactions to them. Proper positioning at the breast can help prevent sore nipples. Soreness can be caused when the baby does not have the nipple far enough back in his or her mouth.
- Watch for infection: Symptoms of breast infection include fever and painful lumps and redness in the breast. These require immediate medical attention.
- Expect engorgement: A new mother usually produces lots of milk, making her breasts big, hard and painful for a few days. To relieve this engorgement, she should feed the baby frequently and on demand until her body adjusts and produces only what the baby needs. In the meantime, the mother can take over-the-counter pain relievers, apply warm, wet compresses to her breasts and take warm baths to relieve the pain.
- Eat right, get rest: To produce plenty of good milk, the nursing mother needs a balanced diet that includes 500 extra calories a day and six to eight glasses of fluid. She should also rest as much as possible to prevent breast infections, which are aggravated by fatigue.

Note: This information adapted in part from the *FDA Consumer* (the magazine of the U.S. Food & Drug Administration).

 CALL YOUR DOCTOR IF

- You have questions about breast-feeding.
- You have a child who is breast-feeding, and you develop signs of breast infection (mastitis). Symtoms include fever; tender, swollen, hard or hot breasts; redness and streaking of the breasts; body aches or a general feeling of illness; purulent drainage (pus) from the affected breast(s).

Breech Presentation

GENERAL INFORMATION

DEFINITION—At birth, most babies are born head first with face down. In a breech position, the fetal buttocks or feet lie nearest the birth canal and are the first part to emerge. Breech presentation occurs in 3%-4% of all births. Types of breech presentations include:
• Frank breech: the baby's thighs are flexed on the abdomen and both legs are extended at the knee so that the feet are near the baby's head.
• Complete breech: the baby's thighs are flexed on the abdomen and both legs are flexed at the knee.
• Footling (or incomplete) breech: one or both legs are extended below the level of the baby's buttocks.

SIGNS & SYMPTOMS—There are no visible signs. The diagnosis can be determined by abdominal or vaginal examination and confirmed by ultrasound.

CAUSES—Before 36 weeks, the fetus may move about from one position to the other. In the later weeks of pregnancy, these changes are more difficult. Sometime between the 32nd and 36th weeks, the fetus will usually spontaneously assume the head down position, but in some instances the breech position occurs. The actual cause of breech presentation is unknown but is probably a combination of one or more of the risk factors listed below.

RISK INCREASES WITH
• Premature labor and delivery.
• Multiple fetuses.
• Uterine abnormalities.
• Fetal congenital malformation.
• Placenta previa.
• Low-birthweight baby.

HOW TO PREVENT
• No known way to prevent the original breech position.
• For some patients, after the breech position is diagnosed, a technique called external version is performed, which attempts to rotate the fetus to the proper position.

PROBABLE OUTCOME
• The decision about delivery will be made on an individual basis. For some, a cesarean birth is recommended for breech babies, while in certain conditions, a vaginal delivery may be recommended.
• In most cases, you and the baby will suffer no complications because of the breech presentation.

POSSIBLE COMPLICATIONS
• Birth injury.
• Compression of the umbilical cord causing lack of oxygen to the fetus.

HOW TO TREAT

GENERAL MEASURES
• Once the diagnosis of breech presentation is made, be sure you understand the options and risks (both to you and to the fetus) involved for each type of delivery (cesarean or vaginal). Discuss any questions or concerns you may have with your physician. Midwives and nurse-midwives usually do not handle breech births. After delivery:
• Showering is fine; delay tub baths for 2 to 3 weeks.
• Some degree of postpartum depression (crying jags and feelings of inadequacy) may occur; this is normal after birth.
• Wear an external pad for the vaginal bleeding that will occur for several weeks. Your first menstrual period should come in 6 to 8 weeks but may be delayed for several months.
• If delivery was by cesarean section, see that topic in this book for instructions on follow-up care.

MEDICATION
• Prescription pain medication should generally be required for only 2 to 7 days following the procedure.
• You may use nonprescription drugs, such as acetaminophen, for minor pain.

ACTIVITY
• You may resume sexual relations after 2 weeks (although for some, 4 to 6 weeks may be recommended).
• Return to normal activity as soon as your health and well-being permit. This will occur more quickly following a vaginal delivery than it will with a cesarean delivery.

DIET—No special diet is usually necessary, but if you are in labor, you should have nothing by mouth until delivery is accomplished.

CALL YOUR DOCTOR IF

Any of the following occurs prior to birth:
• New symptoms develop.
Any of the following occurs following birth:
• Pain, swelling, redness, drainage or bleeding increases in the surgical area.
• You develop signs of infection: headache, muscle aches, dizziness or a general ill feeling and fever.
• Bleeding soaks more than one pad in an hour.
• The urge to urinate frequently persists longer than one month.
• Vaginal discharge persists beyond one month.

Breech Presentation

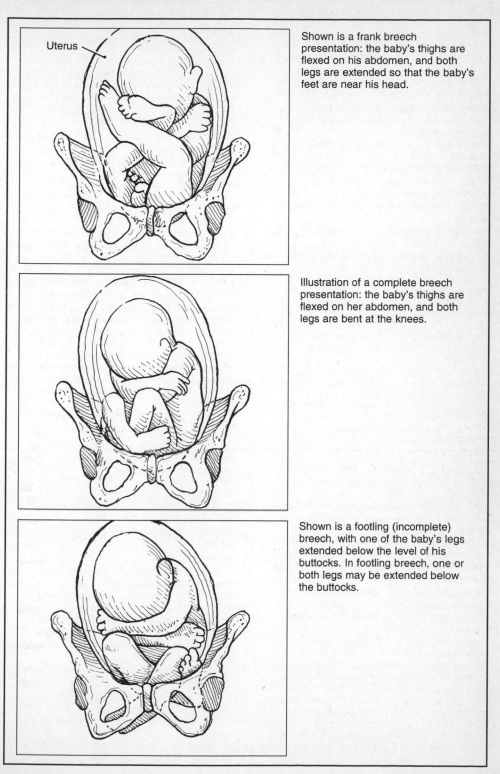

Uterus

Shown is a frank breech presentation: the baby's thighs are flexed on his abdomen, and both legs are extended so that the baby's feet are near his head.

Illustration of a complete breech presentation: the baby's thighs are flexed on her abdomen, and both legs are bent at the knees.

Shown is a footling (incomplete) breech, with one of the baby's legs extended below the level of his buttocks. In footling breech, one or both legs may be extended below the buttocks.

Cesarean Section

GENERAL INFORMATION

DEFINITION—A surgical procedure in which delivery of a baby is accomplished through an incision in the mother's lower abdominal and uterine walls. Cesarean sections account for about 20% of all deliveries in the United States.

REASONS FOR PROCEDURE—Danger to the mother or baby from one or more of many causes, including:
- Baby's head too large to pass through the birth canal.
- Breech presentation.
- Insufficient contractions of the uterus.
- Placenta previa.
- Abruptio placentae with fetal or maternal distress.
- Failure of normal labor in a patient who had a previous cesarean section.
- High blood pressure (hypertension), diabetes or heart trouble in the mother.
- Severe preeclampsia.
- Fetal distress.
- Acute herpes genitalis infection.
- Prior significant uterine surgery.

RISK INCREASES WITH
- Prior cesarean section.
- Obesity.
- Smoking.
- Poor nutrition.
- Excess alcohol consumption.
- Placenta previa with excessive blood loss.
- Preeclampsia or eclampsia in pregnancy.
- Chronic heart or lung disease.
- Use of drugs such as antihypertensives, cortisone, diuretics or insulin.

DESCRIPTION OF PROCEDURE
- The procedure is usually performed in a hospital.
- A urinary catheter is inserted into the bladder before or after anesthesia is administered.
- Anesthesia is administered; in a non-emergency cesarean, the woman's body is usually numbed from the waist down using either an epidural or a spinal anesthesia (see Glossary for both). In cases of an emergency cesarean, or in other special circumstances, a general anesthetic may be used.
- An airway tube is placed in the windpipe if a general anesthesia is used.
- An incision is made in the abdomen.
- Another incision is made in the uterus.
- Baby and placenta are delivered.
- The uterus is closed and the abdominal contents are replaced. Connective tissue, muscles and skin are closed. The skin is closed with sutures or clips, which usually can be removed 2 to 7 days after surgery.
- The urinary catheter will usually remain in place for up to 24 hours following surgery.

PROBABLE OUTCOME—No complications expected. Allow 4 to 6 weeks for recovery.

POSSIBLE COMPLICATIONS
- Excessive bleeding or surgical-wound infection.
- Postoperative anemia.
- Excessive scar formation (keloid).
- Endomyometritis (see Glossary).

FOLLOW-UP CARE

GENERAL MEASURES
- Expect a hospital stay of 3 to 5 days.
- A hard ridge should form along the incision. As it heals, the ridge will gradually recede.
- Move and elevate your legs often while resting in bed to improve circulation and decrease the likelihood of deep-vein clots.
- Use heat to relieve incisional pain.
- Shower as usual. You may wash the incision gently with mild unscented soap. Resume tub baths after 2 to 3 weeks.
- Don't douche unless advised to by your doctor.
- You will experience most of the same postpartum discomforts you would have experienced with a vaginal delivery, including cramping and afterpains; engorgement of your breasts; fatigue; hormonal changes; hair loss; excessive perspiration and postpartum depression or "baby blues." You may also have abdominal discomfort and gas, constipation and referred shoulder pain caused by air in your abdominal cavity.
- You will usually be seen for follow-up at around 2 weeks, and then again at 4-6 weeks, following surgery.

MEDICATION
- Prescription pain medication should generally be required for only 4 to 7 days following the procedure.
- You may use nonprescription drugs, such as acetaminophen, for minor pain.
- Antibiotics, if needed, to prevent or fight infection.

ACTIVITY
- Resume daily activities and work as soon as you are able. Resume driving 2 to 4 weeks after surgery. Full recovery takes about 6 weeks.
- Avoid heavy lifting for 2 to 4 weeks.
- Avoid sexual intercourse for 4 to 6 weeks.

DIET—No special diet.

CALL YOUR DOCTOR IF

- Pain, swelling, redness, drainage or bleeding increases in the surgical area.
- Bleeding soaks more than 1 pad or tampon each hour.
- Vaginal discharge or the urge to urinate frequently persists longer than 1 month.

Cesarean Section

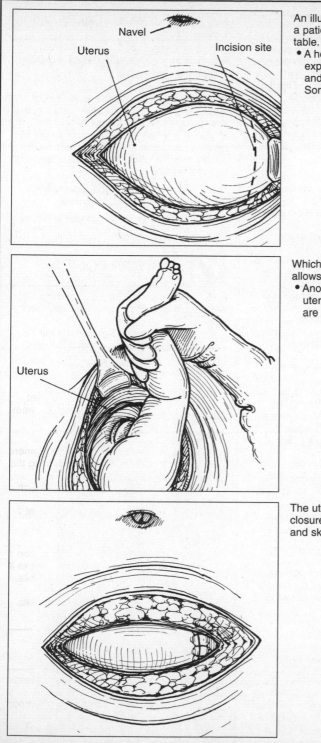

Navel

Uterus

Incision site

An illustration looking from above of a patient lying flat on an operating table.
- A horizontal incision is made, exposing the uterus, musculature and fatty layer below the skin. Sometimes the incision is vertical.

Uterus

Whichever incision site is chosen, it allows exposure of the uterus.
- Another incision is made into the uterus. The baby and the placenta are removed.

The uterus is closed, followed by closure of connective tissue, muscles and skin of the abdominal wall.

Chorionic Villi Sampling (CVS)

 GENERAL INFORMATION

DEFINITION—A prenatal diagnostic test that detects chromosomal abnormalities in a fetus. It involves the villi (hairlike projections) that compose the chorion (the outer layer of the amniotic sac). Cells from the villi provide chromosome information as do the cells from the amniotic fluid. A CVS test can be performed between the 9th and 12th weeks of pregnancy, providing earlier diagnosis than amniotic fluid studies.

REASONS FOR PROCEDURE
• Mother will be over age 35 at time of delivery.
• Pregnancy is considered genetically high risk.
• Either parent has a chromosome abnormality.
• Mother has previously had a child with chromosome abnormality, such as Down syndrome.

RISK INCREASES WITH—None expected.

DESCRIPTION OF PROCEDURE
• The test is usually performed in a hospital or medical center.
• In one technique used, an anesthetic is injected into the abdominal skin and then a long hollow needle is inserted into the abdomen to withdraw the villi.
• The second technique is done through the vagina. A catheter is inserted through the cervix into the uterus and suction is applied to pull the villi into the catheter, which is then removed.
• Ultrasound is used throughout the procedure to determine the location of the fetus and to allow constant viewing of the needle's, or catheter's, path.
• You may experience mild to moderate discomfort during the procedure. Rarely, the pain may be severe.

PROBABLE OUTCOME—You should experience no discomfort once the procedure has been completed. Test results should be available within 2 to 7 days.

POSSIBLE COMPLICATIONS
• In some cases, insufficient villi are obtained and the needle or catheter must be reinserted.
• Slight risk of a miscarriage triggered by the procedure (1%-5%).
• Excessive bleeding (rare).
• Risk of infection.

 FOLLOW-UP CARE

GENERAL MEASURES
• Arrange to have someone drive you home following the procedure.
• Bathe or shower as usual.
• Before you undertake any action based on the results of your genetic CVS, be sure that the results have been evaluated by an experienced physician who specializes in genetics, or by a genetic counselor. If you continue to have doubts after speaking to a genetics specialist, obtain a second opinion.

MEDICATION—Medication is usually not necessary following this procedure.

ACTIVITY—Rest for the remainder of the day.

DIET—No special diet.

CALL YOUR DOCTOR IF

• You experience any pain or cramping.
• You have bleeding or fluid leakage from the vagina.
• You develop signs of infection: headache, muscle aches, fever or a general ill feeling.

Chorionic Villi Sampling (CVS)

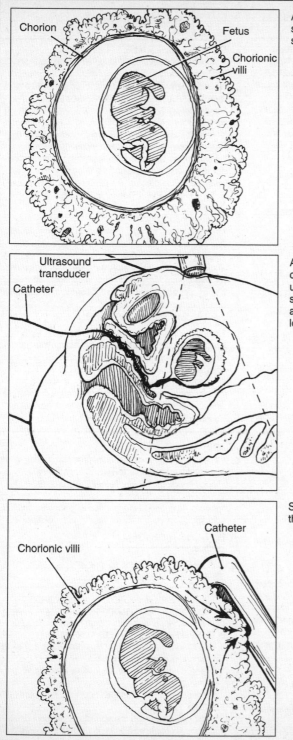

Chorion

Fetus

Chorionic villi

An illustration showing the amniotic sac and the chorionic villi that surround it.

Ultrasound transducer

Catheter

A catheter is inserted through the cervix and into the uterus. An ultrasound transducer, which is shown on the outside of the abdomen, is used to view the location of the fetus and the catheter.

Suction is used to pull the villi into the catheter.

Catheter

Chorionic villi

Ectopic Pregnancy
(Extrauterine or Tubal Pregnancy)

 GENERAL INFORMATION

DEFINITION—A pregnancy that develops outside the uterus. The most common site is in one of the narrow tubes that connect each ovary to the uterus (fallopian tube). Other, more rare, sites include the ovary, outside the reproductive organs in the abdominal cavity, or the cervix. About 1 in 100 pregnancies is ectopic.

SIGNS & SYMPTOMS
Early stages:
• Missed menstrual period or any menstrual irregularity.
• Unexplained vaginal spotting or bleeding.
• Lower abdominal or pelvic pain and cramps.
• Pain in the shoulder (rare).
Late stages:
• Sudden, sharp, severe abdominal pain caused by rupture of the fallopian tube.
• Dizziness, fainting and shock (paleness, rapid heartbeat, drop in blood pressure and cold sweats). These may precede or accompany pain.

CAUSES—An egg from the ovary is fertilized and becomes implanted outside the uterus, usually in the fallopian tube. As the fertilized egg enlarges, the fallopian tube stretches and ruptures, causing life-threatening internal bleeding.

RISK INCREASES WITH
• Previous tubal pregnancy.
• Previous tubal or uterine surgery.
• Use of an intrauterine device (IUD) for contraception.
• Previous pelvic inflammatory disease (PID).
• Previous ruptured appendix.
• Adhesions (bands of scar tissue) from previous abdominal or pelvic surgery.
• History of endometritis.
• Malformed (abnormal) uterus.

HOW TO PREVENT
• Use a contraceptive method other than IUD.
• Obtain prompt treatment for any pelvic infection.

PROBABLE OUTCOME—An ectopic pregnancy cannot progress to full term or produce a viable fetus. Rupture of an ectopic pregnancy is an emergency requiring immediate treatment. Full recovery is likely with early diagnosis and surgery. Subsequent pregnancies are normal in about 50% to 85% of patients.

POSSIBLE COMPLICATIONS
• Infection.
• Diminished fertility.
• Loss of reproductive organs after complicated surgery.
• Shock and death from internal bleeding.

 HOW TO TREAT

GENERAL MEASURES
• Diagnostic tests may include serum pregnancy test, ultrasound, CT scan, MRI, culdocentesis, laparoscopy, D & C and exploratory laparotomy (see Glossary for all of these terms).
• Evaluation and treatment may be done on an outpatient basis.
• Hospitalization may be required for surgery. Blood transfusion may be necessary.
• Surgery to remove the developing embryo, the placenta and any damaged tissue. If the fallopian tube cannot be repaired, it is removed. Future normal pregnancy is possible with one fallopian tube.
Following surgery:
• After 24 hours, you may wash normally over the stitches in your incision.
• Apply a heating pad or hot-water bottle to the abdomen or back to relieve pain. Hot baths also relieve discomfort and relax muscles. Sit in a tub of hot water for 10 to 15 minutes. Repeat as often as needed.

MEDICATION
• In some early, unruptured or chronic ectopic pregnancies, methotrexate (a chemotherapy drug) is effective in devitalizing the pregnancy tissue.
• Following surgery, pain relievers such as nonsteroidal anti-inflammatory drugs (NSAIDs) or narcotics may be prescribed for 2 to 7 days.
• Antibiotics to prevent or treat infection.
• Iron supplements, if necessary, for anemia.

ACTIVITY
• Resume your normal activities, including work, as soon as possible following treatment. Recovery is generally faster with laparoscopy than with laparotomy.
• Avoid sexual relations until a follow-up medical examination determines healing is complete.

DIET—No special diet.

 CALL YOUR DOCTOR IF

• You or a family member has symptoms of ectopic pregnancy, especially a rupture. Call immediately! This is an emergency!
• The following occur after surgery:
    Excessive vaginal bleeding (soaking a pad or tampon every hour).
    Signs of infection: fever, chills, headache or muscle aches.
    Increased urinary frequency that lasts longer than 1 month.
    New, unexplained symptoms develop. Drugs used in teatment may produce side effects.

Ectopic Pregnancy
(Extrauterine or Tubal Pregnancy)

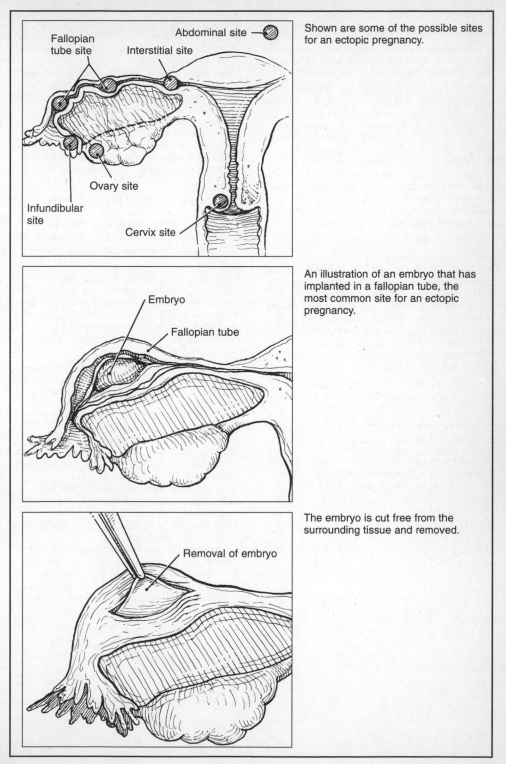

Fallopian tube site

Abdominal site

Interstitial site

Shown are some of the possible sites for an ectopic pregnancy.

Ovary site

Infundibular site

Cervix site

Embryo

Fallopian tube

An illustration of an embryo that has implanted in a fallopian tube, the most common site for an ectopic pregnancy.

Removal of embryo

The embryo is cut free from the surrounding tissue and removed.

Episiotomy
(Perineotomy)

 GENERAL INFORMATION

DEFINITION—Surgical incision at the exterior of the vaginal opening to create enlargement.

REASONS FOR PROCEDURE—Usually performed during childbirth, just before the widest diameter of the baby's head passes through the outlet of the birth canal. This allows easier passage of the baby's head to reduce the potential damage to the mother's vagina, bladder and rectum. Also helps expedite delivery in the case of forceps or vacuum use, or when there is maternal exhaustion or fetal distress, such as in a case of shoulder dystocia (when the shoulders of the baby get stuck after the head has already delivered).

RISK INCREASES WITH—None expected.

DESCRIPTION OF PROCEDURE
• An incision is made in the perineum (the small area between the vaginal opening and the anus), just before the widest part of the baby's head is to be delivered. The size of the incision depends on how large an opening is required for the baby's head to pass through safely.
• The baby and placenta are delivered.
• The surgical area is repaired with sutures that will be absorbed by the body.

PROBABLE OUTCOME—Expect complete healing without complications. Allow about 2 to 4 weeks for recovery from childbirth.

POSSIBLE COMPLICATIONS
• Excessive bleeding.
• Surgical-wound infection (rare).
• Inadvertent injury to sphincter or rectum (rare).
• May lead to increased risk of vaginal injury.

 FOLLOW-UP CARE

GENERAL MEASURES
• Bathe and shower as usual. You may wash the incision gently with mild unscented soap.
• Cleanse the surgical area with warm (not hot) water after urination or bowel movements.
• Take warm baths several times a day to help relieve discomfort.
• Use ice packs made of gauze soaked in ice-cold witch hazel to ease discomfort during the 24 hours after delivery.

MEDICATION
• Stool softener laxative to prevent constipation if needed.
• Antibiotics, if required to fight infection.
• You may use nonprescription drugs, such as acetaminophen or ibuprofen, for minor pain.

ACTIVITY
• Follow doctor's advice on resuming, or beginning, a postpartum exercise program.
• Resume driving 10 days after returning home.
• Resume sexual relations as directed by your doctor, or when a follow-up medical examination determines that healing is complete (usually about 3 to 6 weeks).

DIET—Eating a high fiber diet will help prevent constipation, which is common after childbirth. Increase your fluid intake as you increase your fiber intake.

CALL YOUR DOCTOR IF

• Pain, swelling, redness, drainage or bleeding increases in the surgical area.
• You develop signs of infection: general ill feeling and fever, headache, muscle aches, dizziness.
• You experience nausea, vomiting, constipation or abdominal swelling.
• New, unexplained symptoms develop. Drugs used in treatment may produce side effects.
• You pass uncontrolled urine through the vagina.
• You pass gas (flatus) or stool from the vagina.

Episiotomy (Perineotomy)

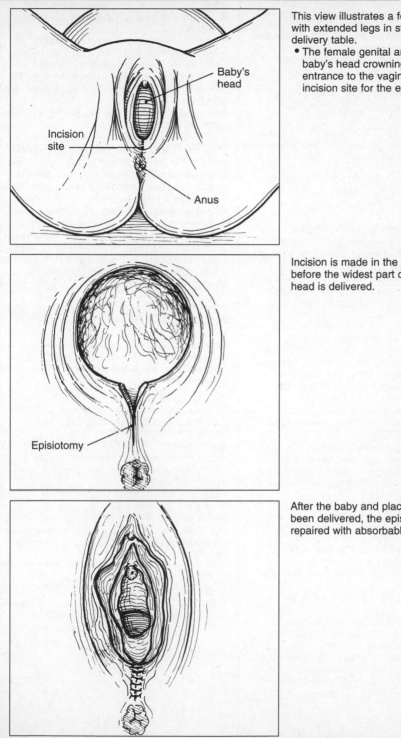

This view illustrates a female patient with extended legs in stirrups on a delivery table.
- The female genital area with a baby's head crowning at the entrance to the vagina and the incision site for the episiotomy.

Baby's head

Incision site

Anus

Incision is made in the perineum just before the widest part of the baby's head is delivered.

Episiotomy

After the baby and placenta have been delivered, the episiotomy site is repaired with absorbable sutures.

Exercises, Postpartum

 ## GENERAL INFORMATION

DEFINITION
• Following childbirth, a woman who gained an average amount of weight (25-35 pounds) during pregnancy can expect to regain her prepregnancy figure and weight in about 6 to 12 weeks.
• Exercising will help tighten the pelvic floor muscles (Kegel exercises), the abdominal muscles and strengthen the back muscles. Exercising for as little as 10 minutes a day and gradually increasing as time permits will help get you back into shape. A daily routine or a minimum of three times a week is better than an intermittent activity (e.g., just on weekends). If the birth was cesarean, consult with your doctor about when to begin an exercise program.
• Recovery time from childbirth will vary among women, depending on prepregnancy fitness condition, amount of weight gained, how much the abdominal wall expanded and how much time and effort a woman is willing to give to improving her body. Additional factors include diet, amount of rest obtained and types of activities involved in.
• Crash dieting is never recommended as a method of losing excess pregnancy weight, even if you are not breast-feeding. It can lead to excessive tiredness, general ill health and even depression. Eating sensibly, with an emphasis on nutrition, will help you return to the peak of fitness.
• Plan an exercise program that includes aerobic activity (walking, biking, swimming or other forms of exercise for which you use special exercise equipment) along with exercises designed to tighten the pelvic floor muscles and abdominal muscles that are loose and soft. Discuss your specific exercise program with the doctor.

ADVANTAGES OF EXERCISING
• Will help flatten the abdomen and tighten the perineum. Promotes healing of uterine, abdominal and pelvic muscles that were involved in pregnancy and childbirth.
• Can help avoid stress incontinence (leakage of urine).
• Helps avoid a dropping (prolapse) of pelvic organs.
• Helps return loosened joints to normal.
• Reduces the risk of backache and edema (excess fluid) in the legs and feet.
• Provides an outlet for stress and lessens the likelihood of postpartum blues or depression.
• A fitness program will condition and tone your body.

EXERCISE SUGGESTIONS
• Any exercise program should be resumed gradually based on your physical capability. Keep routines brief and frequent, rather than one long session.
• Begin a mild exercise program almost immediately following childbirth by performing pelvic tightening exercises (Kegel exercises) in bed. Continue to do these exercises daily. They can be done almost anywhere you are sitting or standing.
• At home, start each exercise program with a warm-up and stretching period.
• Abdominal exercises usually consist of crunches (curl-ups). Lie on a firm surface with legs bent at the knees and feet flat on the floor. Place hands behind head, elbows to the side, and lift head and shoulders a few inches off the floor. You will feel a tightening of the abdominal muscles. Do several, then rest a few seconds and do several more.
• Pelvic tilts can be combined with crunches or done alone. In the same position for crunches, press your back into the floor and lift the pelvis a few inches off the floor and then release. Do several, then rest a few seconds and do several more.
• One of the best options for postpartum fitness is to join an exercise class specifically designed for new mothers. It will not only concentrate on the muscle groups that need strengthening, but will put you in contact with other new mothers going through the same emotional and physical changes as you are.

RESUMING PREPREGNANCY EXERCISE ROUTINE
• It is usually recommended to wait until after your first postpartum checkup (usually 4 to 6 weeks following delivery) to resume a vigorous exercise or fitness routine. Though this medical visit is considered the conclusion of your pregnancy, your body still has physical adjustments to make.
• Discuss your exercise or fitness plan with your doctor. It may involve running, jogging, bicycling, swimming or other strenuous activities. When you resume the activity, do so gradually and build up to your prepregnancy capability.

 ## CALL YOUR DOCTOR IF

You or a family member wants additional information about postpartum exercises.

Exercises, Prenatal

GENERAL INFORMATION

DEFINITION
• Exercising during pregnancy can help minimize minor discomfort associated with the pregnancy, improve posture, make the body more supple, enhance circulation and provide a feeling of general well-being. Pregnancy is a state of health, not of illness. Properly executed exercises can help maintain health and avoid problems. A well-conditioned body will perform better and more reliably during the stress of advanced pregnancy, labor and delivery. Preconditioning will contribute to a more speedy recovery of body contour following delivery.
• Exercise regularly, rather than occasionally. Plan your exercise program with the help of your prenatal medical team. It should be planned around your prepregnancy fitness level. Women who have normally engaged in an exercise program before pregnancy can usually continue it during pregnancy (sometimes modifications are necessary).
• Women who were not exercising prior to pregnancy are usually advised to begin an exercise program. Start slowly, with 10 minutes for warm-up, 5 minutes of strenuous exercise and 5 minutes for cool-down. Over a period of a week, you should gradually increase the period of strenuous exercise to a maximum of 15 minutes per day; be sure to continue to allow time for warm-up and cool-down as well.
• Pregnant women who have a high-risk pregnancy may be advised to eliminate all exercise for the duration of their pregnancy.

CHARACTERISTIC CHANGES DURING PREGNANCY
• The pregnant woman's center of gravity moves forward and downward, altering balance, stability and stance. Backache, a frequent complaint of pregnancy, is directly attributable to poor posture.
• Hormonal changes during pregnancy soften ligaments and connective tissue that can compromise the stability and support of the spine and torso. Proper alignment prevents strain on joints.
• The abdominal muscles are stressed by the weight of the enlarging uterus. Keeping the pelvis in proper position protects these muscles from undue stretching and possible separation.
• Proper posture and alignment will assist with better lung expansion and air exchange, which may become limited by the enlarging uterus.

POSITIVE CHARACTERISTICS TO LOOK FOR IN AN EXERCISE PROGRAM
• Basically, what is needed is a warm-up period that slowly stretches muscles until the limit of range of motion is achieved, and circulation to muscles and heart rate are increased gradually.
• Fifteen minutes is considered a minimum time for the exercises to be effective. Exercising beyond 30 minutes probably provides no additional benefit.
• After exercising, there should be a cooling-down period for muscles and heart rate to return to their pre-exercise state. An exercise routine with the more stressful exercises in the middle helps achieve this goal.
• Exercises should stress control, rhythm, stabilization of the pelvis and proper alignment of the pelvis in a posterior-tilt position.
• Be aware that, as your center of gravity changes with your expanding uterus, your balance will also change. Be careful when engaging in sports that require a good sense of balance.
• Swimming provides rhythm, controlled breathing and water buoyancy.
• Drink plenty of fluids before and after you exercise.
• Compensate for the calories you burn by increasing your intake of nutrients by 100 to 200 calories for every 30 minutes of exercise.
• Most pregnant women are advised to decrease their level of exercise in the third trimester. Stretching routines and brisk walking should provide sufficient exercise until 4 to 6 weeks postpartum.

CAUTIONS
• Do not participate in a strenuous exercise program (such as running a marathon) when pregnant, if you were not doing it regularly prior to pregnancy.
• Do not indulge in rapid exercises with uncontrolled momentum. Sudden or exaggerated motions will severely stress ligaments and joints that are already relaxed under hormonal influence.
• Do not consider any exercises that increase the lordotic (lower back) curve of the spine or cause excessive compression of the uterus.
• Don't exercise outdoors in hot, humid weather.
• Don't bend deeply or greatly extend your joints and don't stand up abruptly.
• Stop any exercise right away if you develop signs of dizziness, bleeding, faintness, significant uterine contractions, abdominal or back pain, overly rapid heart rate or shortness of breath. If symptoms continue, call your doctor.
• Discuss your exercise program with your doctor to ensure that there are no factors that would cause problems. This is especially important if you have any chronic medical disorder or if the pregnancy is considered high risk.

CALL YOUR DOCTOR IF

• You or a family member is pregnant and has questions or concerns about exercising.
• During pregnancy, you are starting a new, or are changing an existing, exercise program.

Fetal Death Syndrome
(Intrauterine Fetal Demise [IUFD])

 GENERAL INFORMATION

DEFINITION—Death of a fetus that occurs for no apparent reason. It happens in about 1% of pregnancies and, in most states, is considered a fetal death when it occurs after the 20th week of pregnancy. The mother's health is usually not jeopardized.

SIGNS & SYMPTOMS
• Signs and symptoms of pregnancy may subside.
• No symptoms may occur in the early stages of pregnancy. The diagnosis is based on the absence of fetal heart tones, the lack of uterine growth, or ultrasound studies during prenatal examinations.
• In later stages of pregnancy, a woman may be aware that the fetal movement has stopped.

CAUSES
• The exact cause of the death is rarely obvious, and 50% of cases are never clearly explained, despite careful evaluation.
• In some cases, examination of the stillborn fetus shows an abnormality in either the umbilical cord, the placenta or the fetus itself. These problems include infections plus a variety of birth defects and genetic disorders.

RISK INCREASES WITH
• Some maternal conditions are known to increase the risk for fetal death (e.g., diabetes, hypertension, severe kidney or liver disease), but in most cases, risk factors are unknown.
• Multiple pregnancy.
• Maternal immunologic disorders.

HOW TO PREVENT—There are no specific preventive measures known.

PROBABLE OUTCOME
• The outcome will vary with the timing of the fetal death. Spontaneous labor often occurs within 2 weeks. Additional treatment options are available.
• Both parents will go through a period of grief. Mothers, sometimes more than fathers, often suffer from feelings of guilt and helplessness.
• If a fetal death has occurred in a multiple pregnancy, careful monitoring and specialized care will be necessary to assure the well-being of the surviving fetus.
• Medical care in subsequent pregnancies will be individualized depending on the needs of the patient and the cause of the previous fetal death, if an explanation was discovered. More frequent office visits and special tests may be indicated to help achieve a normal pregnancy outcome.

POSSIBLE COMPLICATIONS
• Disseminated intravascular coagulation (DIC), a disruption of blood clotting mechanisms that can result in hemorrhage or internal bleeding.
• Infection.

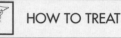 HOW TO TREAT

GENERAL MEASURES
• Diagnostic tests to confirm the fetal death consist of x-rays, ultrasound, amniotic fluid studies and maternal blood studies.
• Most women, upon learning that their fetus is dead, prefer early evacuation of the uterus. In the first trimester, this is usually done with suction curettage. In the second trimester, it is more frequently accomplished with prostaglandin E (Prostin) suppositories, or suction curettage in combination with laminaria (see Glossary). In the third trimester, it may be accomplished with intravenous oxytocin plus prostaglandin medication.
• An additional treatment option is to wait for spontaneous labor, which usually occurs within 2 weeks, but may take longer. This is termed expectant therapy.
• Examination of the stillborn fetus is usually performed to help determine any problems that might prove helpful in consideration and planning of subsequent pregnancies.
• Other issues to be considered include whether or not to see, touch or photograph the infant; whether to name the infant; disposition of the remains (burial or cremation) and holding of religious services.
• Parental feelings of loss, guilt, loneliness, anxiety and hostility should be acknowledged and faced. Family and friends can help with sympathetic listening and comforting. If severe grief lasts longer than several months, professional counseling is recommended. Both parents are urged to join a grief support group.

MEDICATION—Any medicines prescribed will depend on the type of treatment received.

ACTIVITY
• Usually, no restrictions.
• Sexual intercourse should be avoided for 4 to 6 weeks. Consult with your doctor on becoming pregnant again.

DIET—No special diet.

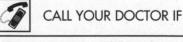 CALL YOUR DOCTOR IF

• You are pregnant and fail to gain weight or your abdomen is not increasing in size.
• Your unborn child appears to have stopped moving.
• Following the death of a fetus, you or a family member need help or emotional support in coping with the grief process.

Genetic Screening & Counseling

 GENERAL INFORMATION

DEFINITION
• Genetics is the study of inheritance and how the characteristics of one generation are passed on to another. Prior to pregnancy, or once pregnancy is diagnosed, a medical and family history of both parents will be taken by the doctor to look for any conditions that could affect, or be inherited by, the fetus. Most couples are at little risk for transmitting a genetic problem. If there appears to be an increased risk, certain screening tests will be recommended and the parents may then be referred to a doctor who is a genetic specialist for further testing and counseling.
• Genetic counseling is used to obtain and provide expectant parents with as much objective information as possible to help them arrive at a decision that is based on their own desires, values and ethics. Counseling is not used to coerce a couple to take or not take any particular tests or to make any reproductive decisions that they are not comfortable with.
• Although some defects are genetically transmitted, others are the result of environmental effects as the fetus develops in the womb. Still other defects that occur are spontaneous and without traceable cause.

POSSIBLE INDICATIONS FOR GENETIC TESTING
• Advanced maternal age (35 or older).
• Parental chromosome abnormality.
• Couples whose blood tests indicate they are carriers of a disorder.
• Couples who have already had a child with a genetic abnormality.
• Closely related couples such as first cousins.
• A pregnant woman whose routine prenatal tests detected a fetal defect.
• One of the partners has a congenital defect such as congenital heart disease.
• Couples who have a family history of a hereditary disorder or mental retardation of unknown origin.
• A woman with a history of multiple miscarriages (generally 3 or more) or stillbirth.
• Either parent belongs to a race or ethnic group at high risk for a specific genetic disease (e.g., sickle cell disease in African-Americans, Tay-Sachs disease in Jews of Ashkenazic background and beta-thalassemia in people of southern European ancestry).
• Either partner has been exposed to high doses of radiation or drugs, or has had occupational exposure to gases, chemicals or other environmental agents that could result in congenital abnormalities.
• A pregnant woman who has been exposed to an infection, such as rubella or toxoplasmosis, that could cause a birth defect.

PRELIMINARY SCREENING TESTS FOR GENETIC (CHROMOSOMAL) DEFECT
• Maternal blood test—measures the serum level of alpha-fetoprotein and other hormones which can identify a fetus with high risk for neural tube defect (cranial and spinal abnormalities) or chromosome abnormality such as Down syndrome. There is a possibility of false-negative or false-positive results.
• Ultrasound—the high-frequency soundwaves produce images of the fetus and placenta. It can detect major defects in the heart, bones, brain, abdomen and spinal cord.

SCREENING TESTS CONCLUSIVE FOR GENETIC (CHROMOSOMAL) DEFECT
• Amniocentesis—a needle is used to take a sample of amniotic fluid (liquid surrounding the baby in the uterus) that is then analyzed for many genetic disorders.
• Chorionic villi sampling (CVS)—a sampling of cells in the chorionic villi (part of the placenta) is analyzed for the presence of various defects or diseases.
• Fetoscopy (rarely used)—an optical instrument with a lighted tip is inserted into the uterus to observe the fetus. A blood sample can be taken at the same time for laboratory analysis.
• Cordocentesis—a sample of fetal blood is obtained from the umbilical cord with a fine needle guided by ultrasound. The blood sample is analyzed for defects or disorders.

OUTCOME OF TESTING
• Tests may indicate no problems.
• Tests may indicate a possible problem that requires further testing.
• Testing may show a definite problem. The parents will need to make a decision about continuing with the pregnancy if the defect is serious. Though the decision is the parents' alone, the health-care team should provide counseling and important information to assist them in a nondirective but understanding manner.
• The determination of serious genetic defects in a couple's history may present problems with future pregnancies and lead to decisions regarding permanent sterilization, as well as discussions about other methods of contraception such as donor insemination. Genetic counseling can assist in determining the best alternative options available.

 CALL YOUR DOCTOR IF

You or a family member has questions or concerns about genetic screening or counseling.

Gestational Diabetes Mellitus
(GDM; Gestational Carbohydrate Intolerance)

 GENERAL INFORMATION

DEFINITION—A type of diabetes occurring only in pregnant women. Gestational diabetes mellitus (GDM) occurs in 2% to 3% of all pregnancies. The percentage is higher in some population groups, such as Native Americans, Mexican Americans, Asians and East Indians.

SIGNS & SYMPTOMS
• Usually no symptoms are apparent. A prenatal examination may find that the fetus is larger than normal for the stage of pregnancy.
• If symptoms are present, they may include excessive hunger or thirst, frequent urination, increased blood pressure or recurring vaginal infections.

CAUSES—Insufficient insulin is produced by the body to keep blood glucose levels normal during pregnancy.

RISK INCREASES WITH
• Previous pregnancy with GDM.
• Obesity (especially in women with an apple-shaped body configuration).
• Marked increase in weight.
• Family history of diabetes mellitus.
• Previous birth of a large-for-date baby.
• Mother over age 25.

HOW TO PREVENT—While there are no specific preventive measures, prepregnancy weight loss in overweight women, as well as prepregnancy evaluation for women considered borderline diabetic or who have a history of GDM, may help reduce maternal or fetal risks.

PROBABLE OUTCOME
• The key to successful treatment and a healthy baby is determined by the mother's motivation and ability to change her lifestyle. For some, dietary control is sufficient, while for others, insulin may be required for treatment.
• Labor is spontaneous and the birth is usually vaginal. Cesarean section may be necessary if the fetus is considered too large for a vaginal birth.
• Gestational diabetes usually disappears following delivery of the baby.

POSSIBLE COMPLICATIONS
• Excess amniotic fluid (polyhydramnios).
• Premature labor.
• Patients with poor glucose control may need to have labor induced.
• Preeclampsia.
• Miscarriage (rare).
• Congenital anomalies (rare) in the newborn, including heart or lung problems, or a larger-than-normal baby. Metabolic disorders of a newborn (low blood sugar, low blood calcium levels) are more likely to occur if the mother has poor glucose control.

• There is an increased risk for the mother of developing diabetes mellitus in the future.

HOW TO TREAT

GENERAL MEASURES
• The diagnosis is based on glucose testing done during the 24th to 28th week of pregnancy for nondiabetic mothers. Earlier testing is often recommended for patients diagnosed with GDM in a previous pregnancy, or for mothers with several risk factors.
• Treatment will include diet changes and a moderate exercise program. Enlist the support of other family members for help in making the necessary changes.
• You will learn how to monitor your glucose levels. At first, glucose checks will need to be done up to 6 times a day on a daily basis. Once glucose levels are in the desired range and diet modifications are understood, glucose checks may be reduced with the doctor's approval.
• See the Resource section of this book for additional information.

MEDICATION
• Medicines are usually not necessary if glucose control is achieved with diet and exercise.
• Insulin may be prescribed for some patients who are unable to control glucose levels through diet and exercise.

ACTIVITY—A program of moderate, nonweight-bearing exercise is usually recommended. Follow any prescribed exercise program carefully.

DIET
• Dietary changes are an important aspect of the treatment and specific diet instructions will be provided. Following the prescribed diet will decrease the risks to mother and unborn child.
• These diet changes will involve increased fiber intake, fat restriction, elimination of concentrated sweets and monitoring of caloric intake to prevent excessive weight gain.
• Consultation with a dietitian is often recommended for educational purposes, to answer your dietary questions and to provide follow-up encouragement.

CALL YOUR DOCTOR IF

• You are 24 to 28 weeks pregnant and have not had a screening test for gestational diabetes mellitus.
• Following diagnosis of gestational diabetes, you develop any new signs or unexplained symptoms, or you have difficulty in following a prescribed diet or exercise program.

Gestational Trophoblastic Disease
(GTD; Hydatidiform Mole; Molar Pregnancy)

 GENERAL INFORMATION

DEFINITION—A disorder that includes hydatidiform mole, choriocarcinoma and invasive mole (chorioadenoma destruens). Hydatidiform mole, the most common, is a tumor of the placenta that is usually benign. It develops, during an early pregnancy, from placental tissue in which the embryo fails to develop normally. The tumor consists of many small vesicles (sacs) and resembles a large cluster of grapes. Invasive mole is a hydatidiform mole that spreads to adjacent structures. Choriocarcinoma is a malignant tumor preceded by hydatidiform mole, abortion or term pregnancy. Although molar pregnancy is fairly rare in the U.S., it is more common in Asia and other parts of the world.

SIGNS & SYMPTOMS
• In early pregnancy, there may be no unusual symptoms.
• Abnormal uterine bleeding, usually during the first trimester.
• Morning sickness that is frequently excessive.
• Passage of vesicle (small, grapelike sac).
• Hypertension or hyperthyroidism.
• Absence of fetal heartbeat.
• Abnormally large or small uterus.

CAUSES—Exact cause is unknown. Genetic factors may be involved.

RISK INCREASES WITH
• Asian race.
• Mother over age 40 or under age 20.
• Diet lacking in protein, folic acid and, possibly, carotene.
• Preeclampsia or eclampsia with onset before the 24th week of pregnancy.
• History of previous hydatidiform mole or other gestational trophoblastic disease (GTD).

HOW TO PREVENT—No specific preventive measures.

PROBABLE OUTCOME
• With early diagnosis and treatment of an uncomplicated hydatidiform, the outlook is excellent.
• Feelings of loss and grief for the terminated pregnancy are common. Feelings of guilt may also be present.
• Reproductive function is generally not affected. A normal subsequent pregnancy is usual, and complications are similar to those in the general population.

POSSIBLE COMPLICATIONS
• Excessive bleeding and/or pulmonary problems following the uterine evacuation procedure.
• There is a small risk that a malignant tumor

may later develop. Follow-up testing is usually necessary for a year to monitor for this possibility. If a tumor does occur, treatment with chemotherapy is usually successful.
• The risk of having a recurrent hydatidiform mole with a future pregnancy is slightly increased.

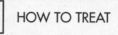 HOW TO TREAT

GENERAL MEASURES
• Diagnostic tests may include ultrasound to assess uterine contents; laboratory studies of blood and/or urine levels of beta-human chorionic gonadotropin (ß-hCG; see Glossary); x-ray and amniocentesis.
• Treatment normally involves suction curettage to evacuate the contents of the uterus. Blood loss is usually moderate and transfusion is rarely necessary.
• Hysterectomy is a treatment option for women not desiring future pregnancy or for older women (who might be more likely to develop a malignancy).
• Regardless of method of treatment, follow-up care is essential to monitor blood and urine levels for the hormone ß-hCG that can indicate a malignancy. These tests will be done weekly for the first 3 months, and then every 3 months for at least a year.
• A new pregnancy must be delayed for a minimum of 1 year, possibly longer if the blood and urine tests indicate the hormone levels are still not within normal range. Effective contraceptive methods should be implemented and maintained throughout this time period.
• Psychological and emotional support are important following diagnosis, as well as during and following treatment for the disorder.

MEDICATION
• Medicines as needed for the selected treatment plan.
• Oral contraceptives are usually the chosen method for contraception purposes.
• Chemotherapy may be recommended as a form of preventive therapy.

ACTIVITY—Any restrictions will be determined by the treatment method.

DIET—No special diet.

 CALL YOUR DOCTOR IF

• You or a family member has symptoms of hydatidiform mole or other GTD.
• You are pregnant and any unusual symptoms occur.
• After treatment, you have excessive vaginal bleeding.

Heartburn during Pregnancy

GENERAL INFORMATION

DEFINITION—Burning pain in the chest and upper abdomen during pregnancy.

SIGNS & SYMPTOMS
• Burning pain in the center of the chest and upper abdomen, frequently accompanied by an unpleasant taste in the mouth.
• Belching (burping).

CAUSES
• Heartburn is not associated with a heart disorder. It is caused by a backflow of acid from the stomach into the esophagus. During pregnancy, the muscles that close off the upper stomach become more relaxed, allowing stomach juices to back up into the esophagus and irritate its lining.
• Changes in gastrointestinal functions (e.g., slower emptying time of the stomach contents, which allows a woman's body to better absorb nutrients for herself and the baby) caused by hormones produced during pregnancy.
• During late pregnancy, the enlarged womb presses on the stomach and may intensify the symptoms.
• Overeating can cause or irritate heartburn.

RISK INCREASES WITH
• Overeating or eating and then lying down.
• Smoking.
• Excess alcohol consumption.

HOW TO PREVENT
• Avoid gaining too much weight; excessive weight gain puts increased pressure on the stomach and its contents.
• Avoid foods which can irritate the gastrointestinal system, such as spicy, fatty or fried foods. Also avoid caffeinated or carbonated beverages (e.g., coffee, soda or tea) and alcohol.
• Eat numerous small meals throughout the day, rather than 3 large ones.
• Eat slowly and chew your food thoroughly.
• Don't eat immediately before bedtime. Try to avoid lying down for at least 1 hour after eating.
• Wearing loose-fitting clothing, especially around the waist and abdomen.
• Don't smoke.

PROBABLE OUTCOME—This is an uncomfortable, but harmless, condition. The heartburn usually disappears after the baby is born unless the cause is not related to pregnancy.

POSSIBLE COMPLICATIONS—Inflammation and ulcer in the lower esophagus (rare).

HOW TO TREAT

GENERAL MEASURES
• Avoid bending over, especially after eating.
• Don't wear tight girdles or belts.
• Sleep with your head and upper body elevated at least 6 inches (use pillows, or place blocks or books under the head of the bed) to help prevent stomach acids from backing up through the esophagus.
• Don't smoke.

MEDICATION—Medication is usually not necessary for this disorder; however, in severe cases, it may be of benefit. The medicines most frequently used include antacids and H2 blockers (acid reduction drugs, such as Tagamet, Zantac and Pepcid). Some patients may want to avoid antacids which contain sodium or sodium bicarbonate. Antacids, and all drugs taken during pregnancy, should be used only with your doctor's approval. As long as you can live with the symptoms, endure the discomfort without drugs or medicines.

ACTIVITY—Stay active. Prenatal exercises can help reduce heartburn by relieving stress, enhancing circulation and minimizing minor discomforts during pregnancy. Avoid abdominal exercises that require bending.

DIET
• Eat small, frequent meals.
• Don't eat before bedtime.
• Avoid highly seasoned food.
• Don't drink alcohol.
• Avoid very hot or very cold beverages.

 ## CALL YOUR DOCTOR IF

• You or a family member has symptoms of heartburn during pregnancy. This should be diagnosed.
• The following occur after diagnosis:
  Simple measures don't bring relief.
  You begin vomiting late in pregnancy.
  You vomit material that has blood in it or looks like coffee grounds.
  You have black or tarry stools.

HIV & AIDS in Pregnancy

GENERAL INFORMATION

DEFINITION—HIV (human immunodeficiency virus) is the infection that leads to AIDS (acquired immunodeficiency syndrome). HIV infection causes a breakdown in the body's immune system. A pregnant woman with HIV may pass the virus to her unborn child. Transmission can occur through the placenta during pregnancy, through blood and bodily fluids during delivery or after the child is born, through breast-feeding.

SIGNS & SYMPTOMS—For HIV infection (some of the symptoms of early HIV infection may mimic those of the first trimester of pregnancy):
- Fatigue.
- Unexplained weight loss.
- Recurrent respiratory and skin infections.
- Fever; night sweats.
- Swollen lymph glands throughout the body.
- Genital changes; enlarged spleen.
- Diarrhea.
- Mouth sores.

CAUSES—HIV is a retrovirus that invades and destroys cells of the immune system, which results in lowered resistance to infections and some types of cancer.

RISK INCREASES WITH
- Injecting drugs of abuse; sharing needles.
- Multiple sexual partners.
- Sexual relations with a man who has had sex with another man.
- Current or past sexually transmitted disease.

HOW TO PREVENT
- If trying to become pregnant, both you and your partner should consider HIV testing before having unprotected sex.
- If artificial insemination is utilized for pregnancy, the donor should be tested first for HIV.
- Avoid intravenous drug abuse. If you do use drugs, never share needles.
- If you are infected with HIV (or at risk of being infected) and become pregnant, seek medical help from a maternal-fetal medicine specialist or an infectious disease specialist.
- Don't breast-feed; this will prevent the possibility of passing HIV to your child through your breast milk.

PROBABLE OUTCOME
- Being infected with HIV or AIDS does appear to have some effect on the pregnancy itself and could cause premature birth or low birthweight.
- Pregnancy does involve your immune system and, therefore, may affect the course of an HIV infection (although the effect is probably small).
- An average of 30% of infants born to HIV mothers become HIV infected, unless the mother is receiving antiviral treatment during pregnancy and delivery.

POSSIBLE COMPLICATIONS—HIV-infected baby.

HOW TO TREAT

GENERAL MEASURES
- Seek early medical help for your pregnancy. Special individualized care will be undertaken with referrals to any necessary support systems (e.g., counseling, social services).
- Screening for other sexually transmitted diseases (e.g., syphilis, gonorrhea, chlamydia and hepatitis B) is important.
- Testing is recommended for other AIDS-related infections, such as tuberculosis, toxoplasmosis and cytomegalovirus (CMV).
- Vaccinations for hepatitis B and pneumococcal and influenza viruses are suggested for susceptible patients.
- Special testing of CD4+ lymphocyte cell count and viral load are usually done each trimester.
- Avoid contact with people who have infections.
- The method used to deliver the baby appears to have no effect on the possible transmission of HIV, however, you should discuss the delivery options with the doctor.
- Research continues into new drugs, treatment methods and a possible vaccine against HIV.
- See the Resource section of this book for additional information.

MEDICATION
- Most of the medications used to fight opportunistic infections in HIV-infected pregnant women have not been shown to cause birth defects. Your doctor will use caution, careful consideration and expert consultation in prescribing any medications. The benefits of the treatment for the mother usually outweigh the possible risks to the baby. Some infections are life-threatening to the mother.
- Antiviral medication (zidovudine) is recommended to reduce the risk of transmitting the HIV infection to the unborn child. This drug is taken during pregnancy and labor and also needs to be given to the newborn.
- Sometimes, a combination of multiple antiviral drugs (an AIDS cocktail) may be prescribed.

ACTIVITY—No specific restrictions. Regular exercise, as permitted by the course of the infection and by the pregnancy, is helpful.

DIET—No special diet unless recommended by the doctor.

CALL YOUR DOCTOR IF

- You have symptoms of HIV infection and/or pregnancy.
- You develop signs of infection: headache, muscle aches, or a general ill feeling and fever.
- New, unexplained symptoms develop. Drugs used in treatment may produce side effects.

Home Pregnancy Tests

GENERAL INFORMATION

DEFINITION—Home pregnancy tests detect the hormone human chorionic gonadotropin (hCG), which is present in the urine of a pregnant woman. These tests are simple to use and almost 100% effective if done correctly, although a positive result is more likely to be correct than a negative result. HCG is produced by the placenta in increasing amounts beginning 7 days after fertilization (conception). An absence of a menstrual period in a sexually active female is usually the first reason a pregnancy test is utilized. Other signs of pregnancy that may occur include:
• Unusually short or light menstrual period.
• Morning sickness (nausea, vomiting, food and smell intolerance).
• Fatigue.
• Frequent urination.
• Tender, swollen breasts.
• Darkening of the area around the nipples (areola).
• Food cravings.
• Blue and pink lines under the skin on the breasts and later on the abdomen.

TYPES OF TESTS—There are a variety of home pregnancy tests that are available without a prescription. Some tests detect pregnancy as early as the first day of a missed period. They all use a urine sample for the basis of the test, and most give results within a few minutes. Home pregnancy tests generally cost between $7 and $14.

USING TESTS WISELY
• Check the expiration date. If the date is past, don't buy the product.
• Follow package directions about storing the test at home.
• Learn about the limitations of the test. Remember, no test is 100% accurate.
• Read the insert to learn how to use the test. Review the instructions so each step is fully understood.
• Don't guess if something is unclear. Consult a pharmacist or call the manufacturer's "800" number if one is listed in the instructions.
• Note any special precautions before using the test.
• Follow instructions exactly. Don't skip a step.
• Note what to do if results are positive, negative or unclear.
• Keep a record of the test results, the date and the brand name of the test to advise the doctor if necessary.
• Discard used materials as directed.

NEGATIVE RESULTS
• If a pregnancy test is negative and the woman is still not menstruating, she should wait the number of days suggested in the instructions and test again, making sure she follows all instructions correctly. If the second test is negative and there is still no menstrual period, she should consult her doctor.
• A false-negative can occur with a home pregnancy test. The result indicates there is no pregnancy when in fact there is. Pregnant women don't always produce the HCG hormone at the same rate, so a woman could be pregnant but not yet producing enough of the hormone to obtain a positive test result. In addition, the levels of the hormone needed to trigger the positive results vary from test to test. One of the problems of a false-negative result is that a woman might continue certain practices that are potentially harmful to the baby's health, such as smoking, excessive drinking or using medications not suitable during pregnancy.

POSITIVE RESULTS—A positive result of a home pregnancy test does not replace the need to schedule an appointment with the doctor. Confirmation of the pregnancy is determined with a physical examination that is combined with a complete prenatal checkup.

CALL YOUR DOCTOR IF

You or a family member has:
• A positive result from a home pregnancy test.
• A negative result from a first or second home pregnancy test and a menstrual period that is a week or more overdue.

Home Pregnancy Tests

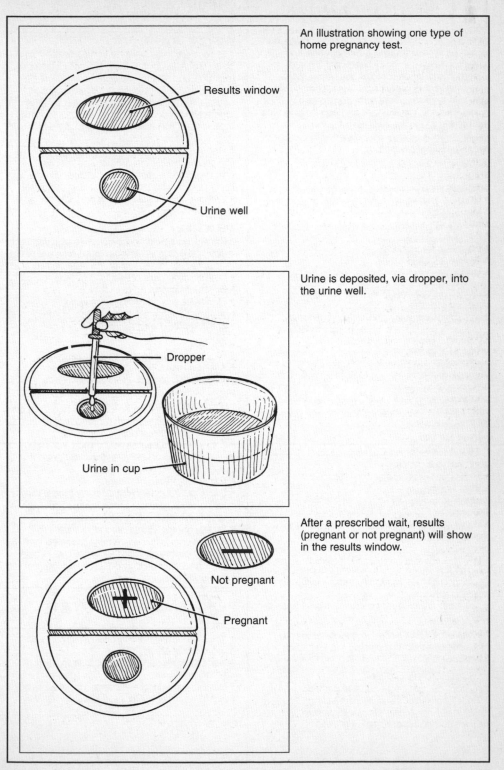

An illustration showing one type of home pregnancy test.

Results window

Urine well

Urine is deposited, via dropper, into the urine well.

Dropper

Urine in cup

After a prescribed wait, results (pregnant or not pregnant) will show in the results window.

Not pregnant

Pregnant

Hyperemesis Gravidarum

GENERAL INFORMATION

DEFINITION—Severe nausea and vomiting in a pregnant woman, causing dehydration and drastic changes in body chemistry. This is different and much more serious than morning sickness during pregnancy; it is a complication that can lead to severe dehydration and malnutrition in the woman, and can threaten the well-being of the fetus. Hyperemesis gravidarum is usually associated with the first 8 to 20 weeks of pregnancy.

SIGNS & SYMPTOMS
- Severe nausea.
- Sustained vomiting (usually 4 to 8 weeks), first of mucus, then of bile and, sometimes, of blood.
- Dehydration.
- Failure to gain weight, or weight loss to less than prepregnancy weight.
- Hypersensitivity to smell.
- Rapid heartbeat.
- Headache, fatigue, confusion or lethargy.

CAUSES—Unknown. The most common theories include:
- Multiple pregnancy (more than one fetus), producing high levels of the hormone HCG (human chorionic gonadotropin).
- Vitamin B6 deficiency caused by a change in protein matabolism during pregnancy.
- Inflammation of the pancreas.
- Bile-duct disease.
- Psychological factors, such as depression, ambivalence about the pregnancy or a poor response to stress.
- Poor nutrition.
- Thyroid disorders.

RISK INCREASES WITH
- Younger maternal age.
- First pregnancy.
- Mother overweight.
- Single marital status.
- Emotional stress.
- Caucasian women.

HOW TO PREVENT
- Don't use any drugs, including nonprescription drugs or alcohol, during pregnancy without medical advice.
- Maintain an adequate diet during all stages of pregnancy.

PROBABLE OUTCOME—Usually curable with time and treatment (replacing the lost fluids in the body).

POSSIBLE COMPLICATIONS
- Severe dehydration and/or malnutrition.
- Poor fetal growth and outcome (rare).
- Sufficient risk to the mother to warrant termination of the pregnancy (rare).

HOW TO TREAT

GENERAL MEASURES
- Diagnostic tests may be conducted to rule out other disorders of the liver, kidney, pancreas, intestine and gastrointestinal tract.
- Hospitalization or outpatient management usually requires replacement of lost fluids and electrolytes (such as sodium and potassium). Intravenous (IV) fluids are necessary when oral intake is not tolerated.
- Reduce stress whenever possible. Psychotherapy is often helpful to resolve emotional problems. If hospitalized, visitors may be limited or restricted to reduce stimulation.
- Weigh yourself daily and report any unusual changes to the doctor.

MEDICATION
- Intravenous fluid and electrolyte replacement if your condition is serious. Intravenous vitamin therapy and antinausea drugs may be required.
- If other drugs are prescribed for you, carefully follow instructions on the label.
- Don't use any medicine, including nonprescription medicine to prevent vomiting, without medical advice.

ACTIVITY
- Bed rest may benefit some patients.
- After recovery, resume activities slowly as your strength allows. Work and exercise moderately. Rest often.

DIET—If the condition has not reached the point to warrant hospitalization for intravenous fluids, follow these instructions:
- If you feel nauseated in the morning, eat dry toast or saltine crackers before you get out of bed.
- Eat small, frequent meals.
- Don't eat fried, high-fat or spicy foods; they can increase nausea. Limit dairy products, especially butter, milk and cheese.
- Sit upright for 45 minutes after eating.
- If intravenous fluids are necessary, you will probably progress from them to a clear liquid diet; a full liquid diet; and then a regular diet with small, frequent meals.

CALL YOUR DOCTOR IF

- You or a family member has symptoms of hyperemesis gravidarum.
- Nausea, vomiting or weight loss worsen, despite treatment.
- New, unexplained symptoms develop. Drugs used in treatment may produce side effects.

Incompetent Cervix

GENERAL INFORMATION

DEFINITION—The cervix is the neck of the womb that connects the vagina with the uterus. Normally, the cervix remains closed throughout pregnancy until labor begins. Women who are diagnosed with an incompetent cervix experience premature opening (dilation) of the cervix, usually in mid-pregnancy (18 to 22 weeks). The condition occurs in about 1 out of every 100 pregnancies and may be responsible for 20% to 25% of second trimester miscarriages. The miscarriage usually occurs after the uterus has enlarged somewhat and the developing fetus becomes heavy enough to press the cervix open.

SIGNS & SYMPTOMS
• No signs and symptoms are usually apparent. In a pregnant woman, there is a gradual thinning and dilatation of the cervix; usually without vaginal bleeding or uterine contractions.
• In some cases, a woman may experience pressure in the lower abdomen or vagina, unusual urinary frequency, vaginal discharge (with or without blood) or a sensation of a lump in the vagina.

CAUSES—The cervix may be weakened by injury, previous childbirth, induced abortion, D & C (dilatation and curettage) surgery, cervical surgery or laser therapy. There are rare conditions in which the substance of the cervix is not strong enough to support a pregnancy.

RISK INCREASES WITH
• Multiple gestation (e.g., twins).
• A woman who was exposed to DES (diethystilbestrol; a drug once used to prevent miscarriage) when she was in her mother's womb.
• Women who have had significant cervical surgery, particularly when portions of the cervix have been removed (e.g., cone biopsy).

HOW TO PREVENT—If a woman experiences a miscarriage that is diagnosed as being caused by cervical incompetence, there are preventive measures that can be taken with a subsequent pregnancy to reduce the risk of another miscarriage.

PROBABLE OUTCOME—If diagnosed with a previous miscarriage, and with proper treatment in the subsequent pregnancy, chances of carrying to term are good.

POSSIBLE COMPLICATIONS—Repeated miscarriages.

HOW TO TREAT

GENERAL MEASURES
• Diagnosis is based on a history of a mid-second trimester miscarriage that was accompanied by painless cervical dilation. This history can be supported by a pelvic examination, and by ultrasound scanning.
• Treatment involves the placing of stitch or suture (cerclage) into the wall of the cervix and drawing it up (similar to a purse string). This helps hold the fetus in the womb. The procedure is normally performed under regional anesthetic or sometimes local anesthetic at about the 12th to 14th week of pregnancy. The stitch is removed shortly before the baby is due or at the time of delivery (depending on the doctor's preference) so that a normal delivery can take place. Stitch removal is simple and does not require anesthesia.
• An incompetent cervix may also be corrected in a nonpregnant woman.
• Rarely, bed rest and use of a uterine support (pessary) for the duration of the pregnancy may be recommended instead of the surgical procedure.

MEDICATION—Medicine is not necessary for this disorder.

ACTIVITY
• Bed rest for 24 hours following the cerclage procedure. Additional restrictions may be recommended by the doctor.
• For some patients, sexual intercourse may be restricted for the duration of the pregnancy.

DIET—No diet restrictions; continue with your recommended pregnancy diet.

CALL YOUR DOCTOR IF

• You or a family member is pregnant and experiences any new or unusual symptoms such as cramping or spotting.
• Any sign of infection develops, such as fever, pain on urination, frequent urination or a general ill feeling.

Intrauterine Growth Retardation (IUGR; Small-for-Gestational-Age [SGA] Pregnancy)

GENERAL INFORMATION

DEFINITION—The fetus is much smaller than would normally be expected for its gestational age. IUGR occurs in 1 in 10 pregnancies. Contrary to the name, babies who are diagnosed with IUGR usually do not have any physical or mental retardation after birth and suffer from growth retardation only while in the womb. There is, however, an increased risk for these children to have developmental delays during early childhood.

SIGNS & SYMPTOMS—Usually no signs or symptoms occur. Diagnosis is based on prenatal physical examinations and ultrasound studies.

CAUSES—Chromosome abnormalities and/or infections of the fetus are often the cause of IUGR. In other cases, the placenta fails to provide adequate nutrients to the fetus. Most often, the placenta is normal, but is functioning abnormally. Abnormal placenta anatomy, such as placenta previa or placental abruption, can result in IUGR. In many cases, the cause of IUGR cannot be identified.

RISK INCREASES WITH
• Multiple fetuses (twins or greater).
• Poor maternal nutrition.
• Maternal illness, such as cyanotic heart disease, hypertension, anemia, chronic kidney disease, diabetes mellitus with vascular involvement or sickle cell disease.
• Smoking.
• Fetal infections.
• Maternal drug addiction or alcohol abuse.
• Placenta previa; placental abruption.
• Fetal congenital abnormalities; chromosomal abnormalities.
• Maternal low prepregnant weight and/or low weight gain with pregnancy.
• Previous pregnancy with an intrauterine growth retardation baby.
• Living at a high altitude.

HOW TO PREVENT
• Avoidance of any of the risk factors that are within the control of the mother, such as smoking or alcohol abuse.
• Genetic counseling prior to pregnancy.
• Good medical care and management of any maternal chronic disorder listed in risk factors.
• Good nutrition during pregnancy.
• Good prenatal care.
• If pregnant, avoid people with infections.

PROBABLE OUTCOME
• For the mother without an underlying condition, the outcome is equivalent to a mother who delivers an average-for-gestational-age (AGA) baby. A cesarean section delivery may be necessary in cases of fetal distress.
• For the vast majority of infants with IUGR, the outlook is generally good for subsequent normal physical development and neurological outcome.

POSSIBLE COMPLICATIONS
• Increased risk for fetal problems prior to and at birth, such as respiratory distress, low birth-weight, prematurity, fetal stress, low blood sugar and temperature instabilities.
• Higher risk exists for congenital defects.
• Risk of SIDS (sudden infant death syndrome).
• Long term, the child may develop physical or neurological handicaps (uncommon).

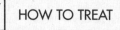

HOW TO TREAT

GENERAL MEASURES
• Any substances being abused by the mother need to be discontinued (smoking, alcohol, drugs).
• Any maternal illness should be stabilized if possible.
• Ongoing testing will be done once or twice weekly to assess the condition of the fetus.
• Hospitalization may be required if outpatient steps are unsuccessful.
• Labor may need to be induced or a cesarean section performed if fetal compromise is diagnosed or it is determined that the optimal time for delivery has been reached (the point at which the baby will do as well outside as inside the uterus).
• Often the baby will need to be delivered in a hospital facility that can provide intensive monitoring during labor and delivery, as well as any critical care of the newborn following delivery (such as in a neonatal intensive care unit).

MEDICATION—Low-dose aspirin may be prescribed for some selected cases.

ACTIVITY—Following diagnosis, complete bed rest is often recommended, while others may be on a limited activity routine. If bed rest is prescribed, lying on the left side helps promote blood flow and nutrition for the fetus.

DIET—If poor nutrition is a problem, a special diet will be prescribed.

CALL YOUR DOCTOR IF

• You are pregnant and have any concerns about the development of your baby.
• During treatment, any new signs or symptoms develop.

Labor & Delivery

GENERAL INFORMATION

DEFINITION
• Normally, labor and subsequent delivery occur 38 to 40 weeks after the start of the last normal menstrual period. If labor occurs before 37 weeks of pregnancy, it is considered premature, and after 42 weeks, is termed postmature (post-term). Labor can be divided into three stages:

The first stage is from the earliest contractions up to the time of birth. It is generally the longest and hardest and involves the effacement (thinning out) and dilation (opening up) of the cervix to 10 centimeters (5 fingerbreadths). Stage 1 has 3 phases.

Stage 2 of labor involves the baby's birth and lasts about 1 to 3 hours.

Stage 3 consists of explusion of the after-birth (placenta) and takes about 30 minutes.

• There is no way to determine how long labor will be for any one woman, but with careful preparation and adequate prenatal care, there is no reason to be afraid. The delivery procedures that you have chosen and practiced will help assure a safe and satisfactory birth experience.

STAGE 1 OF LABOR
Phase 1 (early or latent phase):
• This first phase (early labor) of stage 1 takes about 8 to 12 hours (occasionally longer); the cervix begins to efface and dilates to 3 centimeters. This phase may begin with contractions, the rupture of the amniotic fluid (bag of waters), or the passing of the thick, blood-tinged plug of mucus (bloody show) that protects the mouth of the uterus during pregnancy. This plug may pass hours or some-times several weeks before contractions begin.
• Contractions are the rhythmic, squeezing muscular activity that affects the walls of the uterus during labor. They usually start out lasting 30 to 45 seconds, may be almost imperceptible, and come on an irregular basis (up to 30 minutes apart). As time passes, they become more regular.
• During this first phase of stage 1, a woman usually remains at home.
Phase 2 (active phase):
• This is the active labor phase. Contractions start coming every 3 to 5 minutes and last 40 to 60 seconds. The cervix dilates to 3 to 8 centimeters and is effaced close to 100%.
• At this time, a woman should be at the location chosen for delivery (hospital, birthing center). A physical examination will be done to see how far the cervix is dilated.
• The baby's heart rate will be monitored, usually by Doppler ultrasound or an electronic fetal monitor.
• To help with the discomfort of this phase, a woman should practice relaxation and breathing techniques learned at childbirth classes.

• Depending on the severity of the pain and the doctor's advice, pain medication may be considered, or a regional (epidural) anesthetic may be administered by an anesthesiologist.
• Generally an intravenous drip (occasionally containing glucose) is administered to women in labor. The IV is available for an anesthetic if an emergency cesarean becomes necessary.
• Pitocin, a drug used to stimulate labor, may be used to speed the progression of labor.
Phase 3 (transition phase):
• Transition is probably the most difficult part of labor and lasts about an hour. The cervix usually dilates to 10 centimeters, and the contractions switch from the type that open the cervix to the pushing-down type meant to expel the baby.
• Other symptoms may occur—nausea, vomiting, shivers and irritability. This is often a time of self-doubt when a woman feels she cannot go on through labor. A good supportive birth coach and helpful medical team can aid in overcoming these feelings.

STAGE 2 OF LABOR
• Contractions continue about every 2 to 5 minutes and last 60 to 90 seconds. Pushing down is done between contractions.
• The baby moves down through the birth canal, aided by the mother's pushing. Depending on how the labor is progressing and the baby's position, different positions for the mother might be tried, such as squatting, sitting or kneeling.
• A surgical incision (episiotomy) may be made in the perineum (see Glossary) to widen the birth opening. This procedure may require a local, spinal, epidural, pudendal or paracervical anesthetic.
• Toward the end of this stage, the perineum begins to bulge with the baby's head pushing against it (crowning).
• The baby's head, then the shoulders, emerge; the rest of the body quickly follows.
• The umbilical cord will be clamped and cut.
• The baby's condition will usually be evaluated. The baby will then be dried, weighed and measured; eyedrops will be administered. In many hospitals, these procedures may be done in another area, such as a transitional nursery.
• In some locations, umbilical cord blood is collected and stored so it can be used for a variety of tests and purposes.

STAGE 3 OF LABOR
• The after-birth (placenta) is expelled as it separates from the wall of the uterus.
• A final examination is conducted to be sure the entire placenta is out and there are no tears in the vagina or cervix.

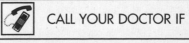 CALL YOUR DOCTOR IF

You or a family member has questions or concerns about labor and delivery.

Miscarriage (Spontaneous Abortion)

GENERAL INFORMATION

DEFINITION—Premature termination of a pregnancy, most frequently in the first trimester. It occurs in about 20% to 30% of pregnancies and frequently occurs so early that the woman is unaware that she is pregnant.

SIGNS & SYMPTOMS
- Uterine cramps.
- Vaginal bleeding which can vary from slight to heavy.
- Dilation of the cervix.
- Many miscarriages are only "threatened," and the pregnancy will continue to term. Symptoms may be the same for threatened miscarriages as for those in progress.

CAUSES
During the first trimester (first 12 weeks of pregnancy):
- Chromosomal abnormalities in the fetus.
- Uterine abnormalities that prevent the fertilized egg from growing normally.
During the second trimester (13 to 28 weeks):
- Uterine abnormalities that cause detachment of the fetus and placenta; incompetent cervix.
- Severe stress (nutritional; psychological).
Anytime:
- Use of substances that harm the fetus (drugs, alcohol, caffeine, tobacco).
- Infections, especially viral infections (e.g., rubella or influenza).
- Trauma or severe medical conditions (e.g., diabetes mellitus, hypertension).

RISK INCREASES WITH
- Smoking; use of alcohol or drugs; excessive caffeine (more than 2 cups of coffee per day).
- Poor nutrition.
- Maternal age under 15 or over 35 years.
- Illness that lowers resistance.
- Recent serious infection.
- Previous abortions.
- History of diabetes mellitus or hypertension.

HOW TO PREVENT
During pregnancy:
- Obtain regular medical checkups.
- Eat a normal, well-balanced diet.
- Don't drink alcohol, smoke cigarettes or use recreational drugs; limit caffeine consumption.
- Don't use any medications, including nonprescription drugs, without medical advice.

PROBABLE OUTCOME
- With treatment, a miscarriage is not life-threatening to the mother. It usually does not affect a woman's ability to carry a healthy baby to term in the future.
- Feelings of loss and grief are common. Feelings of guilt may also be present. If these persist, seek professional psychological help.

POSSIBLE COMPLICATIONS
- Uterine infection, signaled by fever, chills and muscle aches.
- Recurrent or habitual abortion (uncommon).
- Incomplete abortion or missed abortion (see Glossary).
- Disseminated intravascular coagulation (DIC; see Glossary).

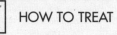

HOW TO TREAT

GENERAL MEASURES
- Ultrasound examination and laboratory blood studies may be needed for diagnosis.
- For a threatened miscarriage, follow your doctor's orders. Bed rest at home is often enough to stabilize the pregnancy. Bleeding is occasionally severe, requiring hospitalization and blood transfusion as indicated.
- Following a miscarriage, expect a small amount of vaginal bleeding or spotting for 8 to 10 days. Don't use tampons for 2 to 4 weeks.
- Generally, women are advised to wait through 2 or 3 normal menstrual cycles before attempting to become pregnant again.
- Surgery (D & C or D & E; see Glossary) may be needed to remove any remaining fetal tissue.
- Psychotherapy or grief counseling for the patient and her partner may be helpful.

MEDICATION
- For a threatened miscarriage: Medicine usually is not necessary. Don't take any medication without medical advice.
- Oxytocin to control bleeding in some patients.
- Pain medication may be prescribed.
- After a miscarriage, antibiotics may be prescribed to fight infection.
- Blood transfusions for severe blood loss.
- An Rh-negative female may be given RhoD (immune globulin).

ACTIVITY
- For a threatened miscarriage: Rest in bed until symptoms disappear. Avoid sexual intercourse until the outcome is known.
- After a miscarriage: Reduce activity and rest often during the next 48 hours.

DIET
- For a threatened miscarriage: Drink fluids only, if bleeding and cramping are severe.
- After a miscarriage: No special diet.

CALL YOUR DOCTOR IF

- Vaginal bleeding occurs during pregnancy.
- Bleeding and cramps worsen during a threatened miscarriage, or you pass tissue.
- Fever and chills occur during a threatened miscarriage or following miscarriage.
- Bleeding (other than vaginal) or unexplained bruising occurs after a miscarriage.
- Infection develops while you are pregnant.

Miscarriage, Habitual
(Recurrent Abortion; Habitual Abortion)

 GENERAL INFORMATION

DEFINITION—Three or more consecutive spontaneous losses before 20 weeks' gestation.

SIGNS & SYMPTOMS—A woman has miscarried 3 or more times, usually without a history of any normal birth.

CAUSES
• Genetic abnormalities in the fetus, which may be hereditary or spontaneous.
• Problems in the immune system.
• An "allergy" to mate's sperm.
• Uterine abnormalities (polyps, fibroids, congenital defects or duplications of the female genital tract).
• Incompetent cervix (inability of the cervix to hold the pregnancy) in cases of second trimester losses.
• Infections.
• Hormonal abnormalities, such as defective corpus luteum function (luteal phase defect) in which inadequate progesterone is produced by the corpus luteum of the ovary.
• Connective tissue disease (e.g., systemic lupus erythematosus, antiphospholipid syndrome).
• Chronic medical conditions (e.g., severe hypertension, diabetes mellitus, hyper- or hypothyroidism, kidney disease).

RISK INCREASES WITH
• Medical history of endocrine diseases, such as diabetes mellitus, hyper- or hypothyroidism.
• A woman who was exposed to DES (diethystilbestrol; a drug once used to prevent miscarriage) when she was in her mother's womb.

HOW TO PREVENT
• Seek expert consultation with a reproductive endocrinologist, or obstetrician specializing in that field, to obtain a thorough evaluation before embarking on a future pregnancy.
• Prevention of another miscarriage in a future pregnancy will depend, in part, on the diagnosis and treatment of any underlying problem.
• Taking prenatal vitamins with folic acid for 3 months prior to conception may help to prevent some genetic problems, which may, in turn, help to decrease the likelihood of miscarriage.
• Wait at least 3 months following a pregnancy before attempting to get pregnant again.
• When pregnancy occurs, seek early prenatal care, schedule more frequent office visits and follow recommended medical advice carefully.

PROBABLE OUTCOME
• In about half of the couples, the cause is undetermined but, even without treatment, there is a 60% chance of a future successful pregnancy. It is not a hopeless situation.
• The prognosis for a successful pregnancy can range from 30% to 90%, depending on the cause of the repetitive miscarriages. Multiple factors may be involved in some couples.

POSSIBLE COMPLICATIONS—Inability to carry a pregnancy to term.

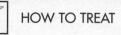 HOW TO TREAT

GENERAL MEASURES
• To aid in finding a cause for the miscarriages, a variety of medical tests will be recommended. These include blood and chromosomal studies of both parents and maternal hormone studies. Physical examinations of the mother, including x-ray imaging of the uterus and fallopian tubes (hysterosalpingography), laparoscopy and hysteroscopy (see Glossary for these terms) will determine any anatomical problems.
• In some cases, medical studies of the aborted material are helpful.
• Surgical procedures on the uterus or cervix (e.g., cerclage; see Glossary) may be required to correct any abnormalities.
• If a serious genetic factor is found in either parent, other fertility options may be considered, such as artificial insemination (for paternal defect) or fertilization of a donor egg by the father's sperm (for maternal defect).
• Repeated miscarriages are very difficult psychologically for both parents. Seek psychotherapy if needed. Support groups are available in some communities.
• See the Resource section of this book for additional information.

MEDICATION
• Medicines will be prescribed for any hormonal deficiencies diagnosed (thyroid dysfunction, progesterone deficiency or diabetes mellitus).
• Antibiotics will be prescribed if infection is confirmed.
• Immunologic abnormalities may require special therapy.
• Medicines as required to treat any systemic disorder, such as hypertension or kidney disease.
• With a subsequent pregnancy, prenatal vitamins and folic acid will usually be prescribed.

ACTIVITY—Normally, there are no restrictions. If pregnancy occurs, some curtailment of activities may be recommended.

DIET—No special diet.

 CALL YOUR DOCTOR IF

Following a surgical procedure, pain, swelling, redness, drainage or bleeding develops in the surgical area.

Monitors, Fetal

GENERAL INFORMATION

DEFINITION—Monitoring of fetal well-being during pregnancy and labor. Sophisticated electronic monitors are used for some prenatal examinations and during labor. A simple form of monitoring is the use of a special fetal stethoscope by medical personnel to listen to the baby's heartbeat.

REASONS FOR PROCEDURE
• In pregnancy, monitoring is often performed to reassure the parents. Extended monitoring is usually only required in mothers who have pregnancy complications.
• During labor, the monitoring is performed to check for abnormalities in the fetal heart rate and detect fetal distress. A drop in the fetal heart rate can indicate that the fetus is not receiving adequate amounts of oxygen. In other cases, drops in the fetal heart rate can be normal and are nothing to be concerned about. The doctor, midwife and nursing staff are critical to the accurate interpretation of the fetal monitoring record.

RISK INCREASES WITH—Conditions or situations that may normally be associated with pregnancy and delivery.

DESCRIPTION OF PROCEDURE
• An electronic fetal monitor attached externally or internally is used to make a continuous recording of the baby's heartbeat. The heartbeat is amplified and heard as a beeping noise or printed as a paper trace.
• With external monitoring, the monitor is placed on the mother's abdomen and held in place by adjustable bands.
• With internal monitoring (done during labor), a wire is inserted through the mother's vagina and attached by an electrode to the surface skin of the baby's head; this can be done only after the membranes have ruptured and the cervix is dilated to at least 1 or 2 centimeters. There may be some mild discomfort felt during placement of the internal monitor (usually no different than that associated with a pelvic examination).
• Electronic monitoring during labor and delivery may also include a pressure gauge that measures and records the mother's contractions using an internal plastic tube inserted through the vagina into the uterus.
• Contractions can also be measured by an external gauge strapped to the mother's abdomen. The belts holding the monitors may have to be adjusted frequently and may be somewhat uncomfortable during labor.

PROBABLE OUTCOME
• Monitoring during pregnancy will help assess the health and well-being of the fetus. The testing is noninvasive and no side effects are expected.

• If the monitoring indicates the baby may be at risk, appropriate action can be taken immediately, such as additional tests and, possibly, cesarean section delivery. If no fetal distress is detected, normal labor and delivery will proceed.

POSSIBLE COMPLICATIONS
• Overdiagnosis of fetal distress and unnecessary cesarean section delivery.
• Internal monitoring may increase the risk of infection during labor.
• The fetus may develop a small rash or a bald spot where the electrode was placed during internal monitoring; usually, this will heal quickly.

FOLLOWUP CARE

GENERAL MEASURES—Follow-up measures will depend on the purpose and time of the fetal monitoring. If done during a prenatal examination, no special measures are necessary. If done during labor, follow-up measures will be determined by the method of delivery.

MEDICATION—Medicine is usually not necessary for the procedure itself. Pain medications may be recommended during labor and delivery.

ACTIVITY—Restrictions as determined by method of childbirth.

DIET—No special diet.

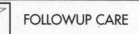

CALL YOUR DOCTOR IF

You or a family member has questions or concerns about the use of fetal monitoring.

Monitors, Fetal

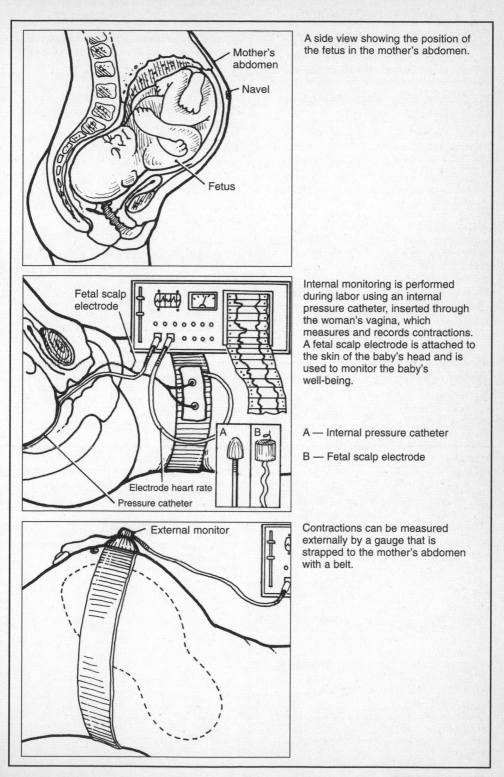

A side view showing the position of the fetus in the mother's abdomen.

Mother's abdomen

Navel

Fetus

Internal monitoring is performed during labor using an internal pressure catheter, inserted through the woman's vagina, which measures and records contractions. A fetal scalp electrode is attached to the skin of the baby's head and is used to monitor the baby's well-being.

Fetal scalp electrode

Electrode heart rate

Pressure catheter

A — Internal pressure catheter

B — Fetal scalp electrode

Contractions can be measured externally by a gauge that is strapped to the mother's abdomen with a belt.

External monitor

Morning Sickness during Pregnancy

 GENERAL INFORMATION

DEFINITION—Nausea during pregnancy. This usually occurs in the morning, but may occur at any time of day or night. Most pregnant women experience at least mild morning sickness.

SIGNS & SYMPTOMS—Mild to severe nausea with or without vomiting that usually occurs during the first 12 to 14 weeks of pregnancy, but may continue throughout pregnancy.

CAUSES
• Major hormonal changes that take place to permit normal growth of the fetus. Progesterone and other hormones cause involuntary muscles to relax, probably slowing movement of food through the stomach and intestines. They may also affect the vomiting center in the brain.
• In addition, blood sugar is lower during early pregnancy in many women, contributing to gastrointestinal upsets.

RISK INCREASES WITH—Unknown.

HOW TO PREVENT—Do not let your stomach get empty; eat something every 2 hours if necessary.

PROBABLE OUTCOME—Morning sickness usually stops after the first 3 to 4 months of pregnancy.

POSSIBLE COMPLICATIONS—Hyperemesis gravidarum, a condition of pregnancy characterized by severe nausea, vomiting, weight loss and electrolyte disturbance (rare).

HOW TO TREAT

GENERAL MEASURES
• Try to identify the particular odors or foods that are most upsetting and avoid them.
• Keep rooms well-ventilated to prevent accumulation of cooking odors or cigarette smoke.
• Don't smoke cigarettes, and ask your family and friends not to smoke while you are experiencing morning sickness.
• Keep a positive attitude. If you have conflicts that you cannot resolve, ask for help from family, friends or professional counselors.
• Keep a daily record of your weight.

MEDICATION
• Medicine is usually not necessary for this disorder.
• Don't take any medications during pregnancy, including nonprescription medicine to prevent vomiting, without medical advice.
• Your doctor may prescribe antinausea medication, usually in suppository form, if nausea and vomiting are severe. Follow your doctor's instructions carefully when using any drugs during pregnancy.
• A trial of vitamin B-6 may be recommended, which appears safe at present.

ACTIVITY—No restrictions.

DIET—The following may help minimize nausea:
• Place a small, quick-energy snack, such as soda crackers, at your bedside. Eat it before getting up in the morning.
• Get up from bed slowly, and avoid sudden movements.
• Eat a small snack at bedtime and when you get up to go to the bathroom during the night.
• Eat a snack as often as every hour or two during the day. Avoid large meals. Snacks should consist of high-protein foods, such as peanut butter on apple slices or celery; nuts; a quarter-sandwich; cheese and crackers; milk; cottage cheese; yogurt sprinkled with granola; and turkey or chicken slices.
• Sit upright for 45 minutes after eating.
• Some women may find that dairy products, such as butter, milk, and cheese, increase their nausea. Limit dairy products if they make you feel more nauseous.
• Avoid foods that are high in fat and salt and low in nutrition.
• Avoid foods that are fried, greasy or spicy; they increase nausea.

 CALL YOUR DOCTOR IF

• You have morning sickness that does not improve, despite the above measures.
• You vomit blood or material that resembles coffee grounds.
• You lose more than 1 or 2 pounds.

Placenta Previa

GENERAL INFORMATION

DEFINITION—A placental attachment that is too low in the uterus and partially or completely covers the cervix. This can result in significant bleeding that, in some cases, can be life-threatening to the unborn child and mother if untreated. Placenta previa occurs to some degree in 1 of 200 pregnancies.

SIGNS & SYMPTOMS
• Sudden, painless bleeding during the second or third trimester of pregnancy is the primary symptom. Bleeding may begin moderately and become severe. Total placenta previa, where the placenta completely covers the cervix, may cause spotting or bleeding in the first trimester.
• Cramping or contractions in some patients.
• Abnormal fetal position in the uterus.

CAUSES—Normally, the placenta attaches high on the uterus wall, away from the cervix. In placenta previa, the placenta covers the cervix partially or completely. Any change in the cervix, such as the softening and dilating that occurs prior to delivery, or pressure placed on the cervix and placenta as the baby grows heavier, can cause the placenta to bleed as it separates from the uterus.

RISK INCREASES WITH
• Previous uterine surgery (e.g., cesarean section, D & C or induced abortion).
• Fibroid tumors of the uterus.
• Smoking.
• Multiple previous pregnancies and deliveries.
• Multiple fetuses (e.g., twins, triplets).
• Mothers over age 35.
• Previous placenta previa.

HOW TO PREVENT
• Get good prenatal care during a pregnancy. It will not prevent previa but can help identify complications early.
• Don't smoke during pregnancy. Smoking also causes a secondary problem that can lead to poor growth of the fetus.

PROBABLE OUTCOME—With prompt care, most mothers and most infants survive without complications. Cesarean section is the preferred method of delivery.

POSSIBLE COMPLICATIONS
• Premature delivery or fetal death may result if extensive bleeding occurs before the expected delivery date.
• Hazardous blood loss, requiring blood transfusions for the mother prior to delivery or following delivery.
• Poor fetal growth due to an abnormal placenta providing a decreased blood flow and oxygen delivery.
• Infection during labor.
• Anemia.
• Maternal shock or death (rare) as a result of

hemorrhage, trauma during surgery, infection or embolism (see Glossary).

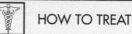

HOW TO TREAT

GENERAL MEASURES
• Diagnostic tests may include laboratory blood studies to determine the amount of blood loss, amniocentesis, and ultrasonography to determine the exact location of the placenta.
• Have regular checkups during pregnancy. If signs of placenta previa appear, be prepared to go to the hospital early for observation and possible delivery. Arrange for fast transportation to the hospital in case of emergency, especially massive bleeding.
• Cesarean delivery is the method of choice with placenta previa.
• A total placenta previa usually requires complete bed rest, usually in the hospital, but sometimes at home. If bleeding stops, you may be allowed to get up, but you will usually need to stay in the hospital until delivery. If you leave the hospital, your life and that of your child will be at risk. Massive bleeding can occur before you can get back to the hospital.
• In determining the best time for delivery, tests of fetal lung maturity, amniotic fluid studies and ultrasonic growth measurements are usually recommended.
• If studies reveal more than a marginal or low-lying placenta, cesarean section is often recommended at 36 to 37 weeks gestation, to reduce complications for both mother and child that could result from an emergency delivery or from massive bleeding later in pregnancy.

MEDICATION
• Only minimal analgesic medications, if any, will be used in delivery so as to increase the child's survival chances. Blood transfusions may be necessary.
• Don't use aspirin during pregnancy unless advised to do so by your doctor (it may increase the risk of bleeding).

ACTIVITY
• Rest in bed until bleeding stops or you deliver your child, depending on your doctor's orders.
• Abstain from sexual intercourse; anything placed in the vagina increases the risk of bleeding.
• Avoid douching, as it can cause bleeding.

DIET—While you are bleeding and as long as surgery is being considered, drink liquids only. Eating solid food before surgery can cause anesthesia problems.

CALL YOUR DOCTOR IF

You have symptoms of placenta previa. Report any bleeding immediately. This is an emergency!

Postpartum Care

GENERAL INFORMATION

DEFINITION
• Though the physical changes that occur with pregnancy usually resolve by the end of 6 weeks, the postpartum period can include the changes in all aspects of the mother's life that occur in the first year following delivery.
• Knowing what to expect once you return home after delivery can help you manage the changes, lessen concerns and develop realistic expectations. Emotional support and help with the baby and housework are related to maternal well-being.

WEIGHT—New mothers generally lose 12 to 13 pounds with the baby's birth and another 3 to 4 pounds the first few days after delivery. Weight loss continues for 6 to 8 weeks, when you should be back to near-normal weight. Breast-feeding mothers usually have more of a dramatic weight loss than non-nursing mothers.

DIET
• In general, you may eat anything you like, observing the dietary guidelines for adults. Naturally, if you gained a bit too much weight during pregnancy, you'll want to stay away from fattening foods until your normal figure has returned.
• If you are breast-feeding, go easy on alcohol and don't smoke. You will need about 600 calories a day more than usual.

BOWEL MOVEMENTS & URINATION
• It may take several days before the first postpartum bowel movement occurs. Abdominal muscles were stretched during delivery and the bowel may have been traumatized also. In many women, there is a psychological fear that the bowel movement will be painful and tear stitches. Try not to worry; eat a high-fiber diet; drink plenty of fluids and start a mild exercise routine. Avoid straining. A stool softener laxative may be prescribed.
• Urination may be painful; there may be no urge, or an urge with no urination. It's important to urinate within 8 hours of delivery to avoid infection. Drinking plenty of fluids and getting up and moving can help. After 24 hours, there is usually an increase in urination as the excess body fluids from the pregnancy are excreted. If this doesn't occur, there may be a bladder infection. If so, antibiotic treatment will begin.

BATHING—You may shower and shampoo any time after delivery, as long as you are steady on your feet. Some doctors may prefer that you put off full tub baths until a few weeks after delivery, but shallow baths in about 4 inches of warm water may be taken as soon as you get home.

BREASTS
• The milk "comes in" on the third or fourth postpartum day. There is often some initial discomfort with the engorgement and fluid retention in the breasts, along with milk leakage. Nursing mothers will be instructed, while in the hospital, on how to breast-feed.
• For non-nursing mothers, the engorgement will start to decrease after 2 to 3 days. Pain and discomfort can be eased with the use of ice packs, mild pain medicine (acetaminophen) and wearing a support bra. Special drugs to suppress lactation are no longer available.

PERINEAL CARE
• Discomfort from an episiotomy or hemorrhoids can be a problem. Symptoms may sometimes persist up to 3 months.
• For relief of discomfort caused by the episiotomy, use ice packs or warm-water cleansing, or apply an astringent, such as witch hazel (Tucks Pads, Tucks Clear Gel) or a topical anesthetic (Americaine, Dermoplast).
• Hemorrhoid or episiotomy discomfort can be treated by taking warm sitz baths for 10 to 20 minutes, twice a day, in water 4 inches deep in the tub. Nonprescription topical hemorrhoid medications and oral medications such as acetaminophen or ibuprofen (little of each of these drugs is excreted in breast milk) may be used.

VAGINAL BLEEDING & MENSTRUATION
• Vaginal bleeding (lochia) will occur for 2 to 6 weeks following delivery. It is leftover blood, mucus and tissue from the uterus. At first, the flow is bright red, heavy and may contain clots, then turns pink to brown and decreases in amount. Use sanitary pads and not tampons.
• If you do not nurse your baby, you can expect to menstruate again within 4 to 8 weeks. The first menstrual flow tends to be heavy and contain clots; it may start, stop, then start again. The second period should be more or less normal. As long as you are nursing, the flow will not ordinarily appear. But if it does, don't worry; it will not interfere with nursing.

EXERCISE & BACK CARE
• You may be concerned about your slack belly muscles. A good way to tighten and tone these muscles is to hold your stomach in. Practice pulling it in while you take several natural breaths; then relax. Repeat this throughout the day. You will be surprised at how effectively this simple practice restores muscle springiness and flattens your stomach.
• A modified postpartum exercise program can begin immediately, and prepregnancy exercise levels can be resumed gradually over a few weeks. Women who had cesarean deliveries should wait at least a week before exercising.
• The changes that took place in your body during pregnancy may have put undue strain on your back. Now is the time to learn how to care for your back to avoid unnecessary back discomfort in the future.
• Never bend from the waist without bending the knees. Avoid any position in which your back is arched. Carry packages and baby high, close

Postpartum Care (cont.)

to your chest. Never twist your body to lift an object or to pick up or put down the baby. When seated, it is often restful to the back to have the knees higher than the hips. You may also find a rocking chair restful, as the back-and-forth motion changes the groups of muscles used.

SEXUAL INTERCOURSE
• There is no specific schedule as to when sexual intercourse can be resumed. If the bright-red bleeding has stopped and the perineum (area between the vagina and rectum) is comfortable for the woman, sexual intercourse is acceptable. Generally, relations can be resumed by the third week postpartum. Women who have had an episiotomy or a tear should wait at least 3 weeks.
• Many women report a low or absent sexual desire during the first few weeks postpartum. Reasons may involve fatigue, weakness, pain with intercourse, vaginal discharge or concern about injury.
• Most couples resume sexual intercourse by 6 to 8 weeks after delivery.
• Sexual intercourse can cause some discomfort for a woman because of vaginal dryness (especially in breast-feeding women). Use of a water-based gel lubricant (K-Y Jelly) will usually help.

CONTRACEPTION
• Because of the wide choice of methods, as well as your individual needs and preference, it is recommended to discuss contraceptive techniques before hospital discharge.
• Breast-feeding usually suppresses ovulation, but mothers who want to minimize their risk of subsequent pregnancy should use another form of birth control while nursing.
• Oral contraceptive use can usually be resumed 2 weeks after birth by nonbreast-feeding mothers. Nursing mothers can be immediately started on progesterone-only pills for the least hormonal impact. If a nursing mother wants added protection, Depo-Provera, an injectable progesterone, can be administered prior to hospital discharge.
• Diaphragm fitting, IUD, hormonal implants or injections can usually be initiated at the 6-week postpartum checkup.

FIRST POSTPARTUM VISIT—Unless you have a problem that requires seeing your doctor earlier, arrange for a follow-up examination 4 to 6 weeks after the baby's birth. At that time, your general physical condition and your urine will be checked, breasts and abdominal wall inspected, and a thorough pelvic examination will be done. You should have a Pap smear and breast examination six months after the baby's birth.

BABY CARE—There are many excellent books available on childcare that have detailed information about the aspects of caring for a newborn. Expectant parents should obtain one or more of these books and read about newborn care in advance of delivery, then refer to this reference as needed to help answer questions and concerns, and for encouragement as to when to seek medical help when you are unsure.

FATIGUE
• Even the fittest of women find they tire easily during the weeks or months after the baby's birth. Trying to take on too much, too soon, can exhaust you and make any emotional letdown even worse. Alternate an hour of activity with an hour of resting with your feet up. Usually, by the end of the fourth week, you should be up to full activity, and in 2 months, you'll feel altogether like yourself again.
• Plan for help when you first bring the baby home. Have your husband take a week off or have another family member help as much as possible.
• Suggestions to give family or friends who offer to help:
  Provide a family meal.
  Watch the baby while you nap or shower.
  Feed the baby (if you are not breast-feeding).
  Babysit while you and your husband go out for a meal.
  Do grocery shopping, run errands, drive you to the doctor.

THE "BLUES"—For 9 months, you and your partner have gone through the many adjustments of pregnancy. He's been through the worry, and you've been through the strenuous physical effort of birth. Now, finally, you're at home with your baby and these should, it seems, be the happiest days of your life. By and large they will be. But don't be surprised if for a time after coming home from the hospital you feel unaccountably depressed. Perhaps you feel let down after the excitement and anticipation of the last few months. Perhaps the feedings are not going well, or you're not getting enough sleep. You may have increasing doubts about your ability to cope with the 24-hour-a-day demands of mothering. You may feel resentful (and guilty about the resentment) at being so tied down. Your husband seems just a little put out at all the time and attention you are lavishing on the baby. You feel discouraged and weepy. Take heart; this postpartum state of mind is normal and very common. It is all part of the tremendous adjustment new parenthood requires. And it doesn't last long. In a month or two, you and your husband will have gotten used to the new routine, you will have returned to a more normal self and the rewards of parenting will start to become obvious.

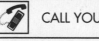 CALL YOUR DOCTOR IF

You or a family member has questions about postpartum care.

Postpartum Depression or Blues ("Baby Blues")

 GENERAL INFORMATION

DEFINITION—Emotional changes following the birth of a baby affect almost half of all new mothers. Baby blues are most common 3 to 10 days following delivery (but can occur anytime in the first year) and usually last anywhere from 48 hours to 2 weeks. In some women, the depression is more pronounced and, rarely, there is extreme depression.

SIGNS & SYMPTOMS—The symptoms vary in intensity, but can include:
• Feelings of sadness, hopelessness or gloom.
• Crying.
• Appetite and weight loss (sometimes a weight gain).
• Sleep disturbances or frightening dreams.
• Loss of energy; fatigue.
• Irritability; anxiety; mood swings.
• Slow speech and thought.
• Frequent headaches and other physical discomfort.
• Fears about personal health and infant's health.

CAUSES
• It's common for mothers to experience some degree of mild depression during the first weeks after birth. Pregnancy and birth are accompanied by sudden hormonal changes that affect emotions.
• Additionally, the 24-hour responsibility for a newborn infant represents a major psychological and lifestyle adjustment for most mothers, even if it is not the first child.
• These physical and emotional stresses are usually accompanied by inadequate rest until the baby's routine stabilizes, so fatigue and depression are not unusual.

RISK INCREASES WITH
• Stress and lack of sleep.
• Poor nutrition.
• Postpartum blues following a previous pregnancy.
• Lack of support from one's partner, family or friends.
• Preexisting mental health problems.

HOW TO PREVENT—Cannot be prevented, but can be minimized with rest, an adequate diet and a strong emotional support system.

PROBABLE OUTCOME—This depression is usually very short-lived. With support from friends and family, mild postpartum depression disappears quickly.

POSSIBLE COMPLICATIONS
• Lack of bonding between mother and infant, which is harmful to both.
• If depression becomes more severe, a mother may not be able to care for herself and the baby, and hospitalization may be necessary (rare). Medication, counseling and support from others usually cure even severe depression in 3 to 6 months.
• Serious depression that may be accompanied by aggressive feelings toward the baby, a loss of pride in appearance and home, loss of appetite or compulsive eating, withdrawal from others or suicidal tendencies.

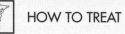 HOW TO TREAT

GENERAL MEASURES
• Diagnosis is usually based on a history of the symptoms. There are no specific diagnostic tests.
• Don't feel guilty if you have mixed feelings about motherhood. Adjustment and bonding take time.
• Schedule frequent outings, such as walks and short visits with friends or family; these help prevent feelings of isolation.
• Have your baby sleep in a separate room; you will sleep more restfully.
• Ask for daytime help from family or friends who will shop for you or care for the baby while you rest.
• If you feel depressed, share your feelings with your partner or a friend who is a good listener. Talking with other mothers can also help you keep problems in perspective.
• Severe postpartum depression requires professional help.

MEDICATION
• A mild sedative may be prescribed temporarily.
• Antidepressant drugs may be recommended for more severe symptoms. These are effective when used for 3 to 4 weeks. Don't stop taking them too early.
• Any medication use must be carefully considered if you are breast-feeding.

ACTIVITY
• No restrictions. Resume your normal activities as soon as possible. Avoid getting fatigued.
• Exercise regularly (as your recovery from childbirth permits).

DIET—Eat a normal, well-balanced diet. Avoid alcohol and caffeinated beverages.

 CALL YOUR DOCTOR IF

• Postpartum depression does not improve after 2 weeks, or the symptom level increases.
• You have postpartum depression and additional life changes occur, such as divorce, career change or moving.
• You have suicidal urges or aggressive feelings towards the baby. Seek help promptly!

Preconception Considerations
(continued on next page)

 GENERAL INFORMATION

DEFINITION—The health of both partners before conception is vital to the development of a healthy baby. The man's sperm and the woman's ovum are the foundation for giving the baby the best start in life. As soon as you decide to have a child, you and your partner should assess your lifestyle to determine if any changes are necessary and should schedule a visit to the doctor for prepregnancy planning, counseling and physical exams.

NUTRITION & DIET
• Both partners should eat a well-balanced diet. Women should include adequate folic-acid intake (spinach, broccoli, kale). Folic-acid supplements are often recommended for all women of childbearing age to prevent certain birth defects. For men, better nutrition helps assure healthy sperm.
• Women should try to get to their normal weight before conceiving. If underweight, a diet to increase weight is appropriate, but keep it healthy. If overweight, try to lose the excess pounds. Don't crash diet. Strenuous dieting can start off a pregnancy with a nutritional deficit.
• To be safe, a woman who takes vitamins or mineral supplements in high doses should discontinue their use or modify the dosages to fall within the recommended daily allowances. Some vitamins and minerals, when taken in high doses, are associated with an increased risk of birth defects.

SMOKING—Both partners need to stop smoking. In addition to a variety of health risks, smoking can lead to decreased fertility in both men and women and is hazardous to the pregnancy and the unborn child. A smoke-free home will provide a more healthy environment for any child.

ALCOHOL USE—Men and women should discontinue alcohol use when trying to conceive. In women, it can contribute to miscarriage, a low-birthweight baby and fetal alcohol syndrome. In men, heavy alcohol consumption may cause sexual problems that make them infertile and possibly damage their sperm, as well as reduce the number of sperm.

DRUGS OF ABUSE—Men and women need to discontinue using any illicit drugs. Drugs of abuse can be dangerous in a pregnancy and can increase the risk of miscarriage, prematurity, and birth defects or death of the fetus. In addition, their use may inhibit conception. For men, drugs of abuse may cause sexual problems.

EXERCISE—A regular exercise routine is important to both men and women. It leads to improved health, decreased stress, helps take off excess weight and improves the quality of life. It also helps a woman prepare for the physical requirements of pregnancy and delivery of a child.

EMOTIONAL HEALTH
• Couples need to assess their emotional health, both as individuals and as a couple. Are both partners emotionally ready for a pregnancy? Are there unresolved psychological problems for either partner such as stress, depression or anxiety? These problems may create difficulties with conceiving and can be heightened during the pregnancy when both a woman and a man go through various mood swings.
• Couples should have an emotionally healthy partnership before trying to conceive. Pregnancy, childbirth and child-rearing bring on a whole new set of stresses to both partners, and if the relationship is already encountering problems, having a child is not the solution. Any domestic violence situations need to be resolved. Seek counseling for unresolved conflicts or if there is an abusive relationship.

GENETIC COUNSELING—If either partner has any genetic disorder, a family history of a genetic disorder or a related child with a birth defect, genetic counseling is recommended to determine the risk of occurrence. Medical tests may be conducted for one or both partners. Other reasons for genetic counseling include habitual abortion (3 or more miscarriages) or previous stillbirth, certain ethnic backgrounds, maternal age over 35 or a previous child with a birth defect.

EXPOSURE TO TOXIC MATERIALS—If either partner works with toxic materials, or if you live or work in a polluted atmosphere, there may be hazards to a pregnancy. Some chemicals, usually in large doses, but occasionally even in very small doses, may be harmful to the ova, to the sperm or to a developing fetus. Discuss any of these concerns with your doctor.

MEDICATIONS—When possible, both partners should avoid taking any medication while trying to conceive. There are a few medications that are linked to birth defects and many others that carry unknown risks. If the medication is taken for a chronic condition, talk to your doctor about its safety during pregnancy and discuss other possible treatment options if there are any risks associated with the medication. Potentially harmful drugs should be discontinued at least a month (and in many cases, 3 to 6 months) before you try to conceive.

Preconception Considerations (cont.)

CONTRACEPTION METHOD CONCERNS—Your present birth control methods should be evaluated before you are ready to conceive. Oral contraceptives (birth control pills) should be discontinued several months before conception so as to allow at least two regular menstrual cycles to occur. An intrauterine device (IUD) needs to be removed. To be extra safe, the use of spermicides alone or with a condom or diaphragm should be discontinued 1 to 2 months before you want to become pregnant (spermicide risk to a subsequent pregnancy is unclear). As a temporary form of contraception, and until you are ready to conceive, use condoms without a spermicide.

AGE
• Most women over age 35 do experience successful pregnancies. Pregnancy-related complications increase gradually with age, but they are still relatively low. A woman over age 35 may have more difficulty in conceiving because of decreased fertility. She is also slightly more prone to problems during the pregnancy, such as high blood pressure, gestational diabetes and miscarriage. In addition, the risk of chromosomal abnormalities, such as having a child with Down syndrome, is increased. In addition to chromosomal abnormalities, advanced age has been associated with several adverse pregnancy outcomes. Maternal age under 15 carries some additional risks also.
• Questions remain unanswered as to whether or not advanced paternal (father's) age can be linked to any birth defects. There may be some small connection, but medical studies have not demonstrated any specific problems and it is not known at what age a problem might begin. Following conception, if there is concern about the effects of the father's age on the fetus, ask about prenatal tests to determine if they are warranted.

MEDICAL CONDITIONS—If you have any chronic medical condition (e.g., asthma, diabetes mellitus, high blood pressure, seizure disorder, thyroid disorder, eating disorder), talk to your doctor about planning for a pregnancy. Find out how the condition will affect the pregnancy, how the pregnancy will affect the condition and if any medications you take might affect the pregnancy. The medical condition needs to be under control before you conceive, and you must continue good self-care throughout the pregnancy.

IMMUNIZATIONS—For the mother-to-be, preconception is a good time to bring immunizations up to date.
• Get a tetanus booster if you haven't had one in the past 10 years.
• A rubella infection (German measles) during a pregnancy can cause birth defects. If you are unsure about your immunity, ask the doctor about a blood test to verify it. If you require a vaccination against German measles, it's recommended that you wait at least 3 months after receiving the vaccination before trying to conceive. It is possible that the vaccination could have an adverse effect on your pregnancy if given too close to conception or during pregnancy.
• You should have immunity against regular measles, either by prior immunization or by having had measles. If unsure, discuss the options with your doctor.
• If you are at high risk for hepatitis B (usually because of a medical work environment), immunization may be recommended. Discuss with your doctor any possible need to delay conception following a hepatitis B vaccination.
• Influenza vaccine may be recommended preconceptually in high-risk patients who might become pregnant during flu season.
• Varicella vaccine (for chickenpox) is now available and should be considered in women who have not had chickenpox (90% of women are immune to chickenpox, even those who don't recall ever having the disorder). Ask your doctor if there is a need to delay conception following vaccination against chickenpox.

REPRODUCTIVE KNOWLEDGE—Partners who want to conceive need to know the basics of the normal menstrual cycle, the timing of ovulation and the timing of intercourse to accomplish fertilization. If you are unsure, talk to your doctor.

PREVIOUS MEDICAL HISTORY—At a prepregnancy doctor's visit, a medical history for both partners will be discussed. It is useful for the doctor to know about any disorders, including infectious diseases and sexually transmitted diseases, in order to determine any possible risks to a future pregnancy. It is also important to advise the doctor of any previous pregnancies that ended in miscarriage or induced abortion, as these may need to be considered in the handling of your pregnancy. The possibility of current or future exposure to infectious disorders is important to know, in addition to any behaviors in either partner that are considered high risk, such as intravenous drug use. Be open and honest in your discussions with your doctor, as it is beneficial for you, and the outcome of your pregnancy, that the doctor be fully aware of any possible risks to a healthy pregnancy.

FINANCIAL CONSIDERATIONS
• Be sure you and your partner discuss the financial responsibilities involved (not only the medical expenses for a pregnancy and delivery, but the substantial costs involved with rearing a

Preconception Considerations (cont.)

child as well). Review any health insurance you have to verify coverage for childbirth. Ideally, you should try to have the financial resources available to pay the expected expenses for prenatal care and delivery if not covered by insurance.
• If both partners work now, you and your partner should discuss whether or not you will be returning to work following delivery. If you will not return to work, you should discuss what the financial impact on the family income and lifestyle will be. If both parents plan to work after the child is born, consider the cost of day care as well (unless a family member will provide it).

EDUCATION FOR PREGNANCY & CHILDBIRTH
• To help prepare you and your partner for the parents-to-be experience, read one or more reference books about pregnancy, childbirth and care of a newborn before you plan to conceive. There are a variety of excellent books available on these subjects. Check your local library, bookstores or borrow books from a family member or friend who has gone through a pregnancy. The information in the books will provide you with an overall perspective of the experience, lessen your confusion, give you reassurance and answer many of your questions. There are also a number of videos on pregnancy, childbirth and care of a newborn available.

• Childbirth classes are available in many communities and are a valuable source of information for expectant parents, particularly for learning ways to cope with labor and birth. Classes will also give you an opportunity to meet other couples with whom you can discuss anxieties and concerns. Classes may be conducted by the hospital, community organizations or by individual instructors. Ask your doctor or a friend who has recently had a child for information on where you might enroll in these types of classes.

 CALL YOUR DOCTOR IF

• You or a family member has questions or concerns about preparing for pregnancy.
• You have reason to believe that you may be pregnant.

Pre-eclampsia & Eclampsia
(Pregnancy-Induced Hypertension [PIH]; Toxemia of Pregnancy)

 GENERAL INFORMATION

DEFINITION—A serious disturbance in blood pressure, kidney function and the central nervous system that may occur from the 20th week of pregnancy until seven days after delivery. Eclampsia is an extension of the pre-eclampsia process, which results in unprovoked seizures.

SIGNS & SYMPTOMS
Mild pre-eclampsia (mild PIH):
• Significant blood-pressure rise, even if still in the normal range.
• Puffiness in the face, hands and feet that is worse in the morning.
• Headache.
• Excessive weight gain (more than 2 to 3 pounds a week during the last trimester).
Severe pre-eclampsia (severe PIH):
• Continued blood-pressure rise.
• Continued swelling and puffiness.
• Blurred vision.
• Severe headache.
• Irritability.
• Abdominal pain.
Eclampsia:
• Worsening of above symptoms.
• Muscle twitching.
• Seizures.
• Coma.

CAUSES—Abnormal placental development that leads to the production of substances or toxins within the woman's body.

RISK INCREASES WITH
• Poor nutrition.
• Diabetes mellitus.
• Prepregnancy high blood pressure.
• History of kidney disease.
• Immune disorders, such as lupus.
• Women under age 20 or over age 35.
• First pregnancy.
• History of pre-eclampsia or eclampsia in a previous pregnancy.
• Obesity.
• Multiple gestation (e.g., twins, triplets).
• Family history of pre-eclampsia or eclampsia.

HOW TO PREVENT
• Obtain good prenatal care throughout pregnancy.
• Eat a normal, well-balanced diet during pregnancy. Take prenatal vitamin and mineral supplements, if prescribed.
• Don't use medications of any kind, including nonprescription drugs, without medical advice.

PROBABLE OUTCOME—If diagnosed early and treated throughout the pregnancy, the problem usually disappears without complications within 7 days after delivery. Severe PIH and hypertensive disease continues to be a significant contributor to maternal mortality. If premature labor occurs, the newborn's survival chances depend on its maturity.

POSSIBLE COMPLICATIONS
• Stroke.
• Increased risk of high blood pressure unrelated to pregnancy after age 30.
• Seizures.
• Pulmonary or cerebral edema.
• Kidney failure.
• Cortical blindness.
• Disseminated intravascular coagulation (DIC; see Glossary).
• Maternal and/or fetal death.

HOW TO TREAT

GENERAL MEASURES
• Diagnostic tests may include laboratory blood studies, 24-hour urine study (to check the protein levels) and others to rule out complications.
• Treatment will depend on severity of the signs and symptoms, and the maturity of the fetus: home care for mild symptoms, hospital care if the condition deteriorates and early delivery if the situation is severe. Eclampsia, because of seizure activity, is more likely to require hospital care and rapid delivery (often cesarean section).
• If you are at home, weigh yourself daily and keep a record. Use a home test to check for protein in the urine (instructions will be provided).

MEDICATION
• Antihypertensive drugs, if needed to lower blood pressure, are generally used only in acute situations, unless you have been on hypertension therapy prior to pregnancy.
• Anticonvulsants to prevent seizures. High-dose magnesium is the most widely used and accepted anticonvulsant.

ACTIVITY—Rest often; this is important in controlling pre-eclampsia. Rest on your left side to help circulation.

DIET—Your doctor will advise you if a special diet is necessary.

 CALL YOUR DOCTOR IF

• You or a family member has symptoms of pre-eclampsia at any stage of pregnancy.
• The following occur during treatment:
  Severe headache or vision disturbance.
  Weight gain of 3 or more pounds in 24 hours.
  Nausea, abdominal pain, vomiting or diarrhea.
  Excessive irritability.

Pregnancy & Alcohol

 GENERAL INFORMATION

DEFINITION—Alcoholic beverages are not healthy for the fetus or the mother-to-be. Since alcohol crosses the placenta and enters the fetal bloodstream at approximately the same level present in the mother's blood, every drink you have while pregnant is shared by your unborn child. In the case of heavy drinking during pregnancy, alcohol can cause fetal alcohol syndrome, a combination of irreversible birth abnormalities. Fetal alcohol syndrome (FAS) has been reported in babies of women who drank 2 mixed drinks, or 2 to 3 bottles of beer or glasses of wine, a day. Lesser degrees of alcohol abuse can result in less severe birth defects (fetal alcohol effect). No safe level of alcohol consumption during pregnancy has been determined.

SIGNS & SYMPTOMS
Of fetal alcohol syndrome: infants with FAS are shorter and lighter in weight and have unusually small heads (microcephaly); abnormal features of the face, head, joints and limbs; heart defects and poor control of movement. There is a high neonatal mortality rate among infants born with this syndrome. As they get older, learning disabilities are common, as is hyperactivity, extreme nervousness and poor attention span. The effects are not reversible.

CAUSES—Chronic (and probably binge-type) alcohol consumption during pregnancy. Alcohol intake can affect the unborn child during the first trimester by interfering with organ development; in the second trimester it is associated with mental retardation; and in the third trimester, retardation of fetal growth.

RISK INCREASES WITH
• The greater the alcohol consumption, the greater the risk for birth defects and their severity.
• Pregnant women not receiving prenatal health care.

HOW TO PREVENT
• Pregnant women (or those likely to become pregnant) should not drink any alcoholic drinks (or use any drugs of abuse). There is not sufficient evidence to indicate that an occasional glass of wine or beer is dangerous, but complete abstinence during pregnancy is best and is recommended by most doctors.
• If you are concerned about your alcohol consumption, seek help from your doctor, Alcoholics Anonymous (see the Resource section of this book for additional information) or other support groups.
• Get early and continuing prenatal care.

PROBABLE OUTCOME
• If maternal alcohol consumption continues, the outcome is unpredictable.
• Discontinuance of maternal alcohol consumption assures the best pregnancy outcome.

POSSIBLE COMPLICATIONS—For the child, the defects are irreversible. The complications may range from mild to severe.

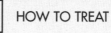 HOW TO TREAT

GENERAL MEASURES
• If you drank a few alcoholic beverages (not heavy consumption) before you learned you were pregnant, it is unlikely that they will affect the unborn child, but do discuss it with your doctor.
• Abstain from drinking alcoholic beverages as soon as you know you are pregnant. The sooner you stop drinking, the less risk there is to the baby.
• If you continue to drink alcohol while pregnant, advise the doctor and discuss the problem.
• Try to determine how you use alcohol in your life and find substitutes. If the alcohol helps you relax, substitute warm baths, exercise, reading or massage; if the drinking is part of a daily ritual, such as wine with dinner, drink a nonalcoholic wine-type drink (unless this triggers a desire for alcohol).
• The stresses or difficult situations that caused you to find comfort and solutions in alcohol will need to be faced or avoided.
• Join a support group in your community or contact Alcoholics Anonymous (see the Resource section of this book for additional information).
• If you know a family member or a friend who is pregnant and continues to drink alcohol, talk to her about your concern and the risks she is taking with her unborn child.
• If you are the parent of a child with fetal alcohol syndrome, get the appropriate help needed for the child's development. Get help for yourself if the alcohol problem is continuing or if you need other psychological or emotional support.

MEDICATION—Medicine is usually not necessary for this problem.

ACTIVITY—Usually no restrictions except those that may be concerned with the pregnancy.

DIET—Eat a well-balanced diet.

 CALL YOUR DOCTOR IF

• You are pregnant or think you might be pregnant and are continuing to drink alcoholic beverages.
• You want to stop drinking alcohol and need help coping.

Pregnancy & Asthma

GENERAL INFORMATION

DEFINITION—Asthma is a chronic disorder with recurrent attacks of wheezing and shortness of breath. The course of asthma in pregnancy is unpredictable. Approximately one-third of women note no change in their asthma; one-third note an improvement in symptoms and for one-third, symptoms worsen. The treatment of asthma in a pregnant woman is similar to the treatment for a nonpregnant woman.

SIGNS & SYMPTOMS
- Chest tightness and shortness of breath.
- Wheezing upon breathing out.
- Dry coughing, especially at night.
- Rapid, shallow breathing that becomes more normal with sitting up.
- Breathing difficulty.
- Tightening of neck muscles.
Severe symptoms of acute attack:
- Bluish skin.
- Exhaustion.
- Grunting respiration; inability to speak.
- Mental changes; restlessness or confusion.

CAUSES—Overactivity and spasm of air passages, followed by swelling of the passages and thickening of lung secretions. This decreases or closes off air to the lungs. These changes are caused by:
- Allergens, such as pollen, dust, animal dander, molds and some foods.
- Infections, especially viral.
- Air irritants, such as smoke and odors.
- Exposure to occupational chemicals or other materials.

RISK INCREASES WITH
- Other allergic conditions, such as eczema or hay fever.
- Family history of asthma or allergies.
- Exposure to air pollutants.
- Smoking.
- Use of some drugs such as aspirin.
- Stresses (viral infection, exercise, emotional upset, noxious odors, cigarette smoke).

HOW TO PREVENT
- Avoid known allergens and air pollutants.
- Follow your doctor's directions carefully for all prescribed preventive medicines. Don't skip your medications when you are feeling well.
- Avoid aspirin.
- Investigate and avoid triggering factors.

PROBABLE OUTCOME
- Symptoms can be controlled with treatment and strict adherence to measures in the How to Prevent section.
- With proper prenatal care and good self-care, you can usually expect a normal pregnancy and a delivery without complications.

POSSIBLE COMPLICATIONS
- With severe asthma, there are increased risks to the fetus, including prematurity, low birth-weight and, possibly, death.
- For the mother, complications of asthma include physical exhaustion, pneumothorax, pulmonary emphysema, collapsed lung and drug hypersensitivity reactions.

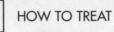

HOW TO TREAT

GENERAL MEASURES
- Eliminate allergens and irritants at home and at work, if possible; keep regular medications with you at all times; sit upright during attacks.
- Obtain good prenatal care.
- Don't smoke.
- Stay indoors as much as possible during high allergen times and avoid exposure to cold, especially if exercising.
- Psychotherapy, if asthma is stress-related.
- Emergency-room care and hospitalization may be required for severe attacks (rare).
- Labor and delivery are monitored carefully to assess pulmonary function. Vaginal delivery is usually considered best, unless circumstances dictate a cesarean section.
- See the Resource section of this book for additional information.

MEDICATION
As needed, the following may be prescribed:
- Expectorants to loosen sputum.
- Bronchodilators to open air passages (e.g., theophylline, terbutaline); best tolerated as inhalers, but can be given orally.
- Intravenous cortisone drugs (emergencies only) to decrease the body's allergic response.
- Cortisone drugs by inhaler or nebulizer, which have fewer adverse reactions than oral forms.
- Antihistamines (e.g., cromolyn sodium or nedocromil) by nebulizer. These are preventive drugs.

ACTIVITY
- Stay active, but avoid heavy exercise. If an attack follows exercise, sit and rest. Sip warm water.
- Bronchodilators often prevent exercise-caused asthma.
- Swimming is usually the best exercise for asthma patients.

DIET
- Avoid foods to which you are sensitive.
- Drink plenty of fluids to keep secretions loose.

CALL YOUR DOCTOR IF

- You or a family member has questions about asthma and pregnancy.
- You have an asthma attack that doesn't respond to treatment. This is an emergency!
- New, unexplained symptoms develop. Drugs used in treatment may produce side effects.

Pregnancy & Chronic Disorders

GENERAL INFORMATION

DEFINITION
• Thanks to medical advances, successful pregnancy is now possible for women who, in the past, might have been unable to have children. However, virtually any chronic medical condition can complicate a pregnancy.
• A woman with any chronic medical condition should consult a doctor before she becomes pregnant. By doing so, she can be instructed on how to attain the best physical and emotional levels possible and control the symptoms of the disorder, and be prescribed medications that are least likely to cause harm to the unborn child.
• Information covered in this instructional sheet is a review of various items you need to consider about a chronic disorder and pregnancy. Understanding, controlling and monitoring these conditions reduces the impact of the pregnancy on your health, and increases your chances of having a healthy, full-term baby.

SIGNS & SYMPTOMS
• Know the signs and symptoms that can be caused by your disorder. Be able to recognize worsening symptoms. If there are no obvious symptoms, find out what you can do to monitor the disorder.
• Know the signs and symptoms caused by a pregnancy (e.g., fatigue, nausea, lack of appetite, frequent urination, tender and swollen breasts, missed period). Often, the pregnancy symptoms may duplicate those of the disorder.

CAUSES
• Learn the history and cause of your disorder.
• Determine if the disorder is hereditary. If so, find out what risks there are to the fetus and what prenatal testing can be done.
• Seek genetic counseling if needed.

RISK INCREASES WITH
• Learn what special risks exist for you as far as the pregnancy and delivery are concerned.
• Determine how the pregnancy will affect your disorder.
• Determine how the disorder will affect the pregnancy and if any precautions are necessary.

HOW TO PREVENT
• Learn what preventive steps can be taken to assure a safe pregnancy and a healthy baby.
• Don't smoke or consume alcohol, whatever the disorder is.

PROBABLE OUTCOME—Learn what the chances are for an uncomplicated pregnancy and delivery of a healthy baby.

POSSIBLE COMPLICATIONS—Determine the type of complications that may occur during the pregnancy, the risk of miscarriage, and the risk to the fetus and to the newborn.

HOW TO TREAT

GENERAL MEASURES
• Keep all medical appointments and follow the doctor's instructions carefully. Supplemental medical tests may be recommended. The tests help evaluate the status of the disorder and the pregnancy and fetus, and determine the optimum time for delivery.
• Your medical care during pregnancy will often involve both the doctor treating the chronic disorder and your obstetrical doctor.
• Wear a medical-alert-type bracelet or pendant that identifies your disorder and medications being taken.
• The emotional aspects of pregnancy (combined with a chronic disorder) may include fear, guilt, pressure, stress and feelings of inadequacy. Seek support from family, friends or counseling.
• Make sure all your vaccinations are current prior to pregnancy.
• Avoid people who have colds or other infections. Wash hands frequently to help prevent infections. Seek medical treatment for any infection. Don't try to treat yourself.
• Find out about your childbirth options and if a normal delivery is possible.
• Weeks or months in bed may be necessary. Hospitalization may be required as a precaution during one or more stages of the pregnancy.
• Elective early delivery is sometimes the recommendation due to complications, or to prevent them. The major concern is that the baby's lungs are developed sufficiently; this can be determined by diagnostic tests.

MEDICATION—Many chronic disorders require continuous medication to control symptoms. Some of these medications carry known risks to the fetus while for others, the safety is not established, and for some, the risks are remote or unknown. For any medication prescribed, learn the risks, benefits and side effects. Follow all instructions for proper use.

ACTIVITY
• Exercise, sexual activity or travel may need to be restricted. Discuss with your doctor any possible restrictions related to your condition.
• Adequate rest during pregnancy is important.

DIET
• A sensible weight gain of 25 to 35 pounds over the course of your pregnancy is important. Don't restrict your diet unless your doctor advises.
• A special diet may be prescribed. Your adherence to any prescribed diet is important.

 CALL YOUR DOCTOR IF

You or a family member has a chronic disorder and is pregnant or planning a pregnancy and would like additional information.

Pregnancy & Diabetes Mellitus, Pregestational

 ## GENERAL INFORMATION

DEFINITION
• A chronic disease of metabolism characterized either by the body's inability to produce enough insulin or by the production of ineffective insulin to process carbohydrates, fat and protein efficiently. Type I diabetes requires injections of insulin, while type II is often diet-controlled.
• Preexisting diabetes complicates pregnancy and requires special medical- and self-care.
• Women with diabetes should seek medical advice before becoming pregnant to help assure a positive outcome.

SIGNS & SYMPTOMS
• Diabetes mellitus: Fatigue; excess thirst; increased appetite; weight loss; frequent urination; genital itching; susceptibility to infections, especially urinary tract infections and yeast infections of the skin, mouth or vagina.
• Some symptoms of pregnancy can duplicate diabetic symptoms (e.g., frequent urination).

CAUSES—For unknown reasons, too little insulin is produced by the pancreas, or there is resistance to the normal ways insulin works in the body.

RISK INCREASES WITH—Family history of diabetes mellitus.

HOW TO PREVENT—Cannot be prevented.

PROBABLE OUTCOME
• Diabetes is incurable, but symptoms and progress of the disease can be controlled with rigid adherence to a treatment program.
• If the diabetes is in good control prior to conception and throughout the pregnancy, the outlook is good for mother and newborn.

POSSIBLE COMPLICATIONS
• For the diabetic: Cardiovascular disease, especially stroke; atherosclerosis and coronary artery disease; urinary tract infection; kidney failure; blindness; peripheral vascular disease; life-threatening hypoglycemia (low blood sugar) if too much insulin is used; life-threatening ketoacidosis (very high blood sugar); pregnancy-induced hypertension; miscarriage. All are more likely to occur with poor control of the diabetes.
• For the fetus or newborn: Excess amniotic fluid (hydramnios); large-for-term size; birth defects; hypoglycemia, hyperbilirubinemia, or hypocalcemia (see Glossary for these terms); fetal death; stillbirth.

 ## HOW TO TREAT

GENERAL MEASURES
• Learn all you can about controlling diabetes and recognizing signs and symptoms of ketoacidosis or hypoglycemia.
• Learn the techniques of home monitoring of blood sugar. Test blood sugar levels a minimum of 4 times a day.
• Women who are on oral hypoglycemics should consider switching to insulin prior to attempting pregnancy.
• Doctor visits and medical testing during pregnancy will be more frequent and more vital than with nondiabetic patients.
• Get regular foot care by a podiatrist and regular eye examinations by a retina specialist.
• Keep a vial of glucagon available at all times to use if hypoglycemia occurs.
• Kidney and cardiac function may need to be monitored during pregnancy.
• Wear a medical-alert-type bracelet indicating the diabetes and any medications you take.
• Avoid people with colds or infections. Seek medical treatment if you develop an infection.
• Testing is usually recommended to assess the growth and development of the fetus.
• Elective early delivery is often recommended due to increased size of the fetus and a deterioration in the placenta. Diagnostic tests may be done to assess fetal lung maturity.
• See the Resource section of this book for additional information.

MEDICATION—Insulin by injection will be prescribed for type I. Dosage must be individualized and occasionally adjusted, especially during pregnancy when insulin requirements change. To avoid risks, patients on oral hypoglycemics are switched to insulin during pregnancy.

ACTIVITY
• Regular daily exercise is an important part of controlling diabetes and will help get you in the best physical condition for delivery. Any exercise program will need your doctor's approval.
• Adequate rest is important during pregnancy.

DIET—A special diet will be prescribed (consult a dietitian or nutritionist). Follow the diet carefully. This is one of the most important aspects of your self-care and can affect the outcome of your pregnancy.

 ## CALL YOUR DOCTOR IF

• You or a family member has diabetes mellitus and wants to become pregnant or is pregnant.
• The following occur during treatment: inability to think clearly; weakness; excessive sweating; paleness; rapid heartbeat; seizures or coma (may indicate hypoglycemia); fruity odor on the breath; changes in breathing pattern or stupor (may indicate ketoacidosis); several days of illness or weakness; numbness, tingling or pain in the feet or hands; chest pain.

Pregnancy & Drug Dependence

 GENERAL INFORMATION

DEFINITION
• Drug dependence is a compulsive and destructive use of mood-altering and perception-altering substances despite adverse medical, psychological and social consequences. These substances can affect the central nervous system, liver, kidneys and blood. Some abused drugs are legal substances such as benzodiazepines, barbiturates, amphetamines and pain-killers. Illegal substances include marijuana, cocaine, crack, heroin, LSD, PCP (angel dust) and volatile substances, such as glue, solvents and paints.
• In pregnancy, the continued use of these substances can cause mild to major problems for the mother and for the unborn child.

SIGNS & SYMPTOMS—Depend on the substance of abuse. Most produce:
• A temporary, pleasant mood.
• Relief from anxiety.
• False feelings of self-confidence.
• Heightened awareness of sights and sounds.
• Hallucinations.
• Stupor; sleeplike states; hyperactivity.
• Unpleasant or painful symptoms when the abused substance is withdrawn.

CAUSES—Substances of abuse may produce addiction (a physiological need) or dependence (a psychological need). Some people seem to be more susceptible to dependency than others.

RISK INCREASES WITH
• The type, frequency and the method of use of certain drugs (e.g., cocaine).
• Illness requiring prescription pain relievers or tranquilizers.
• Family history of drug abuse.
• Genetic factors (possibly).
• Excess alcohol consumption.
• Fatigue or overwork.
• Poverty.
• Psychological problems, including depression, dependency or poor self-esteem.
• Peer pressure.

HOW TO PREVENT
• Don't socialize with persons who use and abuse drugs.
• Seek counseling for mental health problems, such as depression or chronic anxiety.
• Develop wholesome interests and leisure activities.
• After surgery, illness or injury, discontinue the use of prescription pain relievers and tranquilizers as soon as possible. Don't use more than you need.

PROBABLE OUTCOME—Strong motivation, good medical care and support from family and friends offer the best chance for improved maternal and infant outcome.

POSSIBLE COMPLICATIONS
• Maternal: Sexually transmitted diseases, which are more frequent among addicts; severe infections, such as endocarditis (infection of the heart), hepatitis, HIV, or blood poisoning, from intravenous injections with nonsterile needles; malnutrition; accidental injury to oneself or others while in a drug-induced state; loss of job or family; irreversible damage to body organs; death caused by overdose.
• Pregnancy: Preeclampsia; abruptio placenta; premature rupture of the membranes; preterm delivery.
• Fetus and infant: Intrauterine growth retardation; congenital abnormalities (birth defects); medical problems in a newborn, including withdrawal from the drug; death of the fetus; stillbirth or infant death shortly after birth.

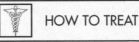 HOW TO TREAT

GENERAL MEASURES
• Acknowledge that you have a problem and seek professional help.
• Advise your doctor about what drugs you use; frequency of use; when last used; how the drug was administered; any history of withdrawals or overdose.
• Appropriate laboratory tests will be obtained and prenatal tests will be performed to determine fetal well-being.
• Be open and honest with your family and close friends, and ask for their help. Avoid friends who tempt you to resume your habit.
• Treatment will involve a coordination of medical, social, nutritional and psychiatric help with long-term follow-up.
• Depending on the specific drug(s) of abuse, outpatient or inpatient withdrawal treatment may be indicated. Patients who are narcotic-dependent can usually be maintained on methadone during the pregnancy and then transitioned to a withdrawal program postpartum.
• Join self-help groups.
• See the Resource section of this book for additional information.

MEDICATION—Methadone for narcotic abuse, a less potent narcotic used to decrease the severity of physical withdrawal symptoms. It can have undesirable side effects on the fetus.

ACTIVITY—A doctor-approved exercise program is recommended.

DIET—Eat a normal, well-balanced diet that is high in protein. Vitamin supplements may be necessary if you suffer from malnutrition.

CALL YOUR DOCTOR IF

• You or a family member abuse or are addicted to drugs and want help.
• New, unexplained symptoms develop. Drugs used in treatment may produce side effects.

Pregnancy & Gaining Weight

 GENERAL INFORMATION

DEFINITION
• Weight gain during pregnancy is made up of several elements. About half of the weight comes from the baby, the placenta and the amniotic fluid; about one third comes from increased weight of the uterus, extra breast weight, and increased blood and tissue in the woman's body. The balance of the weight is stored fat.
• The amount of weight gained in pregnancy varies from one individual to another, and the guidelines discussed are averages. The main concern is to eat a high-quality, well-balanced diet with adequate calories that will ensure good health for you and the baby. If you eat well and nutritiously, the weight gain should take care of itself.
• At the first prenatal visit, your height and weight will be measured and the two compared to help determine if you are starting the pregnancy at about the right weight for your height. At each subsequent prenatal visit, you will be weighed and any concerns you or the doctor has about your weight gain will be discussed.

AVERAGE WEIGHT GAIN GUIDES
• A general recommendation for weight gain in pregnancy is in the range of 25 to 35 pounds. Underweight women may need to gain more. For overweight women, pregnancy is not a time to try and lose weight. However, a special pregnancy diet may be recommended to keep weight gain within certain limits.
• Weight gain should be steady throughout the pregnancy:
  A gain of 3 to 4 pounds the first trimester. Because of morning sickness, many women find it difficult to gain weight during this time; some may actually experience a slight decrease in weight in the first trimester. The fetus needs fewer calories and nutrients during this period than it does later in the pregnancy, so not gaining weight in the first trimester does not usually pose a risk to the baby. However, a weight loss of more than a few pounds can be cause for concern and should be discussed with your doctor.
  About 1 pound every week during the second trimester, for a total of 12 to 14 pounds. Most women are feeling better during this time; morning sickness diminishes and it is usually easier to maintain a healthy diet.
  During the third trimester, the ideal gain of a pound a week continues for the seventh and eighth month. During the ninth month, just 1 to 2 pounds are gained, for a total weight gain in the third trimester of 9 to 10 pounds.
• With each monthly prenatal visit, the expected weight gain is 3 to 4 pounds over the previous visit. If the weight gain is significantly under or over that amount, further evaluation may be necessary to assess nutrition and diet, check for the presence of edema (swelling in the hands, feet and legs), and to screen for hypertension.
• If a woman is pregnant with more than one fetus, the desired weight gain will be higher, but not double or triple. The doctor will discuss a recommended amount.

WEIGHT GAIN CONCERNS
• Excessive weight gain during pregnancy increases a woman's risk of developing gestational diabetes or high blood pressure. In addition, it can cause backache, increase fatigue and contribute to varicose veins. Controlling weight gain is more difficult in late pregnancy, so it is important not to gain most of the total weight during the first months. However, if an excess amount of weight is gained during the first or second trimester, do not diet. Your nutritional intake needs to stay balanced to supply the daily needs for the fetus.
• A lack of adequate weight gain in pregnancy may be due to poor nutrition or an illness in the mother-to-be. It can contribute to intrauterine growth retardation (IUGR), a term used to describe infants whose weights are much lower than expected for gestational age.
• When an obese woman becomes pregnant, there is a somewhat higher risk of gestational diabetes and hypertension than in the average weight mother. It may be more difficult to determine the size of the fetus during prenatal visits because of the fat layers, and delivery is sometimes more complicated because the fetus may be larger than average. A cesarean delivery is also complicated by the amount of fat in the abdomen area. Obese women should not diet during pregnancy but should make every attempt to control weight gain to keep it within recommended guidelines.
• On the average, the larger the weight gain in pregnancy, the larger the baby. However, a woman can gain 35 to 40 pounds and still have a 6- or 7-pound baby.

 CALL YOUR DOCTOR IF

• You or a family member is pregnant and wants additional information on weight gain.
• You are pregnant and your weight increases more than 3 pounds in 1 week, or doesn't increase at all during a 2-week period.

Pregnancy & Medications

GENERAL INFORMATION

DEFINITION

- Medications taken by pregnant women can cross the placenta and reach the fetus, where they can possibly cause birth defects, particularly in the first 3 months when fetal organs are being formed. Therefore, it is important that a pregnant woman take only medications considered essential and that she understand the risks and benefits of any medication used. Sometimes, the risk of the illness has to be weighed against the known or unknown risk of the medication, as illnesses and infections may cause fetal problems also.
- There are many drugs that have been used safely in pregnancy. Once you have made certain a medication is safe and have the doctor's approval, don't hold off taking it. The earlier treatment begins for most infections or disorders, the better the chances are for a faster, uncomplicated recovery.
- Frequently, a woman has taken a prescription or nonprescription medication even before she realizes she has missed a menstrual period and may be pregnant. Always discuss this with the doctor at your first prenatal examination. Be sure you know the name of the medication, the dosage amount, length of time you took it and if you had any side effects. This also includes any herbal products or homeopathic treatments you have used.
- With some chronic conditions, prescribed medications that carry some risks may need to be taken to control the disorder despite the pregnancy. In these situations, doctors will attempt to prescribe the lowest dose possible for effective treatment to reduce risks to the fetus. It is important to adhere to the dosage schedule and to advise the doctor if symptoms are not being controlled.
- There are many herbal remedies on the market that claim to treat a variety of medical problems and prevent others. It is important to recognize that these remedies contain chemicals, just like drugs do, and can present risks to the fetus. The majority of these products are not regulated by the U.S. Food & Drug Administration (FDA). Don't use any of these products without your doctor's approval.

TERATOGENESIS—Teratology is the science dealing with the structural, functional and behavioral abnormalities of offspring. A teratogen is an agent that causes abnormalities (birth defects) in a developing embryo or fetus. Examples are rubella virus (German measles) and the drug thalidomide. If a drug is classified as a teratogen, there is evidence that taking the drug during pregnancy causes congenital abnormalities that cannot be explained by other factors.

HOW DRUGS ARE RATED FOR RISK IN PREGNANCY

- A pregnancy risk category is assigned to individual medications which identifies the potential risk for that particular drug to cause birth defects or death to the unborn child (fetus). These categories are assigned by applying the definitions of the FDA to the available clinical information about the drug. Most drugs are tested only on animals, and not on humans, for safety during pregnancy because such testing would subject unborn human children to unnecessary risks.
- All drugs are best avoided during pregnancy, but this rating system can help your doctor begin to assess the risk-to-benefit ratio should drug treatment become necessary. You and your doctor should discuss these benefits and risks carefully before any drug treatment is initiated.

PREGNANCY RISK CATEGORY

Definition of the drug categories (A, B, C, D and X):

- A: Adequate studies in pregnant women have failed to show a risk to the fetus in the first trimester of pregnancy and there is no evidence of risk in later trimesters.
- B: Animal studies have not shown an adverse effect on the fetus, but there are no adequate studies in pregnant women. Or, animal studies have shown an adverse effect on the fetus, but usually at dosages proportionately much higher than would be consumed by a patient. In these cases, adequate studies in pregnant women have not shown a risk to the fetus.
- C: Animal studies have shown an adverse effect on the fetus, but there are no adequate studies in humans. Or, there are no studies in animals or women. The drug may be used for pregnant women because of the benefits and despite its potential risk.
- D: There is evidence of risk to the human fetus, but the potential benefits of use in pregnant women may be acceptable despite potential risks (e.g., life-threatening situation or for a serious disease for which safer drugs cannot be used or are ineffective).
- X: Studies in animals and humans show fetal abnormalities, or reports of adverse reactions indicate evidence of fetal risk. The risks involved clearly outweigh potential benefits, and the drug is contraindicated for pregnant women.

CALL YOUR DOCTOR IF

- You are pregnant (or trying to conceive) and want to know about taking a prescription or nonprescription drug. This includes headache or pain remedies, laxatives, antihistamines, cold medications, antinausea drugs and any herbal remedies. Don't take any medications while pregnant, even nonprescription medicine, without first consulting your doctor.
- You experience side effects from a prescription or nonprescription medication.

Pregnancy & Nutrition

 GENERAL INFORMATION

PURPOSE—This diet is designed to provide the increased nutrients during pregnancy that are essential for the health of the mother and the well-being of the baby.

DESCRIPTION—Foods from all basic food groups are included in quantities to meet the increased nutrient needs of pregnancy. Nutrient needs that are markedly increased include calories, protein, iron, folic acid and calcium. Alcohol should be avoided during pregnancy.

BASIC INFORMATION
• Weight gain: Recommendations for the range of total weight gain and the pattern of weight gain should be based on prepregnancy weight for height. The pattern of weight gain is as important as total weight gain during pregnancy. Weight gain should be recorded on a chart that shows weight gain by gestational age.
• Pregnancy weight gain recommendations:

Prepregnancy Weight	Total Weight Gain	Rate of Gain 2nd and 3rd Trimesters
Normal Weight	25-35 lbs	1 lb/week
Underweight	28-40 lbs	more than 1 to lb/week
Overweight	15-25 lbs	2/3 lbs/week
Twins	30-35 lbs	1-1/2 lbs/week

NUTRIENT SUPPLEMENTS
• Assessment of dietary intake should be completed for every pregnant woman. The increased nutrient needs of pregnancy can generally be met with slight changes in dietary habits.
• Pregnant women are usually prescribed daily supplementation of 30 mg ferrous iron in the second and third trimester. For those women with limited intakes of fruit, juices, leafy green vegetables or whole grains, folate may be prescribed.
• Prenatal vitamin and mineral supplements should be provided for women with inadequate diets and for high-risk populations. Excessive vitamin and mineral intake should be avoided because of potential toxic effects in pregnancy. Vitamin and mineral supplements for use during pregnancy should not contain more than twice the recommended amount for adults.

ANEMIA
• Iron deficiency is the most common cause of anemia in pregnancy. Iron needs markedly increase in pregnancy. Women taking iron supplements of more than 30 mg per day may be prescribed supplements of 2 mg copper and 15 mg zinc per day.
• Eat foods high in iron such as beef, pork, lamb and organ meats; iron-fortified cereals; dried beans, peas, or lentils; dark green leafy vegetables; peanut butter and molasses. Combine foods high in vitamin C with iron-rich foods. Use cast-iron cookware, if possible.

CAFFEINE—Although data from human studies do not provide significant evidence that caffeine affects pregnancy outcome, the Food & Drug Administration advises that pregnant women eliminate or limit consumption of caffeine-containing beverages such as coffee, tea and colas.

DIABETES MELLITUS—Pregnant women with any type of diabetes need special medical and nutritional care. Women with diabetes mellitus should achieve good blood-sugar control prior to becoming pregnant. All other women should be screened for diabetes at 24 to 28 weeks of pregnancy.

FOOD SAFETY
• Foodborne illness is especially dangerous for pregnant women. To avoid exposure to Listeria, pregnant women should avoid unpasteurized milk and soft cheeses, carefully follow "keep refrigerated" and "use by" dates, and thoroughly reheat processed meats such as hot dogs. To prevent toxoplasmosis, pregnant women should wash hands after handling cats, avoid cleaning cat litter boxes, avoid eating raw or partially cooked meats and wash hands after handling raw meat.
• To avoid other foodborne diseases, proper food-handling procedures should be followed, including storing foods at proper temperatures; washing cutting boards and knives after contact with raw meat, poultry and seafood and careful hand-washing before and after handling food.

HYPERTENSION—Immediate referral for medical treatment is essential for pregnant women with increases in blood pressure. A diet to meet the nutrient needs of pregnancy with ample but not excessive amounts of calories and protein should be encouraged. Sodium intake should not be restricted.

PICA
• Pica is the practice of eating substances with little or no nutritional value. Pica in pregnancy often involves consumption of ice, dirt, clay or cornstarch. Less frequently, matches, hair, charcoal, cigarette ashes, mothballs, baking soda and coffee grounds may be eaten.
• Nutritious food may be displaced by pica substances. Items such as starch that provide calories may result in excessive weight gain. Pica substances may contain toxic elements or interfere with absorption of minerals, such as iron.
• Pica has been associated with iron deficiency. If either iron deficiency or pica is identified during pregnancy, assessment should be initiated to see if the other problem exists.

Pregnancy & Nutrition (cont.)

SODIUM—Normal sodium intake is needed during pregnancy to support the large prenatal expansion of tissues and fluids. Sodium should not be restricted.

TEEN PREGNANCY—Teens should gain weight at the upper end of the appropriate weight for height ranges. Teens are at high risk for iron deficiency and inadequate calorie intake. Eating regular meals and choosing healthy foods are especially important for teenagers.

VEGETARIAN DIETS—Pregnant women consuming vegetarian diets need careful nutritional assessment. The type of vegetarian diet will determine the potential for nutrient deficiencies with increased risk as more foods are excluded. Most pregnant women consuming milk and eggs can meet the increased nutrient needs of pregnancy. Vegan diets will require careful planning to consume adequate protein from complementary plant proteins. Alternate sources of Vitamin B12 and calcium will be needed in a vegan diet. Iron status should be carefully monitored. Low prepregnancy weight and less-than-optimal weight gain are common problems for vegans. High calorie foods such as nuts, nut butter, wheat germ, avocados, dried fruit, coconut, honey and salad dressings may be needed.

Pregnancy-Related Concerns

 GENERAL INFORMATION

ALCOHOL—Don't drink any alcoholic beverages. It is a known fact that alcohol in excess can cause damage to your unborn child. As time goes by, more and more drugs are found to exert harmful effects on the fetus during pregnancy. Remember that alcohol is a drug and that any product that contains alcohol is a drug.

BATHING—You may take tub baths or showers, whichever you prefer. Water generally does not enter the vagina during these activities, so chance of infection is minimal. You may use warm water, but don't use extremely hot water in the bath or shower, as a significant rise in your body temperature can potentially cause damage to the developing fetus. Avoid the use of hot tubs or saunas as well. Keep in mind that your balance may be more difficult to maintain toward the end of your pregnancy, and be careful while getting in and out of your bathtub; make sure it has a nonslip surface on the bottom.

BOWELS—Your regular bowel habits may become disturbed during your pregnancy. Hemorrhoids appear more frequently. These changes probably result from relaxation of the muscle cells in the bowel and pressure on the surface of the bowel wall from the expanding uterus containing the growing baby. Stool-softening laxatives usually provide relief without danger to you or your baby. But don't take a laxative, enema or any drug without consulting your doctor first. Avoid enemas. Some dietary changes can safely prevent constipation; increased quantities of bran, fresh and dried fruits, vegetables, water and other fluids all help.

BREASTS & SKIN—Breasts enlarge during pregnancy because of hormonal changes. The nipple area becomes darker. Other parts of the skin may become discolored, such as the neck and face, and a dark line may appear down the middle or lower part of the abdomen. These changes are temporary and normally disappear after delivery. Use a moistening lotion or cocoa butter around the abdomen and breasts to guard against stretch marks as much as possible. Use sunscreen on skin areas exposed to the sun.

CAFFEINE—Consumption of caffeine in low to moderate amounts is not associated with significant risks during pregnancy. Heavy caffeine use can result in potential problems such as low-birthweight and caffeine withdrawal symptoms in the newborn. Heavy caffeine drinkers need to reduce their caffeine use while pregnant. Other sources of caffeine besides coffee to be alert to are teas, colas and other soft drinks, chocolate and some nonprescription drugs.

CLOTHING & SHOES
• Maternity clothes are available in a wide range of prices and styles. In addition, some regular clothing with a loose fit can be worn during and after a pregnancy. Outer clothing should be practical and nonconstrictive. Because a pregnant woman may feel the cold less and perspire more, cotton and natural fibers may be more comfortable than synthetic fabrics. Borrow maternity clothing from a family member or a friend. Keeping up your appearance can help boost your spirits.
• Wear maternity pantyhose or special support hose. Regular pantyhose may constrict blood flow. Wear well-fitting maternity bras that give good support.
• Shoes should be low- or medium-heeled and as comfortable as possible with nonskid soles. Swollen feet are common during pregnancy due to normal fluid retention. There may be extra fat in the feet if weight gain is excessive. The shoe size may increase and sometimes becomes a permanent change.

DOUCHING—Don't douche.

EMOTIONS—You may experience more emotional ups and downs than usual. This is quite normal during pregnancy. Urge those close to you to understand and to be supportive.

EMPLOYMENT
• Usually, you may safely continue working throughout your pregnancy for as long as you remain comfortable at your job and avoid severe physical strain.
• Some jobs that involve physical exertion may need evaluating by your doctor. There are no set guidelines regarding work during pregnancy as expectant mothers have differences in levels of capability, prepregnancy conditioning, exercise tolerance and physique.

EXERCISE—Continue to enjoy fitness and recreational activities as you did before pregnancy if your doctor has given the go-ahead. Some physically strenuous activities may need to be moderated. Pregnancy is not the time to try a new sport or physical activity. Exercise classes designed for pregnant women are helpful. Avoid activities such as horseback riding, skydiving, motorcycle-racing, fast running, water-skiing and others that carry undue risks.

COSMETICS & HAIR CARE PRODUCTS
• There is no specific evidence that cosmetics and other personal care products (soaps, lotions, deodorants) affect pregnancy outcomes. There should be no need to limit their use unless your doctor advises differently.
• Hair care products such as dyes, straighteners (relaxers) and permanent wave solutions have been studied in pregnant women and have not shown any specific risks. Exposure to these products should not pose a risk to the fetus. During pregnancy, hair reacts differently

Pregnancy-Related Concerns (cont.)

to a tint or permanent, so it might be best to wait until after delivery. Hair care products such as sprays and shampoos carry no evidence that they do or don't cause any adverse outcomes for a pregnancy. Most women continue to use their prepregnancy hair products and experience no problems.

INSECTICIDES—Avoid the use of, or contact with, pesticides for the yard, pets or the home (including pesticide strips and flea collars). Little information is available about the risks of exposure during pregnancy to these products, so it is best to keep them out of your household.

MEDICATIONS—Don't take any drug without checking with your doctor first. This includes all prescription drugs, nonprescription drugs, vitamins, laxatives, cold remedies, simple pain remedies and others. For the sake of your unborn child as well as for your own welfare, completely avoid marijuana, cocaine, tobacco, alcohol, narcotics, tranquilizers, sleeping pills or any other mind-altering drugs.

PAINTS—Avoid painting and inhaling toxic fumes in confined areas. Medical studies on paint exposure and fetal harm are inconclusive. Oil-based paints and paint thinners contain different solvents that should be avoided, especially in the first trimester of pregnancy.

REST PERIODS—Include rest periods in your routine, several times a day for short periods. Lie on your left side during these rest periods, rather than flat on your back, because blood flow through the placenta is increased when lying on your left side and is decreased when lying on your back.

SEAT BELT USE   The use of seat belts is recommended to decrease maternal and fetal trauma in the event of a motor vehicle accident. Use a diagonal shoulder strap and a lap belt. The diagonal strap should pass over the shoulder and across the chest between the breasts. The lap strap should lie across the upper thighs. The straps should be above and below the "bump" of pregnancy, not over it. If your vehicle is equipped with a driver's-side air bag, position the seat as far back from the steering wheel as possible, to help prevent injury to the fetus in the event of an accident.

SEXUAL INTERCOURSE—Usually, you may enjoy sexual intercourse, as long as it is not uncomfortable or contraindicated because of a complication of pregnancy (e.g., placenta previa). There may also be restrictions on sexual intercourse during the last few weeks of pregnancy. Follow your doctor's advice regarding sex during your pregnancy.

SMOKING—There can now be no doubt that smoking is injurious to both you and your unborn child. So don't smoke! If you are a smoker and need help stopping, speak to your doctor about methods, support groups, etc.

TEETH—Pregnancy puts an extra strain on dental health. Be particularly careful about brushing and flossing during your pregnancy. Routine dental examinations and preventive and restorative procedures should be provided when necessary. Local anesthetics used for dental procedures are considered safe. If dental x-rays (or other kinds of x-rays) become necessary, make sure that your abdomen is shielded by a standard lead apron.

TRAVEL
• If possible, plan your trip for the second trimester of pregnancy. The risk of miscarriage is greatest during the first trimester, and in the third trimester, early labor could begin.
• Travel does not adversely affect pregnancy. Avoid sitting for many hours without getting up and moving around. Empty your bladder frequently to avoid an increased risk of bladder infections caused by retained urine. Don't take any antinausea travel medications without your doctor's approval. Carry a record of your medical history with you.
• Avoid travel if you have a threatened miscarriage or a history of miscarriage. Avoid travel to areas at high altitudes or areas where certain vaccinations (that may be hazardous during pregnancy) would be necessary.
• Airlines will not allow you to fly late in pregnancy (usually, the last month) without a letter stating your doctor's approval.

VIDEO DISPLAY TERMINALS (COMPUTERS)
• Medical studies to date have not demonstrated a convincing association between use of these devices and an increased rate of miscarriage, low birthweight or birth defects.
• Sitting for long periods in front of a computer does cause other symptoms that can compound the normal discomforts of pregnancy. These include back, neck, wrist, arm and eye strain, dizziness and headaches. Be sure to take frequent breaks from the sitting position and do stretching or relaxation exercises. Use an adjustable-height chair with good back support and have the keyboard and monitor at a comfortable height.

ADDITIONAL NOTES
Consider these suggestions to help you have a healthy and emotionally rewarding pregnancy:
• Define and resolve areas of concern or conflict involving family, occupational, civic, spiritual, emotional or recreational activities. If you cannot resolve these problems alone, seek help from family, friends or competent counselors.
• Be moderate in all activities. Seek a balanced lifestyle of work, intellectual pursuits, recreation, reflection and rest.

 CALL YOUR DOCTOR IF

You or a family member has questions about pregnancy.

Pregnancy & Seizure Disorder, Pregestational

 GENERAL INFORMATION

DEFINITION
• Seizure disorder or epilepsy is characterized by sudden seizures, bizarre movements, brief attacks of inappropriate behavior or change in one's state of consciousness. Seizures (also called convulsions) are a symptom, not a disease. Seizure disorders are not contagious.
• The effect of pregnancy on seizure activity varies; approximately 50% of patients show no change in frequency, 40% show an increase, and 10% have decreased seizure activity.
• In general, the course of a pregnancy is not affected by the seizure disorder, though it may affect the newborn.
• A woman with a history of seizure disorder should seek medical advice prior to any planned pregnancy. Since most anticonvulsants have some effect on the developing fetus, talk to a geneticist, before conception, about the risks.

SIGNS & SYMPTOMS—There are several forms of epileptic seizures (some listed below), each with its own characteristics:
• Petit mal (or absence), which mostly affects children. The person stops activity and stares blankly around for a minute or so, unaware of what is happening.
• Grand mal, which affects all ages. The person loses consciousness, stiffens, then twitches and jerks uncontrollably. He or she may lose bladder control. The seizure lasts several minutes and is often followed by deep sleep or mental confusion. Prior to the seizure, the person may have warning signals: a tense feeling, visual or auditory disturbances or smelling a bad odor.
• Focal epilepsy, in which a small part of the body begins twitching uncontrollably. The twitching can spread to involve the whole body.
• Temporal-lobe epilepsy, in which the person suddenly behaves out of character or inappropriately, such as becoming suddenly violent or angry, laughing for no reason or making agitated or bizarre body movements.

CAUSES—More than 50 brain disorders, but the organic cause can be determined in only 25% of cases. Common causes include brain damage at or before birth; drug or alcohol abuse; chemical poisoning; severe head injury; brain infection or brain tumor (occasionally).

RISK INCREASES WITH
• Family history of seizure disorders.
• Use of alcohol or mind-altering drugs.
• Exposure to toxic fumes.
• Low blood sugar.
• History of prior head injury.
• Certain medications which cause seizures.

HOW TO PREVENT—No way to prevent.

PROBABLE OUTCOME
• Adequately controlled seizures are not likely to worsen during pregnancy. Mothers-to-be with frequent, uncontrolled seizures before pregnancy will likely experience no change.
• Depending on the type of drug being taken, a pregnant women taking an anticonvulsant medication usually has at least a 70% chance of having a normal baby.

POSSIBLE COMPLICATIONS
• Continuing seizures (despite treatment).
• Possible birth defects in the newborn due to anticonvulsant medications or to seizure activity.

 HOW TO TREAT

GENERAL MEASURES
• Treatment for epilepsy consists of medications specific to the type of seizure. Routine prenatal care will be provided with careful monitoring of blood levels of anticonvulsant drugs.
• Avoid any circumstance that has previously triggered a seizure.
• Make sure your family knows what to do should a seizure occur: Loosen the clothing, lay the person flat and protect her from injury.
• Wear a medical alert bracelet that shows you have epilepsy and any medications being taken.
• See the Resource section of this book for additional information.

MEDICATION
• Anticonvulsant medications that are used to treat seizures are teratogenic (can cause congenital abnormalities). It is best to use the lowest dose of your medicine that controls seizures. Seizure activity itself can possibly cause birth defects, so it is not recommended to avoid anticonvulsant medication unless seizure activity is known to be controlled without it.
• Folic-acid or vitamin D supplements are often prescribed.
• Vitamin K is usually prescribed in late pregnancy, and to the newborn at delivery, to prevent hemorrhage. Anticonvulsant drugs can affect blood clotting factors in the fetus.

ACTIVITY—If seizures are under control, there are usually no restrictions. Avoid overfatigue.

DIET—No special diet. Avoid alcohol; it may decrease the effectiveness of your medication and provoke seizures.

 CALL YOUR DOCTOR IF

• You or a family member has a seizure disorder and is planning to become pregnant.
• You are pregnant and have a seizure.
• New, unexplained symptoms develop. Drugs used in treatment may produce side effects.

Pregnancy & Smoking

GENERAL INFORMATION

DEFINITION—Smoking is associated with numerous medical and health disorders, including cancer, heart disease and lung disorders. In addition, smoking causes many complications in pregnancy. Pregnant woman who smoke endanger not only themselves, but also their unborn child. Infants born to mothers who smoke have more respiratory infections; when they get older, they also have more ear infections and asthma. Pregnancy is a good time for both parents to stop smoking. The medical and economical benefits gained by the family will outweigh any stress or inconvenience caused by the smoking cessation.

FERTILITY EFFECTS—Smoking in either partner may lead to problems even before pregnancy. Studies have shown that smoking can reduce fertility in both men and women and make it more difficult to conceive or cause delays in conceiving (smokers may take more than one year to conceive). Smoking is associated with higher miscarriage rate.

EFFECTS ON THE FETUS
- The various by-products and additives in cigarettes reduce the amount of oxygen and nutrients available to the fetus.
- Nicotine slows fetal breathing and causes the arteries in the placenta and cord to contract, which in turn reduces the flow of oxygen; fetal heartbeat quickens to try to increase the oxygen supply.

POSSIBLE COMPLICATIONS
- Ectopic pregnancy (see Glossary).
- Spontaneous abortion (miscarriage).
- Intrauterine growth retardation (IUGR).
- Low newborn birthweight.
- Placenta previa or abruptio placentae.
- Vaginal bleeding.
- Preterm birth.
- Perinatal death (see Glossary).

POSSIBLE BIRTH DEFECTS
- Cleft palate.
- Cardiovascular or urogenital abnormalities.

COMPLICATIONS IN INFANTS
- More risk of severe respiratory disorders.
- Increased risk of sudden infant death syndrome (SIDS).
- In general, babies of smokers aren't as healthy as babies of nonsmokers.

PROBABLE OUTCOME
For discontinuing smoking:
- Quitting smoking as soon as you know you are pregnant can usually substantially reduce the risks to a fetus.
- Can reverse the majority of other health risks, some in one year, others within 10 to 15 years.
- Expect withdrawal symptoms to occur. The intensity varies from person to person.

HOW TO TREAT

GENERAL MEASURES
- The majority of smokers who quit do it on their own; others are helped by a variety of methods. No one way works for everyone.
- Self-help steps for quitting:
1) Analyze your smoking habits by determining when and why you smoke. 2) Make up your mind to quit. 3) Choose the day and quit on that day. 4) Use a substitute (gum, hard candy). 5) Temporarily give up those activities that you associate with smoking. 6) Reward yourself for not smoking. 7) During the first few weeks, eat plenty of low-calorie snacks; drink lots of water.
- Join a support group or a formal smoking cessation program.
- See the Resource section of this book for information on where to get help quitting.
- Hypnosis or acupuncture may be helpful.
- Concerns about quitting: 1) Weight gain—average amount is 5 to 8 pounds over 5 years; this extra weight is not a health threat. 2) Stress—may occur; get counseling or help with stress management. 3) Withdrawal—physical symptoms subside in 10 to 14 days; psychological symptoms may persist for months or longer. 4) Fear of failure—relapse is common; if it happens, try again immediately.
- If quitting seems impossible, cut down on the amount smoked.

MEDICATION—The safety of prescription smoking cessation aids, including nicotine gum and transdermal nicotine patches, has not been established in pregnancy. There is concern about the effects of the nicotine on the fetus. These aids may be prescribed for a mother-to-be who has failed a smoking cessation program and understands the risks and benefits involved. The effects of continued smoking on the pregnancy may be more risky than the nicotine replacement therapy.

ACTIVITY—Establish a regular prenatal exercise routine. It will help control weight, combat restlessness and make you feel better mentally and physically. Lung capacity improves when smoking is discontinued, so there is less shortness of breath during physical activities.

DIET—No special diet. Maintain good prenatal nutrition. Metabolism rate tends to slow when you quit smoking and a moderate weight gain is common, but will not adversely affect a pregnancy.

CALL YOUR DOCTOR IF

You or a family member is a cigarette smoker and is pregnant or wants to become pregnant and needs help to quit smoking.

Pregnancy & Work

GENERAL INFORMATION

DEFINITION
• Women continue to work during pregnancy for a variety of reasons. The money earned and/or health benefits are needed, they don't want to interrupt careers any longer than necessary, they want to stay busy or they enjoy their work.
• In a normal pregnancy, there are few restrictions concerning work, although it is beneficial to moderate activity and to allow for additional periods of rest. If you are not at risk for complications, you can probably continue to work up to your delivery date. In one large medical study, it was found that demanding and stressful work with long hours did not have an adverse effect on the pregnancy outcome.
• A pregnant woman will need to make the decision about working and for how long, based upon her needs, the needs of her family, her health, the type of work being performed and the input from her doctor.

MATERNITY LEAVE—Maternity leave traditionally runs from one month before the expected delivery date extending to 6 weeks after birth. These dates can vary depending on health, well-being and desires of the mother-to-be; the work involved; the employer's attitude and any guidelines established by the health benefit provider. Some women work right up to the delivery date, while others feel that they want some transition time between their work and the baby's birth.

PHYSICAL DEMANDS OF WORK
• The physical requirements of the work will play a role in determining how long to work. How physically demanding is the job and does the pregnancy interfere with accomplishing the work? Are there some modifications that can be made to accommodate the physical demands of the pregnancy?
• Advise the doctor if the work involves:
Heavy lifting, pulling or pushing.
Climbing (stairs, poles or ladders).
Bending below the waist.
Shift changes.
An added risk of accidents or falls.
• If you do continue working, there are some steps you can take to help reduce physical stress while pregnant:
Use your lunch hour as a rest period; lie on your left side, if possible, or sit with your feet elevated. Rest more when you are not at work, and decrease strenuous activities such as jogging, biking, tennis, etc.
Take frequent bathroom breaks; try to empty your bladder every 2 hours to avoid an increased risk of bladder infections caused by retained urine.

Avoid chemicals, noxious fumes, smoke-filled areas and extremes in temperature.

HAZARDOUS SUBSTANCES AT WORK—Some work involves being around hazardous substances. Always discuss these possibilities with the doctor on your first prenatal visit. It may be recommended that you transfer to a less hazardous work area.

WORK THAT REQUIRES STANDING
• For pregnant women who stand for long periods, there are no set times for discontinuing the work. There are some concerns about the effect of standing for long periods during the last months of pregnancy. In some cases, a woman may be permitted to work to delivery time, while others are advised to quit anywhere from the 24th to the 32nd week of pregnancy.
• If you do need to stand for long periods, keep one foot on a low stool with knee bent. This takes some of the pressure off the back. Wear support hose.
• Consider cutting back on your hours, if possible, and/or increase the frequency and duration of your rest periods.

SEDENTARY WORK
• A woman in a sedentary job can usually work up to the delivery date without any threat to her well-being or the baby's health.
• While sitting at your desk, use a stool or a low box to elevate your legs whenever possible.

CALL YOUR DOCTOR IF

You or a family member is pregnant and working and has concerns about the effect the work may have on the pregnancy.

Premature Labor & Premature Birth

GENERAL INFORMATION

DEFINITION—Labor that begins after the 20th and before the 37th week of pregnancy. Premature birth frequently follows premature labor.

SIGNS & SYMPTOMS
- Menstrual-like cramps, or uterine contractions at regular intervals, that begin before the fetus is mature.
- Passage of bloody mucus (sometimes).
- A sensation of pelvic pressure.
- Flow of fluid (amniotic fluid) from the uterus (sometimes). This may occur with a gush or may be only a continuous watery discharge.
- Some degree of vaginal bleeding or spotting.
- Dull, lower backache, pain or pressure.

CAUSES—In most cases, the exact mechanisms that cause premature labor are not well-identified. Many obstetric, medical and anatomic disorders are associated with premature labor.

RISK INCREASES WITH
- Premature rupture of the membranes.
- Illness of the mother, including preeclampsia, high blood pressure or diabetes mellitus.
- Abnormal shape or size of the uterus.
- Weak (incompetent) cervix.
- Fetal abnormalities.
- Vaginal infection that spreads to the uterus.
- Large fetus or more than one fetus.
- Abnormalities of the placenta, such as placenta previa.
- Excessive amniotic fluid.
- Poor nutrition, especially if associated with weight loss.
- Previous premature labor.
- Smoking; excess alcohol consumption.
- Injury (trauma) to the uterus.
- Urinary tract infection, especially kidney infection (pyelonephritis).
- Use of mind-altering drugs (e.g., narcotics, psychedelics, hallucinogens, marijuana, sedatives, hypnotics or cocaine).
- Adolescent mothers.
- Significant prior cervical procedure(s) such as cone biopsy.
- Multiple abortions; particularly second trimester procedures.

HOW TO PREVENT
- Obtain good prenatal care throughout your pregnancy.
- Don't smoke, use mind-altering drugs or drink alcohol during pregnancy.
- Eat a normal, well-balanced diet during pregnancy. Take prescribed prenatal vitamin and mineral supplements.
- Don't use medications of any kind, including nonprescription drugs, without medical advice.
- If you have a weak cervix, which is sometimes evident before pregnancy, get medical advice about a minor operation to strengthen the cervix.
- Rest more and decrease activity in the third trimester, especially if you have spotting of blood or irregular contractions.

PROBABLE OUTCOME
- In about 80% of cases, the premature labor ceases, either spontaneously or with treatment.
- Labor can often be stopped with treatment to allow more time for the fetus to mature. However, if the membranes have ruptured or the placenta has separated from the uterus, often labor must proceed or delivery must be accomplished by cesarean section. The outcome depends on fetal maturity.

POSSIBLE COMPLICATIONS
- Premature infant.
- Uterine infection after delivery.
- Fetal death.

HOW TO TREAT

GENERAL MEASURES
- Diagnostic tests may include amniocentesis to determine fetal maturity and to check for infection inside the uterus that could be causing the symptoms. Ultrasound is used to determine fetal weight, age, growth and position. Laboratory blood and urine studies on the mother are used to check for infection. Samples of fetal protein from the mother's genital tract, or hormones in the mother's saliva, may be collected and tested for indications of impending premature birth.
- Hospitalization and treatment may be necessary for any underlying risk factors.

MEDICATION
- Medications to stop labor include terbutaline, ritodrine and magnesium; less frequently used are indomethacin and nifedipine.
- Antibiotics to fight or prevent infection in the mother, or to protect the fetus from infection.
- Corticosteroids are recommended to accelerate fetal lung maturity in fetuses between 24 and 34 weeks who are likely to be delivered soon.
- Sedatives and pain relievers if needed.

ACTIVITY—Complete bed rest, possibly in the hospital, is necessary once signs of premature labor begin. Discontinue work or other physical activities. Avoid any sexual activity.

DIET—Once labor begins, drink only clear liquids until after the delivery.

CALL YOUR DOCTOR IF

- You or a family member has symptoms of premature labor. Call immediately. This is an emergency!
- During pregnancy, you think you have a urinary tract infection.
- New, unexplained symptoms develop. Drugs used in treatment may produce side effects.

Premature Rupture of the Membranes (PROM)

GENERAL INFORMATION

DEFINITION—A spontaneous break or tear in the amniotic fluid sac before the onset of labor. It may happen at any time during a pregnancy and occurs in approximately 10% to 15% of all pregnancies, and in 0.5% of women who undergo amniocentesis. When PROM occurs following genetic amniocentesis early in pregnancy, there is often resealing of the membranes.

SIGNS & SYMPTOMS
• A leakage or a gush of blood-tinged amniotic fluid from the vagina.
• Fever or foul-smelling vaginal discharge associated with uterine tenderness (often indicates an infection in the amniotic cavity).

CAUSES—The exact cause is unknown. There is often a combination of PROM, preterm labor and infection involved.

RISK INCREASES WITH
• Poor nutrition and poor hygiene.
• Lack of proper prenatal care.
• Weak (incompetent) cervix.
• Increased intrauterine pressure due to excessive amniotic fluid or multiple pregnancies.
• Defect in the strength of the membrane itself.
• Uterine infection; urinary tract infection.
• Presence of sexually transmitted disease.

HOW TO PREVENT—No specific preventive measures other than to avoid risk factors when possible.

PROBABLE OUTCOME
• In a term pregnancy, labor and delivery usually occur within 24 hours following the rupture. In some preterm pregnancies, the period between the rupture and delivery may extend into weeks, or even months.
• Outcome for a preterm rupture varies depending on the length of the pregnancy. If prior to 24 weeks' gestation, the outlook is poor.
• On rare occasions, the leakage will cease, and the membranes are said to "seal over." The amniotic fluid reaccumulates.

POSSIBLE COMPLICATIONS—Extensive intra-amniotic infection, which will generally result in intensive uterine tenderness, fever and accelerated heart rates for both mother and fetus. If this occurs, intravenous antibiotics and induction of labor are necessary regardless of gestational age. In some cases, intra-amniotic infection can lead to serious consequences for both mother and child.

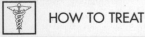

HOW TO TREAT

GENERAL MEASURES
• Hospitalization is normally required in order to conduct further diagnostic studies and to make determinations about treatment and delivery.
• Tests may include characterization of the fluid which has been allowed to dry on a microscope slide (ferning). Your physician may perform a pelvic examination with a speculum in order to try to visualize the fluid as it emerges from the cervix. Ultrasound and amniocentesis may also be used in diagnosis.
• With a pregnancy longer than 36 weeks or when fetal lung maturity has been established, treatment leans toward delivery; 80% of patients go into spontaneous labor within 12 to 24 hours. For some patients, labor may be induced immediately, particularly if there are any signs of infection. If there is concern about fetal well-being or fetal position (breech), cesarean birth is sometimes necessary.
• For a pregnancy of longer than 24 to 26 weeks' duration, hospitalization until delivery is usually recommended. Careful monitoring of vital signs and laboratory blood studies will continue to check for infections and fetal distress. Labor will need to be induced if problems develop. Avoid any vaginal douches and sexual intercourse if you are at home.
• For a pregnancy of less than 24 to 26 weeks, the fetal risks increase significantly. These include compression deformities due to the collapse of amniotic membranes around the fetus and pulmonary hypoplasia (inadequate development of the fetal lung tissue). In the case of PROM occurring before 24 weeks, the fetal survival rates are less than 20%; among those fetuses that survive, there is a high frequency of developmental defects. Termination of the pregnancy may need to be discussed.

MEDICATION
• Oxytocin may be used to induce labor.
• Antibiotics may be given to fight or prevent infection.
• Steroids may be prescribed prior to delivery to enhance fetal pulmonary maturity.

ACTIVITY—Bed rest while awaiting labor and delivery. You may be allowed some walking around with medical approval.

DIET—No special diet unless labor and delivery are immediate.

CALL YOUR DOCTOR IF

• You or a pregnant family member has a leakage or gush of amniotic fluid (water) from the vagina. Call immediately. This may be an emergency!
• If you are being treated as an outpatient for PROM and any new signs or symptoms develop, or there is further leakage of the fluid.

Rh Isoimmunization
(Erythroblastosis Fetalis)

 GENERAL INFORMATION

DEFINITION—Incompatibility between an infant's blood type and that of its mother, resulting in destruction of the infant's red blood cells (hemolytic anemia) during pregnancy and after birth by antibodies from its mother's blood.

SIGNS & SYMPTOMS
Signs during pregnancy:
• Decreased fetal growth.
• Decreased fetal movement.
Signs in a newborn:
• Paleness.
• Jaundice (yellow skin and eyes).
• Unexplained bruising or blood spots under the skin.
• Tissue swelling (edema).
• Breathing difficulty.
• Seizures.
• Lack of normal movement.
• Poor reflex response.

CAUSES—The fetus of an Rh-negative (blood type) mother and an Rh-positive father may be Rh-positive. If the father is known to be Rh-negative, there is no concern. During delivery, a small amount of the infant's blood is absorbed by the mother through the placenta, stimulating her body to produce antibodies against Rh-positive blood. The antibodies are produced after delivery, so the first infant is not affected. With succeeding pregnancies, the antibodies in the mother's blood cross the placenta and can potentially destroy fetal blood cells. The resulting anemia can be severe enough to cause fetal death. If the fetus survives, antibodies can cross to the baby during birth, causing jaundice and other symptoms shortly after birth.

RISK INCREASES WITH
• Each pregnancy after the first involving different blood types.
• Previous blood transfusions that might have contained incompatible blood types.

HOW TO PREVENT
• Obtain prenatal care throughout pregnancy. Medical supervision early in pregnancy is essential to determine the risk of Rh incompatibility.
• Special anti-Rh gamma globulin (RhoGAM) is given to the mother at 28 weeks' gestation and within 72 hours after delivery, miscarriage, ectopic pregnancy or abortion. This prevents formation of antibodies that might affect future infants. In women who are already producing antibodies, there is no benefit to using RhoGAM.
• Amniocentesis beginning at 16 to 20 weeks if indicated by elevated antibody concentration in the mother. Amniocentesis can now be used to determine the fetal blood type.
• Cordocentesis (percutaneous umbilical blood sampling or PUBS) may be recommended, despite some risks, to determine fetal blood type and the degree of anemia.

PROBABLE OUTCOME—With prompt recognition of the disorder, damage to the infant can be prevented with exchange transfusions. These transfusions are administered directly into fetal circulation by PUBS.

POSSIBLE COMPLICATIONS
• Permanent neurological damage to the infant, such as cerebral palsy or hearing loss (rare).
• Blood-transfusion reaction.
• Fetal distress requiring emergency delivery.
• Fetal death in utero.

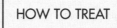 HOW TO TREAT

GENERAL MEASURES
• Blood tests to type the mother's, father's and infant's blood, measure the mother's Rh-positive antibodies and detect hemolytic anemia in the infant's blood.
• Amniocentesis (see Glossary) to evaluate fetal lung maturity or determine fetal blood type.
• Intrauterine blood transfusions (sometimes).
• Transfusion to completely exchange the infant's blood after birth.
• Hospitalization. The newborn child will remain in the hospital up to 2 weeks after an exchange transfusion.
• If you have an Rh-negative blood type, tell any doctor or medical professional who treats you. Make sure this information is in your medical records. Wear a medical-alert-type bracelet or pendant identifying your blood type.

MEDICATION—If you are pregnant and have Rh-negative blood type, you will be given an anti-Rh gamma globulin injection (RhoGAM) at 28 weeks and again within 72 hours after delivery, termination of a pregnancy for any reason, or trauma. You may also have an antibody titer drawn during pregnancy to see if you are producing anti-Rh antibodies.

ACTIVITY—No restrictions after treatment.

DIET—No special diet. The infant may be breast-fed or bottle-fed normally.

 CALL YOUR DOCTOR IF

Your baby has any of the following symptoms after returning home:
• Fever.
• Jaundice.
• Poor appetite or poor weight gain.

Urinary Tract Infection in Pregnancy (UTI in Pregnancy)

 GENERAL INFORMATION

DEFINITION—Urinary tract infections (UTIs) can involve the bladder, kidneys, ureters (tubes connecting kidneys to bladder) and urethra (vessel that leads from bladder to external opening through which urination occurs). Pregnant women have a greater risk of developing urinary tract infections. Disorders include:
• Asymptomatic bacteriuria (presence of multiplying bacteria in the urinary tract without obvious symptoms).
• Cystitis, which is an infection of the urinary bladder.
• Pyelonephritis, which is a kidney infection that can arise from cystitis. It is a significant and potentially dangerous infection.

SIGNS & SYMPTOMS
• Sometimes, no symptoms are obvious.
• Painful, burning sensation during urination.
• Increased urge to urinate.
• Frequent urination, although the urine amount may be small.
• Painful sexual intercourse.
• Blood or pus in the urine.
• Pain in the lower abdomen over the bladder.
• Cloudy and unpleasant-smelling urine.
• Low fever.
• Lower back pain.
• With pyelonephritis, there may be fever, chills, nausea, vomiting and flank pain.

CAUSES—A breakdown in the body's defense mechanisms that allows bacteria from the vagina, perineum, rectum or a sexual partner to invade the urinary tract system. Women are more vulnerable to these infections than men, due to shortness of the urethra. Infection ascends from the urethra to the bladder. Various changes in the urinary tract in pregnant women increase the risk of infection.

RISK INCREASES WITH
• A history of urinary tract infections.
• Diabetes mellitus.
• Sickle cell anemia trait.
• Underlying abnormalities of the urinary tract.
• Poor hygiene.
• More than 3 previous pregnancies.
• Presence of renal stones (nephrolithiasis).

HOW TO PREVENT
• Drink 8 glasses of water a day.
• Empty bladder immediately before, and right after, sexual intercourse.
• Wipe from front to back after a bowel movement.
• Urine studies during prenatal office visits.
• Don't postpone urination.
• Drinking 10 ounces of cranberry juice a day can significantly reduce a woman's chance of developing a UTI.

PROBABLE OUTCOME—With early diagnosis and treatment, symptoms usually resolve in a few days. Recurrence is not uncommon.

POSSIBLE COMPLICATIONS
• Pyelonephritis, that may become chronic.
• Untreated urinary tract infections can progress to pyelonephritis, which is associated with premature labor and poses a serious risk to the unborn child and mother.

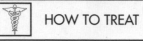 HOW TO TREAT

GENERAL MEASURES
• Diagnostic laboratory tests will include a urinalysis and urine culture. You will be advised on how to collect a clean, midstream urine sample.
• For an asymptomatic infection or cystitis, medication is generally all that is required for treatment. Follow-up urine cultures are important to ensure that the infection is eradicated.
• Treatment for pyelonephritis normally requires hospitalization for intravenous medications and careful monitoring for complications, such as dehydration. If there is no improvement in symptoms, further diagnostic testing is considered.

MEDICATION—Antibiotics will be prescribed. It is important to complete the full dosage even if the symptoms disappear. In some cases, when a UTI recurs, antibiotic treatment may be recommended for the remainder of the pregnancy. In cases of pyelonephritis, antibiotic therapy is often continued to suppress future infections, a preventive strategy referred to as antibiotic prophylaxis.

ACTIVITY—Avoid sexual intercourse until you have been free of symptoms for 2 weeks.

DIET—No special diet. Drink plenty of fluids, especially water and cranberry juice. Avoid caffeine, which irritates the bladder.

 CALL YOUR DOCTOR IF

• You or a family member has symptoms of a urinary tract infection.
• Symptoms do not disappear following the first 2 days of treatment.
• You have not had a follow-up urine test to be sure the infection is eradicated.
• You develop fever, chills or flank pain, or blood appears in the urine.
• New, unexplained symptoms develop. Drugs used in treatment may produce side effects.

Vaginal Bleeding during Pregnancy

 GENERAL INFORMATION

DEFINITION—Vaginal bleeding that occurs at any time during a pregnancy. It is a common problem, with the bleeding ranging in severity from mild to life-threatening for both mother and infant. Any bleeding should be reported promptly to your prenatal health-care provider.

SIGNS & SYMPTOMS
- Vaginal bleeding that can vary from hardly more than spotting to light or heavy.
- Color of blood varies from brown to bright red.
- May be painful or painless.

CAUSES
- Vaginal infection or trauma.
- Disorders of the cervix.
- Light bleeding may occur after sexual intercourse, possibly due to a small injury to the surface of the cervix.
- Complications of pregnancy.
- Ectopic pregnancy.
- "Bloody show" (bloody discharge that normally precedes labor).
- In the third trimester, bleeding may be a sign of preterm labor.
- Can include unlikely diseases and medications.
- If the bleeding is in the first trimester, no cause is found in over 50% of the cases.

RISK INCREASES WITH—Varies depending on the cause.

HOW TO PREVENT
- In most cases, no preventive measures are known. Obtaining proper prenatal care will help guarantee that all measures are being taken to achieve a successful pregnancy.
- If bleeding is determined to be a result of sexual intercourse, avoid deep penetration.
- Avoid situations or unsafe activities that could result in accidents or trauma. Avoid smoking, drugs of any kind and alcohol.

PROBABLE OUTCOME
- Will depend on the cause, the severity of the bleeding and how quickly it is diagnosed and treated. For some patients, the pregnancy can proceed normally to term.
- Bleeding in early pregnancy may result in miscarriage in up to 50% of the cases.
- An ectopic pregnancy will always result in death of the fetus.
- The two causes of bleeding in the second half of pregnancy that require greatest attention are placenta previa and abruptio placenta.
- In some cases, the patient has mistaken bleeding from hemorrhoids or even blood in the urine for vaginal bleeding. A medical examination will verify the source of the blood.

POSSIBLE COMPLICATIONS
- Anemia due to blood loss.
- Shock.
- Infection.
- Premature delivery of the baby and complications associated with premature delivery.
- Bleeding disorders.
- Death of the infant or mother.

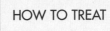 HOW TO TREAT

GENERAL MEASURES
- Laboratory studies, such as blood tests, blood clotting studies and hormone tests will often be necessary. A sample of fluid may be withdrawn from the womb. A pelvic examination will usually be performed by the doctor. An ultrasound exam may also be required to make a diagnosis. Occasionally, a laparoscopic examination may be performed.
- Treatment methods will depend upon diagnosis.
- For threatened miscarriage in early pregnancy, bed rest is the most common treatment. Avoid douching and sexual intercourse. If the bleeding is severe, hospitalization may be required.
- During late pregnancy, most patients need to be hospitalized for observation. Conservative treatment measures are often appropriate. The amount of bleeding and the status of the mother and baby may indicate the need for an urgent cesarean section.
- Blood transfusion may be ordered if the blood loss is severe.
- Surgery may be necessary for ectopic pregnancy or for an incomplete miscarriage.
- Grief counseling is appropriate if pregnancy loss is unavoidable.
- Save any tissue that is passed vaginally and bring it to your doctor for examination.

MEDICATION—Usually no medications are necessary. Antibiotics may be prescribed if there is an infection.

ACTIVITY—Restrictions are usually required and will be determined by the severity of the problem. Always follow the medical advice provided by your doctor.

DIET—No special diet.

 CALL YOUR DOCTOR IF

- You or a family member is pregnant and any vaginal bleeding occurs.
- Bleeding or pain worsens despite treatment.
- Tissue is passed vaginally.

Infertility

Infertility Problems in Men

GENERAL INFORMATION

DEFINITION—Infertility is described as an inability to achieve pregnancy after 1 year of sexual activity without contraception. Infertility occurs in 10% to 15% of all couples. Fertility depends on the production of normal quantities of healthy sperm, ability to achieve an erection, and ejaculation of sperm into the vagina during sexual intercourse. About 30% to 40% of infertility causes can be attributed to male partners.

SIGNS & SYMPTOMS—Failure to impregnate a fertile woman.

CAUSES
- Azospermia: complete absence of sperm (uncommon).
- Low sperm count (not enough sperm).
- Low motility (slow-moving sperm).
- Misshapen or immature sperm.
- Anatomical abnormalities of the penis or testicles, including undescended testicles.
- Excessive alcohol intake.
- Urinary tract infection.
- Hormone disturbance.
- Endocrine disorders.
- Severe chronic or metabolic disorders (such as uremia or cirrhosis).
- Mumps.
- Use of some drugs, such as antihypertensives, cytotoxic drugs, male hormones and MAO inhibitors.
- Sexually transmitted disease, especially syphilis and nonspecific urethritis that causes scarring.
- Injury to the genitals.
- Varicose veins in the testicles (varicocele).
- Psychological reasons, such as fear of infertility.
- Overheating of the testicles caused by vigorous, repetitive exercise or underwear that is too tight and holds the testicles too close to the body (possibly).
- Intercourse problems (e.g., premature withdrawal, poor timing with ovulation, too infrequent).
- Ejaculatory dysfunction.
- Exposure to insecticides or industrial chemicals.

RISK INCREASES WITH
- Diabetes mellitus.
- Poor nutrition and poor general health.
- Smoking.

HOW TO PREVENT—Any specific preventive measures depend on the cause.

PROBABLE OUTCOME—Some fertility problems are minor and reversible. Often, no clear cause for infertility is found. Approach treatment with optimism.

POSSIBLE COMPLICATIONS—Psychological distress in your partner, caused by feelings of guilt, inadequacy, and loss of his self-esteem.

HOW TO TREAT

GENERAL MEASURES
- Consultation with a reproductive endocrinologist is often helpful in identifying the underlying problem and guiding therapy.
- Laboratory studies, such as blood studies of hormones and semen analysis (to determine quality, quantity, form and motility). Your partner will need to abstain from ejaculation for 4 days prior to semen analysis, to help ensure an accurate test result.
- Surgical diagnostic procedures such as testicular biopsy.
- Special tests of sperm function and quality are available at major infertility centers.
- Psychotherapy or counseling for sexual therapy techniques, marital problems or alcoholism.
- Surgery to correct anatomical abnormalities of the reproductive system (e.g., surgery for varicocele).
- Heat may decrease sperm production in the testicles. To prevent this, your partner should avoid wearing tight underwear or athletic supporters that hold the testicles too close to the body; avoid hot baths; avoid long bicycle rides.
- Have sexual intercourse during the time you are ovulating. Your partner should not ejaculate for 3 days prior to intercourse. Intercourse should occur every 36 hours during the fertile period.
- Consider other methods for initiating a pregnancy, including artificial insemination of washed concentrated sperm; donor insemination if no remedy is presently available; or direct intracytoplasmic sperm injection (ICSI), whereby a single sperm is injected into a single egg and the resulting zygote is transferred to the uterus.
- See the Resource section of this book for additional information.

MEDICATION—Medication may be prescribed depending on the cause of infertility.

ACTIVITY—Your partner should work and exercise moderately and rest when he tires. Overexercising can be a factor in infertility.

DIET—Have your partner eat a normal, well-balanced diet. Increased intake of zinc, vitamin C and vitamin E is sometimes recommended.

CALL YOUR DOCTOR IF

- You or a family member has symptoms of infertility and wants help.
- Conception doesn't occur within 6 months, despite recommendations and treatment.

Infertility Problems in Women

GENERAL INFORMATION

DEFINITION—The inability to become pregnant after 1 year of sexual activity without contraception. Infertility occurs in 10% to 15% of all couples. Female fertility depends on normal functioning of the reproductive tract and the production of hormones necessary for normal sexual development and functioning. About 40% to 50% of all infertility is attributed to the female.

SIGNS & SYMPTOMS—Inability to conceive.

CAUSES
- Anatomic abnormalities of the reproductive system; tubal obstruction.
- Emotional stress.
- Repeated weight gain/weight loss cycles.
- Hormone dysfunction, especially thyroid disorders; absent or infrequent ovulation.
- Vaginitis.
- Disorders of the cervix, such as infection (cervicitis), laceration or tearing from previous childbirth or narrowing of the cervix (stenosis) for any reason.
- Amenorrhea (lack of menstrual periods) caused by strenuous exercise programs or nutritional disorders (bulimia or anorexia nervosa).
- Chemical changes in the cervical mucus.
- Tumors; ovarian cysts.
- Pelvic adhesions; endometriosis.
- Smoking.
- The use of some medications, including oral contraceptives. Many women cannot conceive for several months after discontinuing use.
- Intrauterine device (IUD) (possibly).
- Disorders probably not related to infertility include a tilted uterus, small fibroid tumors of the uterus or inability to achieve orgasm.

RISK INCREASES WITH
- Stress.
- Diabetes mellitus.
- Marital discord and infrequent sexual intercourse.
- Genital disorders.
- Smoking; drugs of abuse, such as heroin.

HOW TO PREVENT
- Obtain treatment for any treatable disorder that causes infertility.
- Avoid preventable causes of infertility.

PROBABLE OUTCOME
- Some fertility problems are minor and reversible. Approach treatment with optimism.
- Research continues into new options.

POSSIBLE COMPLICATIONS
- Psychological distress, including feelings of guilt, inadequacy and loss of self-esteem.
- Treatment costs are high and often not covered by insurance.
- The unknown and possible long-term effects of medications used to increase fertility.

HOW TO TREAT

GENERAL MEASURES
- Consultation with a reproductive endocrinologist is often helpful in identifying the underlying problem and guiding treatment.
- Diagnostic tests may include laboratory blood tests; pelvic examination; hysterosalpingogram (see Glossary); postcoital test (PCT) (see Glossary); endometrial biopsy to rule out luteal phase defect (a defect in hormone production) and possibly others.
- Surgical diagnostic procedures, such as laparoscopy (see Glossary), to examine reproductive organs.
- Psychotherapy or counseling, if marital problems exist.
- Surgery to correct any reproductive system abnormalities.
- Keep a basal body-temperature chart to become familiar with your ovulation pattern. Have intercourse just before ovulation.
- Don't use a lubricant during sexual relations. Lubricants may interfere with sperm mobility.
- Your partner should withdraw his penis quickly from your vagina after ejaculation. If left in, it reduces the number of sperm that can swim toward the egg.
- After your partner's ejaculation, place pillows under your buttocks to provide an easier downhill swim for the sperm.
- Maintain a positive attitude. Worry and tension may contribute to infertility.
- Alternate pregnancy methods include in-vitro fertilization (IVF); gamete or zygote intrafallopian transfer (GIFT or ZIFT); and intracytoplasmic sperm injection (ICSI) (see Glossary for these terms).
- See the Resource section of this book for additional information.

MEDICATION
- Hormones for a hormone imbalance.
- Gonad stimulants such as clomiphene, menotropins (Pergonal), human chorionic gonadotropin (hCG), leuprolide (Lupron) or urofollitropin. Fertility drugs may cause multiple births.

ACTIVITY—Exercise moderately. Overexercising may contribute to infertility.

DIET—Eat a normal, well-balanced diet. If you are overweight, try to achieve your ideal weight.

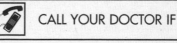

CALL YOUR DOCTOR IF

- You or a family member is concerned about infertility.
- Conception does not occur within 6 months, despite recommendations and treatment.
- New, unexplained symptoms develop. Drugs used in treatment may produce side effects.

Infertility Tests

GENERAL INFORMATION

DEFINITION
• Tests that are done to determine the cause of infertility in an individual or a couple who has been unable to achieve pregnancy after 1 year of sexual activity without contraception. Some infertility tests are for women only, others are for men only and still others cannot be performed without the cooperation of both partners.
• An initial work-up for a woman can take as little as six to eight weeks, or as much as three months or longer because some of the tests may have to be repeated for verification at different specific times in her menstrual cycle.
• The initial work-up of a man usually can be done faster because men have no monthly hormonal cycles, and because there are fewer tests for men.
• Diagnostic surgical procedures may be suggested for both men and women in order to look directly at reproductive structures and to obtain small tissue samples for laboratory analysis.

FEMALE'S TESTS—These tests are more varied and extensive than for males and generally begin with an analysis of if and when the woman is ovulating.

Basal body temperature:
One of the most popular techniques for pinpointing ovulation relies on the typically slight rise in a woman's resting body temperature midway in the menstrual cycle, signaling that ovulation has recently occurred. A woman's body temperature fluctuates throughout her menstrual cycle, and she is instructed to record these fluctuations on a chart after taking her temperature each morning before getting out of bed. If the chart, called a basal body temperature, or BBT, chart, indicates that the woman has been ovulating, it can often be used to predict when ovulation will happen during subsequent menstrual cycles. The couple can then use the information to attempt to time conception. Several urine-test kits for sale over the counter can be used to supplement the temperature chart.

Hormone tests:
Laboratory blood and urine studies to measure hormones that play a role in fertility. Tests may be done at the start of the menstrual cycle, in the middle or at the end. Progesterone increases in plasma after ovulation; it can be measured to confirm that ovulation has occurred. Luteinizing hormone (LH) and follicle-stimulating hormone (FSH) help stimulate ovulation. If their levels are low or high, or if they do not fluctuate properly, infertility can occur. Other hormones measured include prolactin, testosterone and thyroid-stimulating hormone (TSH). In addition, blood studies can detect the presence of antibodies to sperm.

Cervical mucus:
Other methods widely used to predict ovulation rely on examinations of the cervical mucus, which undergoes a series of hormone-induced changes at various times in the menstrual cycle. Some versions of these tests require a health professional's expertise. There are, however, versions of them that some women, with a physician's guidance, can learn to do themselves. Cultures of the cervix may also be performed to eliminate the possibility of infection.

Endometrial biopsy:
A long, hollow tube is passed into the patient's uterus late in her menstrual cycle, and a little of the lining is scraped off and examined with a microscope. The examination helps the physician tell whether the development of the egg and lining are in proper phase with each other. In most cases, the scraping is done in a physician's office and, because it is only very briefly painful, no anesthetic is used.

Ultrasound:
This technology relies on sound waves to produce images of internal structures. It is used, often in combination with one or more of the tests already discussed, to find the presence or absence of follicles that contain and release the eggs. Ultrasound is also used to detect abnormalities in the ovaries or uterus.

Hysterosalpingogram:
This is an x-ray study of the uterus and fallopian tubes. It is done just after a woman's menstrual period so there is no danger of her being pregnant and thereby exposing the fertilized egg or embryo to radiation. A dye containing iodine (technically called a contrast medium) is injected through the cervix. It spreads into the uterus and the fallopian tubes, allowing them to be visualized on x-ray. Among other things, this study often enables the physician to determine if the fallopian tubes are open. It is usually done, without an anesthetic, in the x-ray department of a hospital or clinic.

Hysteroscopy:
The patient's uterus is filled with a liquid or gas, instilled through the cervix. A small lighted telescope called a hysteroscope is then inserted into the uterus through the cervix, enabling the surgeon or physician to look directly inside. Many hysteroscopes have a separate channel through which instruments can be passed, often making it possible to immediately correct any abnormalities. Patients undergoing hysteroscopy are usually given an anesthetic, which may be local or general.

Laparoscopy:
A laparoscope, like a hysteroscope, is a small lighted telescope. It is slipped into the abdominal cavity through a small incision in or near the navel. For a clearer view of the

Infertility Tests
(cont.)

woman's reproductive tract, the cavity is filled with gas during the procedure and a colored solution (usually blue) is injected into the uterus and fallopian tubes. A general anesthetic is required. Advanced operative techniques may allow the repair of any defects in the reproductive tract to be made at the same time as the examination.

MALE'S TESTS
Semen analysis:
Semen analysis is almost always the first test done on men, and it is usually repeated several times. After abstaining from intercourse for 48 to 96 hours, depending on the doctor's recommendation, the man collects a semen sample in a container. The sample is microscopically examined to determine the number, activity and shape of individual spermatozoa (sperm cells), as well as the characteristics of the fluid part of the semen. A healthy, potent ejaculate typically contains 1.5 to 5 cubic centimeters (5 cc = I teaspoon) of semen and each cc will contain an average of 70 million sperm that look to be of normal size, shape and behavior. If the specimen markedly differs on any of these factors, further tests may be done to determine whether infection, hormonal imbalance or another problem could be the cause of the low sperm count. Cultures of the male urethra may also be performed in order to eliminate the role of infection.

Testicular biopsy:
This is a minor operation, performed with a local or general anesthetic, in which a small amount of tissue from the testes is removed for laboratory studies. Since even men with sperm counts well below 70 million per cubic centimeter sometimes father children, this test is ordinarily done only when the sperm count is zero. If damage to one or both of the vas deferens is known or suspected, an x-ray examination may also be ordered. The patient is first given a local or general anesthetic, so that an iodine-containing solution can be injected into the tubes to make them visible on x-rays. If the examination discloses damage, surgical repairs are often attempted at the same time the diagnosis is made.

Other special tests:
May be ordered if none of the tests already mentioned seem to explain the man's infertility. They may help in some cases, but results are uncertain in others. In the bovine (cow) mucus test, bovine mucus from the cervix or neck of the uterus (where it opens into the vagina) is placed in a special glass column. Samples of the man's semen are applied to the column, and measurements are made of how well the sperm are able to enter and swim through the mucus, giving some indication of their ability to swim through human cervical mucus. In the hamster-oocyte penetration test, some of the man's semen is mixed with hamster egg cells that have had their outer shells (membranes) removed. If the sperm are functioning normally, they will penetrate the hamster eggs, an indication that they are also capable of fertilizing human eggs. However, failure of the sperm to penetrate the hamster eggs does not always mean that they are incapable of fertilizing human eggs.

COUPLE'S TESTS
Postcoital test:
This test requires participation of both partners, as it has to be done after intercourse, which has to take place at the most fertile time in the woman's cycle. During the test at a doctor's office, which is performed 2 to 12 hours after intercourse, several samples of cervical mucus are taken. Laboratory analysis determines whether sperm and mucus have been able to properly interact.

Other tests:
There are also a variety of tests that are used when the doctor suspects that infertility may be due to the man's forming antibodies against his own sperm, or to the woman's forming antibodies against them. The exact nature of these immunological problems is not yet well understood, but their detection is sometimes helpful in explaining why a couple is having reproductive difficulty. Some of these tests require the participation of both partners; others require either one partner or the other.

Note:
A final word about all infertility tests: It is always best to ask in advance why they are being suggested, what they may show, how definitive they are, what the possible remedies are for any problem they may disclose and what side effects or complications are possible from a given test. Many of these tests have potential risks as well as potential benefits.

 CALL YOUR DOCTOR IF

You are interested in more information about infertility tests.

Infertility Treatments

 GENERAL INFORMATION

DEFINITION—Deciding what to do, if anything, when a fertility evaluation is complete may not be easy. Assuming these problems are treatable (and not all of them are), there is a bewildering array of choices, especially for women, and there are no guarantees that any of them will work. So it is that specialists in this field (called reproductive endocrinologists) speak of "maximizing fertility potential" rather than "curing infertility."

FERTILITY DRUGS
• When blood and urine tests from an infertility work-up suggest some sort of hormone imbalance in one or both partners, corrective therapy with so-called "fertility drugs" is frequently prescribed. The most popular of these drugs are Clomid and Serophene (both are clomiphene citrate in tablet form), which act on the hypothalamus, and Pergonal (human menopausal gonadotropin), which acts on the pituitary gland. A newer drug to treat infertility is Humegon, which is the equivalent of generic Pergonal.
• Because these powerful drugs have a wide range of side effects, patients should always discuss the pros and cons of their use with the physician in advance. Clomid and Serophene, for example, can prolong the menstrual cycle and make a woman mistakenly think she has conceived. Moreover, there is a risk of multiple births with some fertility drugs. Even if the couple would welcome several babies, multiple births complicate pregnancy and delivery, and can endanger infant survival.

SURGERY IN THE MALE
• Many men have a varicocele, a collection of swollen veins in the scrotum that often looks and feels like a bag of worms but may be less obvious. Some men with a varicocele easily sire children and so are clearly fertile. For those who seemingly are not and whose sperm are sluggish, surgical repair of the varicocele may better their chances of fatherhood. However, there is some debate about when the operation is appropriate. It may not be recommended unless other reasons for infertility are not found.
• Another male infertility problem often treated by surgery is damage to the vas deferens, through which sperm must pass for ejaculation. A common cause of such damage is vasectomy (male sterilization). Though it should be considered irreversible, some men later wish to have it reversed. This is sometimes possible through microsurgery. Other candidates for such surgery are men whose vas deferens have been blocked by scar tissue caused by earlier unrelated surgery, a sexually transmitted disease or other infection.

• Microsurgery is not a cure-all. Men with extensive damage to these structures, and many with limited damage, may not be able to father a child, despite the operation's apparent success.

SURGERY IN THE FEMALE
• A sterilization procedure for women, tubal ligation, involves tying, cutting or burning the fallopian tubes and thereby scarring them. Damage to the tubes by earlier unrelated surgery or infection—again, sometimes sexually transmitted—can also cause female infertility. In both cases, corrective surgery is sometimes, but not always, a possibility. Nor do seemingly successful surgical repairs of damaged fallopian tubes necessarily mean that any eggs fertilized in them will be able to make their way to the uterus. Sometimes, an ectopic (literally, out-of-place) pregnancy occurs, in which the fertilized egg gets trapped in the tube where it cannot survive when it grows. Any woman can have an ectopic pregnancy, but those whose tubes have been damaged are at greatest risk, even after corrective surgery. Although surgical repair of the damage lowers the risk of having an ectopic pregnancy, it remains higher than for women with tubes that have never been damaged.
• Endometriosis, a common disorder in women, also can cause or contribute to infertility when small pieces of the uterine lining escape and take up residence on the surfaces of organs in the abdominal cavity. Inflammation and consequent chronic irritation from the misplaced tissue can result in significant internal scarring of the ovaries, fallopian tubes, inner or outer walls of the uterus or other nearby structures, so that the woman cannot conceive. Both surgery and drug treatments (sometimes combined) are used to treat endometriosis. Success rates in treating this disorder are in the 50 to 60 percent range and depend on several factors, including the patient's age and disease severity.

ARTIFICIAL INSEMINATION
• Some infertility treatments attempt to get a pregnancy started without intercourse. Artificial insemination, the oldest of these treatments, has been used for more than a century. A hollow, flexible instrument—called a catheter—is used to place the donor's washed semen into the woman's uterus or vaginal canal.
• All inseminations are performed around the time the woman should be ovulating, either naturally or after priming with a fertility drug. The semen may be from the woman's husband ("artificial insemination-husband," or AIH) or from an anonymous donor ("artificial insemination-donor," or AID).
• A recent advance for AIHs is for men who—because of spinal cord injury, cancer surgery or other reasons—can't ejaculate normally. Electrical stimulation can be used to help them

Infertility Treatments (cont.)

overcome this problem and the ejaculate is collected and inseminated in their partner.
• Fresh semen was once used for all inseminations and still is, as a rule, for AIHs, but because of concern about AIDS and other sexually transmitted infections, it is now recommended that anonymous-donor semen be frozen for at least 180 days before use. The delay allows the donor to be retested for possible occult (undiagnosed) HIV infection at the time of the donation.
• Some women become pregnant with one insemination. More often, repeat inseminations over the course of four to five menstrual cycles are required. And there are women who, after a year or more of periodic insemination, still do not conceive. Depending on the nature of the couple's infertility, studies show success rates between 50% and 65%.

IN-VITRO FERTILIZATION
• Much newer than artificial insemination is in-vitro fertilization (IVF), an option when various other treatments have failed or are inappropriate. It can be used, for example, in women who have a uterus and at least one ovary, but whose fallopian tubes are damaged, missing or diseased.
• The woman is prepared for this procedure with fertility drugs that ready several of her eggs for fertilization and the lining of her uterus to support a pregnancy. The eggs are then taken from her by one of several methods and placed in a laboratory dish where they are incubated with her partner's sperm for about 18 hours.
• Assuming that some eggs are fertilized and continue to develop normally for two days or so, one or more (usually several, for insurance) are transferred by instrument into the woman's uterus. If at least one implants there within about 2 weeks, the woman is pregnant. Implantation can often be determined at that time by a blood test. However, this chemical assessment is sometimes misleading. Therefore, a conclusive diagnosis cannot be made until a week or more has passed when— if the pregnancy is real, rather than just chemical—a sac will have formed around the embryo that can be detected by ultrasound. As with other infertility treatments, couples undergoing IVF should recognize that positive outcomes are never guaranteed.

GAMETE INTRAFALLOPIAN TRANSFER (GIFT) OR ZYGOTE INTRAFALLOPIAN TRANSFER (ZIFT)
• GIFT is similar to IVF except that sperm and eggs (gametes) are collected and immediately inserted into one or both fallopian tubes, where conception occurs.
• With ZIFT, instead of placing the sperm and egg immediately into the fallopian tubes, they will be placed into an incubator for 24 hours. Then the fertilized eggs are put into the fallopian tubes. Zygote is the term for the cell produced by fertilization.
• These procedures require that the woman have at least one healthy fallopian tube.
• Success rate for either GIFT or ZIFT is around 25%.

INTRACYTOPLASMIC SPERM INJECTION (ICSI)— Can be used for male infertility problems. A single sperm is taken from the male and injected into a single egg from the female; the resulting zygote is then transferred into the uterus. The success rate is about 24%.

TUBAL OVUM TRANSFER—The woman's eggs are retrieved and put into the fallopian tube close to where it opens into the uterus. The couple then has intercourse or the woman is artificially inseminated. Since this method allows the eggs to be placed beyond the parts of the tube that may be damaged or blocked, it can often be used when GIFT or ZIFT cannot.

EMBRYO LAVAGE—A fertile female donor provides the eggs. At the proper time in her menstrual cycle, she is artificially inseminated. If the donor conceives, the early embryo is washed out of her reproductive tract and transferred to the uterus or a fallopian tube of the woman who is to bear the child. The recipient, meanwhile, has been hormonally treated with fertility drugs to make her uterus receptive to the embryo. This technique allows women who have no eggs of their own to become pregnant—provided they have a uterus.

SURROGATE MOTHERHOOD
• This is an option for women who do not respond to ovulation induction therapies or who have no ovaries or lack a uterus. It also may be an option for those for whom pregnancy might be life-threatening or those who have good reason to worry that they might transmit a serious genetic disorder to the child.
• A healthy, fertile woman agrees to be artificially inseminated and also agrees to let the infertile couple adopt the baby. If the female member of the infertile couple can safely provide eggs of her own, these can be fertilized by the IVF process and then transferred to the surrogate woman who carries the fetus to term. In that case, the surrogate mother takes fertility drugs to prepare her uterus. Surrogate motherhood is controversial and has resulted in court cases about custody and parentage, which are rare with other forms of fertility treatment.

 CALL YOUR DOCTOR IF

You or a family member is interested in additional information about infertility treatments.
Note: This information is adapted in part from the *FDA Consumer* (the magazine of the Food & Drug Administration).

General Health

Alcoholism

GENERAL INFORMATION

DEFINITION—A psychological and physiological dependence on alcohol, resulting in chronic disease and disruption of interpersonal, family and work relationships. It affects both sexes but occurs more often in men than women. Rough estimates indicate that one in 50 of the U.S. population is alcohol-dependent.

SIGNS & SYMPTOMS
Early stages:
• Increased tolerance to the effects of alcohol.
• Need for alcohol at the beginning of the day, or at times of stress.
• Anxiety; depression; insomnia; nightmares.
• Habitual Monday-morning hangovers, and frequent absences from work.
• Preoccupation with obtaining alcohol and hiding drinking from family and friends.
• Guilt or irritability when others suggest drinking is excessive.
Late stages:
• Frequent blackouts; memory loss; depression.
• Delirium tremens (tremors, hallucinations, confusion, sweating, rapid heartbeat).
• Liver disease (jaundice, internal bleeding, bloating); anemia.
• Neurological impairment (numbness and tingling in hands and feet, declining sexual interest and potency, confusion, coma).
• Congestive heart failure.

CAUSES—Not fully understood, but include:
• Personality factors (possibly), especially dependency, anger, mania or introversion.
• Family influences, especially alcoholic or divorced parents.
• Social and cultural pressure to drink.
• Abnormal metabolism of alcohol (perhaps).

RISK INCREASES WITH
• Genetic factors. Some ethnic groups have high alcoholism rates for either social or biological reasons.
• Use of recreational drugs.
• Crisis situations, including unemployment, frequent moves or loss of friends or family.
• Insecure and immature personality types.
• Environmental factors such as ready availability, affordability, social acceptance of alcohol in the cultural, work or social group.

HOW TO PREVENT
• Keep to safe limits of alcohol intake as recommended by medical authorities.
• Drink slowly; never gulp alcoholic drinks. Do not drink on an empty stomach.
• Do not drink to relieve stress, anxiety, tension or depression. Do not drink alone.
• Counseling for people at risk of alcoholism, such as those with a family history of the disorder.
• Provide children with a loving, stable family environment. Use alcohol in moderation, if at all, to provide a healthy role model for children.
• Encourage a spouse, friend or co-worker to admit when an alcohol problem exists, and to seek professional care.

PROBABLE OUTCOME
• Without treatment, alcoholism can lead to progressive brain and liver disease, job loss, divorce and premature death.
• With abstinence (absence of alcohol or drugs), sobriety is a way of life. The change in lifestyle is difficult and relapses occur. If you are determined to give up alcohol, you can.

POSSIBLE COMPLICATIONS
• Chronic and progressive liver disease.
• Gastric erosion (raw area in stomach lining) with bleeding; stomach inflammation.
• Neuritis; tremors; seizures; brain impairment.
• Inflammation of the pancreas and/or heart.
• Mental and physical damage to the fetus if a woman drinks during pregnancy.

HOW TO TREAT

GENERAL MEASURES
• Recognize the existence of the problem and be willing to overcome it.
• No single form of treatment works for all alcoholics. Psychological, social and physical treatments may be combined.
• Some patients may require detoxification (medical help in getting over the physical withdrawal symptoms when drinking stops).
• Sometimes requires inpatient care at a special treatment center.
• Keep appointments with doctors and counselors.
• Join and regularly attend a local Alcoholics Anonymous group or other support group.
• Reassess your lifestyle, friends, work and family to identify and alter factors that encourage drinking.
• Family members of alcoholics may benefit from support groups such as Al-Anon.

MEDICATION
• Disulfiram (Antabuse), which causes several extremely unpleasant physical symptoms when alcohol is consumed, may be recommended.
• Other medications to help control withdrawal symptoms may be prescribed.

ACTIVITY—There are usually no restrictions. Discuss physical activities with your doctor.

DIET—Eat a normal, well-balanced diet. Vitamin supplements, such as thiamine and folic acid, are often necessary.

CALL YOUR DOCTOR IF

You or a family member has symptoms of alcoholism.

Alopecia Areata

GENERAL INFORMATION

DEFINITION—Sudden and rapid hair loss in circular patches, usually from the scalp but occasionally from other areas of the body. The hair loss is not accompanied by other visible evidence of scalp disease. It can involve hair on the scalp, eyebrows, eyelashes, genital area and underarms (sometimes).

SIGNS & SYMPTOMS
- Sudden hair loss in sharply defined circular patches. In rare cases, body hair loss may be total (alopecia universalis).
- Easily removable hairs at the outer edges of the bald patches.
- No pain.
- No itch.

CAUSES
- Unknown, but heredity and emotional factors, such as anxiety, may contribute to hair loss. The autoimmune system (misdirected immune response in which the body's defenses become self-destructive) may also be involved.
- Occasionally due to thyroiditis or pernicious anemia.

RISK INCREASES WITH
- Physical or psychological stress.
- Family history of alopecia areata.

HOW TO PREVENT—Cannot be prevented at present.

PROBABLE OUTCOME—Usually curable, with spontaneous new growth, in 18 months to three years. Persons with a few small patches are generally cured completely. The disorder recurs in 25% of cases.

POSSIBLE COMPLICATIONS
- Loss of all hair.
- Slow or incomplete regrowth.

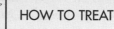

HOW TO TREAT

GENERAL MEASURES
- Consider wearing a hairpiece or wig during the acute phase.
- In a simple, self-limited case when the alopecia is not noticeable, no treatment may be necessary.
- Continue to bathe and shampoo as usual. The disorder is not contagious.
- Don't tug on normal hair close to areas of hair loss.
- See the Resource section of this book for additional information.

MEDICATION
- Topical steroids may be prescribed. Apply topical steroid once or twice a day unless directed otherwise. Apply immediately after bathing or shampooing for better spreading and penetration. For scalp and groin, use only low-potency steroid products without fluorine. In special cases, you may have injections of steroids into affected areas and be prescribed oral cortisone drugs to take on alternate days.
- Topical minoxidil (Rogaine), a drug used for hair growth, may help. However, its effectiveness is highly variable.
- Injections of triamcinolone into the scalp may be used for some patients.
- Photochemotherapy with PUVA may be recommended. This treatment combines the use of a drug that sensitizes the skin along with a controlled dose of ultraviolet light.

ACTIVITY—No restrictions.

DIET—No special diet.

CALL YOUR DOCTOR IF

- You or a family member has symptoms of alopecia areata.
- The following occurs during treatment:
  Hair loss increases.
  Hair loss doesn't diminish in 4 weeks.
  Areas show signs of infection (redness, swelling, tenderness, warmth) after injections.

Anemia, Folic-Acid Deficiency

 GENERAL INFORMATION

DEFINITION—Anemia that is caused by a deficiency of folic acid. It is often accompanied by iron-deficiency anemia.

SIGNS & SYMPTOMS
• Fatigue and weakness.
• Red, sore tongue.
• Mouth ulcers.
• Paleness.
• Numbness and tingling of fingers and toes.
• Irritability.
• Shortness of breath.
• Nausea, vomiting and diarrhea (rare).

CAUSES
• Complication of pregnancy, when the body needs 8 times more folic acid than usual.
• Inadequate intake or absorption of foods with a high folic-acid content, such as meat, poultry, fish, cheese, milk, eggs, green vegetables, yeast and mushrooms.
• Alcoholism.
• Overcooking foods, which destroys folic acid.
• Deficiency of vitamin B-12 or vitamin C.

RISK INCREASES WITH
• Adults over 60, especially those who have poor nutrition.
• Pregnancy.
• Recent surgery.
• Illness such as tropical sprue, psoriasis, acne rosacea, eczema or dermatitis herpetiformis.
• Fad diets or general poor nutrition, especially vitamin C deficiency.
• Chronic illness.
• Surgical removal of a portion of the stomach.
• Alcohol or drug abuse.
• Smoking, which decreases vitamin C absorption. Vitamin C is necessary for folic-acid absorption.
• Use of certain drugs, such as oral contraceptives, anticonvulsants, methotrexate, triamterene or sulfasalazine.

HOW TO PREVENT
• Don't drink alcohol.
• Have regular medical checkups during pregnancy. Take prenatal vitamin supplements, if they are prescribed.
• Eat well. Include fresh vegetables, meat and other animal proteins. Avoid fad diets. Don't overcook food.
• Don't smoke. Smoking increases vitamin requirements.

PROBABLE OUTCOME—Usually curable in 3 weeks with an adequate folic-acid intake.

POSSIBLE COMPLICATIONS
• Infertility.
• Increased susceptibility to infection.
• Congestive heart failure (severe cases only).
• Folic-acid deficiency can increase the risk of conceiving a child with a neural tube defect.

 HOW TO TREAT

GENERAL MEASURES
• Diagnostic tests may include laboratory blood studies, a Schilling test to measure vitamin B-12 levels and a therapeutic trial of vitamin B-12.
• Treatment consists of folic-acid supplements and elimination of contributing causes.
• If you smoke, stop smoking.
• If you take oral contraceptives, consider using another form of contraception.

MEDICATION
• Folic-acid supplements.
• Iron supplements to take orally.

ACTIVITY—Anemia does cause fatigue. Schedule regular rest periods until you are able to resume normal activity.

DIET—No special diet. Eat foods daily that are high in folic acid. The liver can store folic acid for a limited time only. Foods high in folic acid include asparagus spears, beef liver, broccoli spears, collards (cooked), mushrooms, oatmeal, peanut butter, red beans, wheat germ.

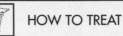 CALL YOUR DOCTOR IF

• You or a family member has symptoms of anemia.
• Symptoms don't improve in 2 weeks, despite treatment.
• Symptoms of infection (fever, chills and muscle aches) occur during treatment.

Anemia, Iron Deficiency

GENERAL INFORMATION

DEFINITION—Anemia due to a decreased amount of iron stored in the blood, or insufficient hemoglobin in the cells. Anemia is a symptom of other disorders. This is the most common type of anemia in the U.S.

SIGNS & SYMPTOMS
- Initially, there may be no symptoms.
Signs of pronounced anemia:
- Fatigue; weakness; listlessness.
- Headache.
- Inability to concentrate; irritability.
- Tiredness and weakness.
- Paleness, especially in the hands and lining of the lower eyelids.
Less common signs:
- Tongue inflammation.
- Fainting.
- Breathlessness.
- Rapid heartbeat.
- Appetite loss.
- Abdominal discomfort.
- Cravings for ice, paint or dirt.
- Susceptibility to infection.

CAUSES—Decreased absorption of iron, poor iron intake or increased need for iron.
Causes in adolescents and adults:
- Rapid growth spurts.
- Heavy menstrual bleeding or other blood loss.
- Pregnancy.
- Malabsorption.
- Gastrointestinal disease with bleeding, including cancer.

RISK INCREASES WITH
- Poor nutrition.
- Age over 60.
- Recent illness, such as an ulcer, diverticulitis, colitis, hemorrhoids or gastrointestinal tumors.

HOW TO PREVENT
- Maintain adequate iron intake through a well-balanced diet or iron supplements.
- Correct gynecologic or other problems causing excess blood loss.

PROBABLE OUTCOME—Usually curable with iron supplements if the underlying cause can be identified and cured.

POSSIBLE COMPLICATIONS
- Failure to diagnose a bleeding malignancy.
- Angina pectoris (pain or pressure beneath the breastbone caused by inadequate blood supply to the heart) or congestive heart failure (pumping action of the heart is insufficient) may develop as a result of marked iron deficiency.

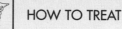

HOW TO TREAT

GENERAL MEASURES
- Diagnostic tests may include laboratory blood studies and bone marrow aspiration; sigmoidoscopy, gastroscopy or colonoscopy (see Glossary for these terms) may be done to rule out internal bleeding or malignancy.
- The most important part of treatment for iron-deficiency anemia is to correct the underlying cause. Iron deficiency can be treated well with iron supplements.
- Avoid risk of infections.
- Blood studies may be repeated after treatment to detect recurrences.
- See the Resource section of this book for additional information.

MEDICATION
Iron supplements are usually prescribed:
- Take iron on an empty stomach (at least 1/2 hour before meals) for best absorption. If it upsets your stomach, you may take it with a small amount of food (except milk).
- If you take other vitamins or medications, wait at least 2 hours after taking iron before taking them. Antacids, tetracyclines and calcium especially interfere with iron absorption.
- Iron supplements may cause black bowel movements, indigestion, diarrhea or constipation.
- Continue iron supplements until 2 to 3 months after blood tests return to normal.
- Too much iron is dangerous; an overdose is highly toxic. Keep iron supplements out of the reach of children.

ACTIVITY—No restrictions. You may need to pace activities until symptoms of fatigue are gone.

DIET
- Limit milk to 1 pint a day. It interferes with iron absorption.
- Eat protein- and iron-containing foods, including meat, beans and leafy green vegetables.
- Increase dietary fiber to prevent constipation.

CALL YOUR DOCTOR IF

- You have symptoms of anemia.
- Nausea, vomiting, severe diarrhea or constipation occur during treatment.

Anorexia Nervosa

GENERAL INFORMATION

DEFINITION—A psychological eating disorder in which a person refuses to eat adequately in spite of hunger and loses enough weight to become emaciated. The person eats very little, and refuses to stop dieting after a reasonable weight loss. The body perception is distorted; person sees self as "fat" when she or he is at normal weight or emaciated. Anorexia nervosa primarily affects teenage and young adult females and occasionally young men.

SIGNS & SYMPTOMS—Symptoms may vary, depending on length and severity of the disorder:
• Weight loss of at least 15% of body weight without physical illness.
• Reduction in total food intake; refusal to eat.
• High energy level despite body wasting.
• Extensive exercise.
• Intense fear of obesity.
• Preoccupation with body size, weight control.
• Depression.
• Appetite loss.
• Constipation.
• Cracked, dry skin; sparse scalp hair.
• Fine, downy hair on face, extremities and trunk.
• Cold intolerance.
• Refusal to maintain a minimum standard weight for age and height.
• Distorted body image. The person continues to feel fat even when emaciated.
• Cessation of menstrual periods.

CAUSES—Unknown. Suggested causes include family and internal conflicts; sexual conflicts; phobia about putting on weight; changes in fashion in U.S. (being slim is identified with beauty); depression or personality disorder.

RISK INCREASES WITH
• Peer pressure to be thin.
• History of slight excess weight.
• Perfectionistic, compulsive or overachieving personalities.
• Low self-esteem.
• Stress due to multiple responsibilities, tight schedules.
• Dancers, models, cheerleaders and athletes.

HOW TO PREVENT
• Confront personal problems realistically. Try to correct or cope with problems, such as stress, with the help of counselors, family and friends.
• Develop a rational attitude about weight.

PROBABLE OUTCOME
• Treatable if the patient recognizes the emotional disturbance, wants help and cooperates in treatment.
• Without treatment, this can cause permanent disability and death. Persons with anorexia nervosa have a high rate of attempted suicide due to low self-esteem.

POSSIBLE COMPLICATIONS
• Chronic anorexia nervosa caused by patient's resistance to treatment.
• Bulimia nervosa (see Glossary), due to feelings of shame and the fear of weight-gain caused by eating (especially binging).
• Infertility.
• Electrolyte disturbances or irregular heartbeat. These may be life-threatening.
• Osteoporosis.
• Death as a result of starvation or suicide.

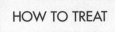

HOW TO TREAT

GENERAL MEASURES
• Diagnostic tests will include laboratory blood studies and psychological screening.
• The goal of treatment is for the patient to establish healthy eating patterns to help regain normal weight. The patient can accomplish this with behavior-modification training supervised by qualified professionals.
• Treatment may often be done on an outpatient basis, but sometimes inpatient treatment in a hospital or clinic is recommended.
• A successful treatment program usually includes a multidisciplinary approach, involving the physician, a nutritionist and psychotherapy or counseling for the patient and family.
• Hospitalization during crises for intravenous or tube feeding, to correct electrolyte imbalance or if patient is suicidal.
• Therapy may continue over several years. Relapses are common, especially when stressful situations occur.
• See the Resource section of this book for additional information.

MEDICATION—Lithium or other antidepressants, or antianxiety medications may be prescribed on a temporary basis.

ACTIVITY
• Increase activity as weight is gained back.
• Focus on playful, rather than goal-oriented, activities.

DIET
• A controlled diet program will be established.
• Vitamin and mineral supplements may be prescribed.

CALL YOUR DOCTOR IF

• You have symptoms of anorexia nervosa or observe them in a family member.
• Life-threatening symptoms occur, including rapid, irregular heartbeat, chest pain or loss of consciousness. Call immediately. This is an emergency!
• Weight loss continues, despite treatment.

Anxiety

GENERAL INFORMATION

DEFINITION—A vague, uncomfortable feeling of fear, dread or danger from an unknown source. For some it may be a one-time episode; other persons become constantly anxious about everything. A certain amount of anxiety is normal, helps improve performance and allows people to avoid dangerous situations. Several types of anxiety are recognized, including acute situational anxiety, which is usually a short-term response to a recent stressful event; adjustment disorder with anxious mood, which is a persistent, maladaptive reaction to stress that lasts up to 6 months; and generalized anxiety disorder, which is defined as unrealistic or excessive anxiety, often without an identifiable cause, which lasts for 6 months or longer. Other types of anxiety include panic disorder, post-traumatic stress disorder, phobias and obsessive-compulsive disorders. Anxiety is the most common mental health problem in the U.S.

SIGNS & SYMPTOMS
- Feeling that something undesirable or harmful is about to happen.
- Dry mouth; swallowing difficulty or hoarseness.
- Rapid breathing and heartbeat.
- Twitching or trembling.
- Muscle tension; headaches.
- Sweating.
- Nausea; diarrhea; weight loss.
- Nervousness; restlessness; irritability.
- Feeling of tightness or pressure in the chest.
- Sleeplessness.
- Fatigue.
- Nightmares.
- Memory problems.
- Sexual impotence.
- Dizziness or faintness.

CAUSES—Activation of the body's defense mechanisms for fight or flight. Excess adrenaline is discharged from the adrenal glands, and adrenaline breakdown products (catecholamines) stimulate the nervous system, causing quickened heart rate, increased alertness and tensed muscles. Attempts to avoid the anxiety often leads to more anxiety.

RISK INCREASES WITH
- Stress from any source (such as social or financial problems).
- Family history of anxiety.
- Fatigue or overwork.
- Recurrence of situations that have been previously stressful or harmful.
- Medical illness.
- Unrealistic perfectionism.
- Withdrawal from drugs or alcohol.
- Lack of a strong social or family support system.

HOW TO PREVENT
- Determine what stressful or potentially harmful situation is causing the anxiety. Deal directly with it.
- Consider lifestyle changes to reduce stress.
- Learn relaxation techniques.

PROBABLE OUTCOME—Anxiety, especially short-term anxiety and panic disorders, can often be controlled with treatment. Obsessive-compulsive disorder and post-traumatic stress disorder are more difficult to treat, and often require long-term psychotherapy and medication. Overcoming anxiety often results in a richer, more satisfying life.

POSSIBLE COMPLICATIONS
- Untreated anxiety may lead to neuroses, such as phobias, compulsions or hypochondriasis.
- A sudden increase in anxiety may lead to panic and violent escape behavior.
- Anxiety is often associated with depression.
- Dependence on drugs.
- Heart arrhythmias.

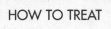

HOW TO TREAT

GENERAL MEASURES
- Some laboratory studies may be done to rule out medical conditions that produce anxiety, such as hyperthyroidism. Laboratory tests are usually normal.
- Obtain psychotherapy or counseling to understand the specific, but unconscious, threat or source of stress.
- Learn stress reduction techniques, including biofeedback and relaxation therapy.
- Follow a regular, energetic fitness routine using aerobic exercise.
- See the Resource section of this book for additional information.

MEDICATION
- Antianxiety drugs may be prescribed on a short-term basis.
- Antidepressants may be prescribed for panic disorders.

ACTIVITY—Stay active. Physical exertion helps reduce anxiety.

DIET
- No special diet.
- Avoid caffeine and other stimulants.
- Avoid alcohol.

CALL YOUR DOCTOR IF

- You or a family member has symptoms of anxiety and self-treatment has failed.
- You develop sudden feelings of panic.
- New, unexplained symptoms develop. Drugs used in treatment may produce side effects.

Bone-Density Testing
(Bone-Mass Measurement)

 GENERAL INFORMATION

DEFINITION—These tests are performed to measure the density of bones, usually in postmenopausal women. Bone density decreases in both men and women as they age, but in women, the decrease is more rapid and more severe once estrogen production ceases. Bone-density tests can show a bone loss of as little as 1% and can indicate whether a woman's bones are healthy or that moderate to severe bone loss exists. Low bone mass is a major cause of osteoporosis and of bone fractures (particularly of the hip, spine or forearm) in women over age 50.

REASONS FOR PROCEDURE
• As an aid in diagnosing osteoporosis.
• Woman with family history of osteoporosis, or other risk factors for osteoporosis.
• Follow-up of a previous bone-density test to determine effectiveness of any treatment.
• As a predictor of fracture risks.
• Low estrogen levels in a woman who has no symptoms of menopause.
• After menopause, to help in making decisions about hormone replacement therapy or bone-building drug therapy.
• Long term use of corticosteroids, thyroid hormone or Dilantin; all of these medications can lead to osteoporosis.
• Follow-up testing for osteopenia (a term used to describe bone density that is lower than that seen in healthy young adults).
• Though some medical experts recommend a bone-density test for every woman after menopause, official guidelines for this type of screening test have not yet been established.

RISK INCREASES WITH—Usually no risks associated with these tests.

DESCRIPTION OF PROCEDURE
• Several types of bone-density tests are available. Machines called densitometers can detect a 1% bone loss. The test selected depends on available equipment, the part of the body to be tested and the costs involved.
• The most accurate is the dual energy x-ray absorptiometry (DXA or DEXA). This test uses very little radiation. You sit or lie comfortably during the 5- to 15-minute procedure. No needles or injections are used. It can measure the bone density of the spine, hip, forearm or entire body.
• Dual photon absorptiometry (DPA) measures the total calcium and mineral content of the hips and spine. It takes about 20 to 40 minutes, and delivers more radiation than DEXA.
• Single photon absorptiometry (SPA) measures the bone density in the wrist or heel. It usually takes only a few minutes to perform.

• Quantitative computed tomography (QCT) measures the mineral content of the bone; it is used to assess loss of bone mass, particularly in the lower spine. QCT delivers more radiation than the other available tests and is generally more expensive. It takes 15 to 20 minutes to perform.
• Radiographic absorptiometry (RA) measures bone density in the hand. It takes only 3 to 5 minutes to perform.
• Additional bone density tests are being developed and may be recommended.

PROBABLE OUTCOME—Tests are completed without any complications. The test results will be reported to you in 2 numbers—age-matched and young-normal (called the T-score). The first compares your results to other women of the same age as you; the second number (T-score) compares your results to a healthy 30-year-old female (the norm). Results indicate if your bones are more dense (+), or less dense (–) or the same density as the healthy 30-year-old female (this is when peak bone density is achieved, which should be maintained for life). General ranges for interpreting bone mass T-scores are:
• Optimal = above +1.0 SD (standard deviation).
• Borderline = between a +1.0 SD and a –1.0 SD.
• Low = between a –1.0 SD and a –2.5 SD.
• Osteoporosis = below a –2.5 SD.
Note: The norm 0.0 is the healthy 30-year-old.

POSSIBLE COMPLICATIONS—None expected from the testing.

FOLLOW-UP CARE

GENERAL MEASURES—No specific measures necessary following the testing.

MEDICATION—One or more medications or supplements may be prescribed depending on test results. These include hormone replacement therapy, bone-building drugs, vitamin D and calcium.

ACTIVITY—No restrictions immediately before or after testing. Exercise is important in developing and maintaining bone density. Follow a regular fitness program that includes aerobic activity and weight-bearing exercises, such as brisk walking, stair climbing, weight training, etc.

DIET—No special diet is required prior to testing.

CALL YOUR DOCTOR IF

You or a family member has any questions about bone-density tests, their results or recommended follow-up.

Bone-Density Testing
(Bone-Mass Measurement)

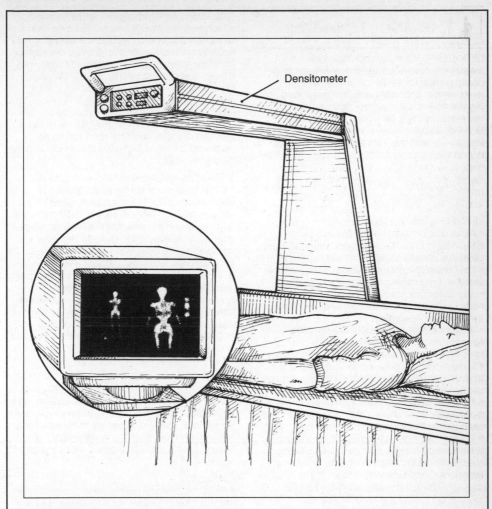

Densitometer

An illustration that shows a woman lying on her back while a densitometer is used to determine bone density in her body.

Inset shows the image seen by the technician performing the procedure.

Bone-Mass Building Treatment (Osteoporosis Therapy)

 GENERAL INFORMATION

DEFINITION—When osteoporosis (the progressive disease in which bone breakdown increases faster than bone formation) is diagnosed, a combination of treatment methods are available to stop or slow down the loss and help rebuild bones. Maintaining bone health is an important step in preventing bone fractures and subsequent disability that often occurs in women over age 50.

MEDICATIONS
• Hormone replacement therapy (HRT), consisting of estrogen plus a progestin or estrogen alone, is currently recommended (to prevent and treat osteoporosis) for all post-menopausal women, unless the medication is not tolerated or contraindications exist. HRT also offers protection against heart problems and some cancers. For most women, the benefits of hormone replacement will outweigh the possibility of any risks. For best results, the therapy should be started right after menopause and continue indefinitely.
• Alendronate (brand name, Fosamax) is a nonhormonal drug that slows down the loss of bone tissue and increases bone mass in women with osteoporosis. Take it in the morning at least 30 to 60 minutes before eating. The tablet should be swallowed with 6 to 8 ounces of water. To help the medicine reach the stomach faster and to prevent throat irritation, don't lie down for 30 minutes after taking it. Don't take any other medication for at least 30 minutes after taking alendronate. Side effects may include stomach, muscle or joint pain and other gastrointestinal symptoms. Long-term safety has not been established and medical studies are continuing.
• Calcitonin (brand name, Miacalcin) is a treatment for postmenopausal osteoporosis. The exact mechanism of how it works is not fully understood. It slows down the loss of bone tissue and increases bone mass in women with osteoporosis. It comes in the form of a nasal spray. Use one spray per day in a nostril, alternating nostrils daily. Side effects can include nasal symptoms such as dryness, stuffiness or runny nose.
• Other drugs undergoing testing with approval pending include:
  Slow-release sodium fluoride, a mineral encapsulated in a wax tablet. In medical studies, this drug therapy appears to slow down bone loss and to help build bone. In the past, high doses of sodium fluoride have caused some unwanted side effects, but this new slow-release formula appears to avoid them. Once approved, women taking this drug will need to have an annual blood test to check levels of fluoride to be sure it remains under toxic levels.

Calcitriol, a hormone drug, helps with the absorption of calcium and slows bone loss. It is used in many other countries for osteoporosis but has not been approved for this disorder in the U.S. Approved and used for the treatment of a bone disorder caused by kidney dialysis, it can cause kidney stones when taken in high doses.

Other agents are being investigated for use in the treatment of osteoporosis. Some of these are new drugs and others are existing drugs approved for other purposes but which also may help bone loss.

DIETARY SUPPLEMENTS
• Calcium is essential for development of normal bone. The recommended dietary allowance (RDA) for calcium is 1000 mg. Many health experts believe that the RDA for women over 40 should be 1000 to 1500 mg. This amount can be achieved with diet and/or supplements. Sufficient calcium intake is necessary, in addition to any type of prescription medication that is taken for bone loss.
• Vitamin D is also necessary for maintaining bone density. It is often difficult to get sufficient vitamin D in unfortified foods or sunlight exposure. Daily supplementation of 400 to 800 international units (IU) is usually recommended for postmenopausal women.

DIET
• Eat a healthful diet that follows the adult diet guidelines established by the U.S. government. Your doctor may recommend dietary restrictions for salt, fat, animal protein, alcohol or caffeine.
• If you are overweight or underweight, try to reduce health risks through better eating and exercise habits.

EXERCISE
• Physical exercise is important in developing and maintaining bone strength. Exercise also aids in strengthening back muscles, improves flexibility and mobility (which can reduce the risk of falls and bone fractures) and helps one's sense of well-being.
• A basic exercise routine should consist of 30 minutes of aerobic activity (such as brisk walking) and weight-bearing activity (such as weight lifting) at least 3 times a week, more often if possible. Choose an exercise program that you will follow regularly and faithfully.

 CALL YOUR DOCTOR IF

• You or a family member wants more information about bone-building treatment.
• New unexplained symptoms develop. Drugs used in treatment may cause side effects.

Bulimia Nervosa
(Binge-Eating Syndrome)

 GENERAL INFORMATION

DEFINITION—A psychological eating disorder characterized by abnormal perception of body image, constant craving for food and binge eating, followed by self-induced vomiting or laxative use. It affects adolescents or young adults, usually female.

SIGNS & SYMPTOMS—Recurrent episodes of binge eating (rapid consumption of a large amount of food in a short time, usually less than 2 hours) combined with any number of the following:
• Preference for high-calorie, convenience foods during a binge.
• Secretive eating during a binge. Patients are aware that the eating pattern is abnormal, and they fear being unable to stop eating.
• Termination of an eating binge with purging measures, such as laxative use or self-induced vomiting.
• Depression and guilt following an eating binge.
• Repeated attempts to lose weight with severely restrictive diets, self-induced vomiting and use of laxatives or diuretics.
• Frequent weight fluctuations greater than 10 pounds from alternately fasting and gorging.
• Eroded teeth and/or scarred hands from frequent self-induced vomiting.
• No underlying physical disorder.

CAUSES—Unknown; thought to be largely emotional.

RISK INCREASES WITH
• Strict, compulsive, perfectionistic family environment.
• Anorexia nervosa.
• Depression.
• Stress, including lifestyle changes, such as moving or starting a new school or job.
• Neurotic preoccupation with being physically attractive.

HOW TO PREVENT
• Raise children in a wholesome family environment with emphasis on caring and good communication rather than on external appearances.
• Encourage rational attitude about weight.
• Avoid stress.

PROBABLE OUTCOME—Outcome is variable; patients can learn to control the behavior with counseling, psychotherapy, biofeedback training and individual or group psychotherapy.

POSSIBLE COMPLICATIONS
• Fluid and electrolyte imbalance from vomiting; dental disease; stomach rupture (rare).
• Relapse.
• Cardiac arrhythmia; cardiac arrest.
• Without treatment, complications can be fatal.
• Suicide.

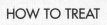 HOW TO TREAT

GENERAL MEASURES
• Diagnostic tests may include laboratory blood studies and electrocardiography (see Glossary).
• Therapy will consist of assessing nutritional status, establishing target goals, identifying triggers, improving relationships and overall well-being, techniques to avoid stress, etc.
• Treatment in an eating disorder facility may be recommended.
• Hospitalization in severe cases.
• Psychotherapy or counseling that may include hypnosis or biofeedback training.
• See the Resource section of this book for additional information.

MEDICATION—Antidepressants may be prescribed. They are sometimes helpful for some patients.

ACTIVITY—No restrictions.

DIET
• If hospitalization is necessary, intravenous fluids may be prescribed. During recovery, vitamin and mineral supplements will be necessary until signs of deficiency disappear and normal eating patterns are established.
• For outpatient therapy, supervision and regulation of eating habits; a food diary may be maintained and feared foods will be reintroduced.

 CALL YOUR DOCTOR IF

• You have symptoms of bulimia or you suspect a family member has bulimia.
• The following occur during treatment:
  Rapid, irregular heartbeat or chest pain.
  Loss of consciousness.
  Cessation of menstrual periods.
  Repeated vomiting or diarrhea.
  Continued weight loss, despite treatment.

Chronic Fatigue Syndrome

 GENERAL INFORMATION

DEFINITION
• Chronic fatigue syndrome (CFS) is characterized primarily by profound fatigue. There is usually an abrupt onset of symptoms that come and go for at least six months. It is unknown whether it represents one or many disorders. It is difficult to diagnose because there is no specific laboratory test, or a defined set of signs and symptoms. It is observed primarily in young adults between 20 and 40 years of age, and women outnumber the men by about two to one.
• The major criteria used to define cases currently are 1) persistence of relapsing fatigue that does not resolve with bed rest and is severe enough to reduce average daily activity by at least 50% for at least 6 months, and 2) other chronic clinical conditions have been satisfactorily excluded, including preexisting psychiatric disease. Additional symptoms and physical criteria aid in the diagnosis.

SIGNS & SYMPTOMS
• Fatigue.
• Sore throat.
• Mild fever.
• Lymph node pain.
• Muscle weakness, stiffness and discomfort.
• Headache.
• Sleep disturbances.
• Mood swings; irritability.
• Depression.
• Confusion; forgetfulness.
• Inability to concentrate.
• Vision changes; sensitivity to light.
• Dry eyes, mouth.
• Diarrhea.
• Loss of appetite.
• Night sweats.

CAUSES—Unknown. Immunological abnormalities may be involved. Many theories center on an infectious agent, but no such agent has been identified. Epstein-Barr (a virus that causes mononucleosis) and others have been implicated.

RISK INCREASES WITH—Unknown.

HOW TO PREVENT—Unknown.

PROBABLE OUTCOME—Symptoms will usually come and go over a long period of time. Generally there is very slow improvement over months or years.

POSSIBLE COMPLICATIONS—None specific to the disorder. Symptoms are usually most severe during the first 6 months.

 HOW TO TREAT

GENERAL MEASURES
• No specific diagnostic tests to identify CFS. Laboratory blood studies may be done to rule out other causes.
• Basic management involves four areas: 1) validation of the diagnosis and education of the patient, 2) general therapeutic measures, 3) symptomatic therapy, 4) experimental therapy.
• Join a local or national support group.
• Psychotherapy or counseling may be helpful for some patients.
• Be patient; recovery takes time.
• See the Resource section of this book for additional information.

MEDICATION
• Medications must be individually tailored but may include pain medicine, local injections, antidepressants and others.
• Other experimental medication therapies are being studied and may prove to be more helpful.

ACTIVITY—Strenuous exercise can exacerbate symptoms and should be avoided. Moderate exercise, however, is important; most doctors recommend limbering or stretching, rather than aerobic exercises. Begin a gradual program that may be just 3-5 minutes a day to start with. Increase the activity by about 20% every 2-3 weeks. Setbacks will occur, so don't be discouraged.

DIET—Try to maintain good nutrition, even if appetite is decreased.

CALL YOUR DOCTOR IF

• You or a family member has signs and symptoms of chronic fatigue syndrome.
• Symptoms worsen after treatment is started.
• New, unexplained symptoms develop. Drugs used in treatment may produce side effects.

Constipation

GENERAL INFORMATION

DEFINITION—A combination of changes in the frequency, consistency and ease of bowel movements. Difficult, uncomfortable or infrequent bowel movements that are hard and dry. In most people, constipation is harmless, but it can indicate an underlying disorder.

SIGNS & SYMPTOMS—People vary widely in bowel activity. Normal bowel movements may occur as often as 3 times a day or as infrequently as 3 times a week. Any of the following may be a sign of constipation:
- Decreased frequency of bowel movements, sometimes accompanied by abdominal swelling.
- Harder or smaller feces then normal.
- Straining during bowel movements.
- Pain or bleeding with bowel movements.
- Sensation of continuing fullness after a bowel movement.

CAUSES
- Inadequate fluid intake.
- Insufficient fiber in the diet. Fiber adds bulk, holds water and creates easily passed, soft feces.
- Inactivity; depression.
- Hypothyroidism.
- Electrolyte abnormalities; hypercalcemia; hypokalemia.
- Anal fissure.
- Chronic kidney failure.
- Back pain.
- Irritable bowel syndrome.
- Chronic abuse of laxatives.
- Colon or rectal cancer (uncommon).

RISK INCREASES WITH
- Stress.
- Illness or injury requiring complete bed rest.
- Use of certain drugs, including belladonna, calcium-channel blockers, beta-adrenergic blockers, tricyclic antidepressants, narcotics, atropine, iron or antacids.
- Sedentary lifestyle.

HOW TO PREVENT
- Eat a well-balanced, high-fiber diet.
- Exercise regularly.
- Drink at least 8 eight-ounce glasses of water a day.

PROBABLE OUTCOME—Usually curable with exercise, diet and adequate fluids.

POSSIBLE COMPLICATIONS
- Hemorrhoids.
- Laxative dependency.
- Hernia from excessive straining.
- Uterine or rectal prolapse.
- Spastic colitis.
- Fecal impaction; bowel obstruction.
- Chronic constipation.

HOW TO TREAT

GENERAL MEASURES
- Diagnostic tests including laboratory blood studies, abdominal x-rays, barium enema, colonoscopy or sigmoidoscopy (see Glossary for these terms) may be performed to rule out other disorders that can cause constipation.
- Set aside a regular time each day for bowel movements. The best time is often within 1 hour after breakfast. Don't try to hurry. Sit at least 10 minutes, whether or not a bowel movement occurs.
- Drinking hot water, tea or coffee may help stimulate bowel.
- If constipation persists for 3 or 4 days, despite other measures, you may use a nonprescription disposable enema for temporary relief. If you prefer not to use a commercial enema preparation, you may give yourself an enema as follows:
  Spread a bath mat on the bathroom floor or in the tub.
  Fill an enema bag with lukewarm water.
  Hang the enema bag no higher than 30 inches from the floor.
  Lie on your left side on the mat.
  Insert the nozzle gently inside the rectum.
  Let the water flow in slowly, a little at a time. If it hurts, stop the water flow until the pain subsides, then start the flow again.
  Use the entire quart of water.
  Hold the fluid inside until you are uncomfortable, then sit on the toilet for a bowel movement.

MEDICATION—For occasional constipation, you may use a stool softener laxative, mild nonprescription laxatives or enemas. Don't use laxatives or enemas regularly as this can cause dependency. Avoid harsh laxatives and cathartics, such as Epsom salts. The best laxatives are bulk-formers, such as bran, psyllium, polycarbophil and methylcellulose.

ACTIVITY—Exercise and good physical fitness help maintain healthy bowel patterns.

DIET—Drink at least 8 eight-ounce glasses of water each day. Include bulk foods, such as bran, whole grain cereals, and raw fruits and vegetables, in your diet. Avoid refined cereals and breads, pastries and sugar.

CALL YOUR DOCTOR IF

- Constipation persists, despite self-care and especially if the constipation represents a change in your normal bowel patterns (may be an early sign of cancer).
- Constipation is accompanied by fever or severe abdominal cramping.
- New, unexplained symptoms develop. Drugs used in treatment may produce side effects.

Depression

GENERAL INFORMATION

DEFINITION—A continuing feeling of sadness, despondency or hopelessness with accompanying symptoms. Major depression occurs in about 1 in 10 Americans. It affects both sexes but is more common in women. It can be difficult to treat, but there is continued improvement in effectiveness of treatment.

SIGNS & SYMPTOMS
- Loss of interest in life; boredom.
- Listlessness and fatigue.
- Insomnia; excessive or disturbed sleeping.
- Social isolation.
- Appetite loss or overeating; constipation.
- Loss of sex drive.
- Difficulty in making decisions or concentrating.
- Irritability; unexplained crying bouts.
- Intense guilt feelings over minor or imaginary misdeeds.
- Various pains, such as headache or chest pain, without evidence of disease.

CAUSES
- A truly depressive illness has no single obvious cause. Biological factors (e.g., physical illness, hormonal disorders, certain drugs), social and psychological factors can all contribute to depression.
- Inherited disorders may also contribute (manic-depression runs in families).

RISK INCREASES WITH
- Unexpressed anger or other emotion.
- Compulsive, rigid, perfectionistic or highly dependent personalities.
- Family history of depression.
- Alcoholism.
- Failure in occupation, marriage or other interpersonal relationships.
- Death or loss of a loved one; loss of something important (job, home, investments).
- Job change or move to a new area.
- Major illness, surgery or disability.
- Passing from one life stage to another, such as menopause or retirement.
- Use of some drugs, such as reserpine, beta-adrenergic blockers or benzodiazepines.
- Withdrawal from mood-altering drugs, such as narcotics, amphetamines or caffeine.
- Diabetes mellitus; cancer; hormonal abnormalities.

HOW TO PREVENT
- Maintain good communication with family and close friends.
- Raise children with love and reasonable expectations in school and home.
- Anticipate and prepare for major life changes when possible.

PROBABLE OUTCOME—Spontaneous recovery in many cases, but professional help can shorten the duration of the depression and help you learn to cope in the future. The recovery rate is high, but recurrence is common.

POSSIBLE COMPLICATIONS
- Hallucinations or psychotic behavior.
- Manic behavior, characterized by inappropriate overactivity and comic or irresponsible behavior.
- Suicide. Warning signs include:
  Withdrawal from family and friends.
  Neglect of personal appearance.
  Mention of wanting "to end it all" or being "a burden to others."
  Evidence of a suicide plan (e.g., buying or cleaning a gun).
  Sudden cheerfulness after prolonged despondency.

HOW TO TREAT

GENERAL MEASURES
- Therapy consists of treating acute symptoms, avoiding a relapse, and maintenance therapy to prevent recurrence.
- Psychotherapy or counseling along with drug treatment appears to obtain the best results. Different types of psychotherapy are available, including cognitive therapy, behavioral therapy and interpersonal therapy.
- Hospitalization at a special treatment center may be required for severe depression.
- Seek support groups. See the Resource section of this book for additional information.
- Call your local suicide-prevention hot line if you feel suicidal.

MEDICATION
- Antidepressant drugs for some persons with prolonged or moderately severe depression.
- Specific drugs are used for alternating mania and depression.
- Antianxiety drugs may be prescribed.
- Sedatives may be prescribed for insomnia.
- Hormone therapy, if needed, to correct hormonal imbalances.

ACTIVITY
- No restrictions. Maintain daily activities and interests. Attend social functions, athletic events, concerts, plays and movies. Keep in touch with friends and loved ones.
- A regular exercise program can help relieve depression.

DIET—Eat a normal, well-balanced diet even if you have no appetite. Vitamin and mineral supplements may be necessary.

CALL YOUR DOCTOR IF

- You or a family member has symptoms of depression.
- You feel suicidal or hopeless.
- Symptoms of depression recur after treatment.

Domestic Violence
(Battering; Spousal Abuse)

GENERAL INFORMATION

DEFINITION—Abuse includes different behaviors (physical, sexual, psychological and emotional forms) that are used to establish power and to control the victim, who is most frequently a woman. Often, because of shame and guilt, the victim does not report the abuse to authorities or talk about it with family or friends. Abuse can occur in any race, age group, nationality, economic or educational level. Over 2 million women in the U.S. are battered by a male partner each year; some studies have shown that 1 in 4 pregnant women are battered.

SIGNS & SYMPTOMS
In female victims:
- Physical injuries to the body, including broken bones, bruises, burns, choking, bites and rape. Most injuries are inflicted on the head, neck, chest, breasts and abdomen. Injuries also occur on the arms, which are used to deflect blows.
- Other symptoms may include chronic pelvic pain, sexual dysfunction, feelings of anxiety, sleep disorders, depression, post-traumatic stress disorder (PTSD), eating disorders, psychological problems and thoughts of suicide.
In the male abuser:
- Angry, suspicious, tense and moody behaviors. Sometimes the abuser can be extremely charming. They often alternate periods of abuse with periods of affection.
- May demonstrate pathological jealousy, fear of abandonment, lack of assertiveness, possessiveness and fear of dependence.
- Watches wife closely; keeps her away from her friends and sometimes her family.
- Makes threats of violence; may play with guns or knives.

CAUSES—There are a number of theories as to why domestic abuse occurs and how it evolves. Researchers are still looking for answers. The same characteristics and risk factors that describe abusers also describe many men who do not become abusive.

RISK INCREASES WITH
- A history of family abuse. The male abuser, and often the female victims, witnessed abuse as they grew up.
- Abusers are often men who tend to use alcohol or drugs, frequently are unemployed and are often less educated (however, many educated professional men are abusers).
- Males who are dependent on women, have financial worries, have feelings of inadequacy and have traditional attitudes, particularly about sex.
- Females lacking self-esteem or who feel dependent and useless.
- Pregnant females. Abuse is often a factor in miscarriages.

HOW TO PREVENT
- To stem domestic violence, society must deal with the roots of the problem.
- Women should seek help at the first sign of abuse and not assume that the abuser will change or the abuse will stop.

PROBABLE OUTCOME—With the increased public awareness of the problem and availability of support systems, more women are seeking help early.

POSSIBLE COMPLICATIONS
- Years of emotional and physical abuse.
- Death of the abused woman.
- Killing of abuser.

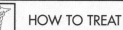

HOW TO TREAT

GENERAL MEASURES
If you are abused:
- Protect yourself, especially the head and abdomen. Get help; if you can, get away from the abuser. Document the abuse with pictures, by telling someone or by calling 911.
- Have a personal safety plan established (place to stay, money necessary to get there, survival funds, transportation and clothing and personal essentials packed).
- Seek legal help. Police departments and prosecutory practices are rapidly improving in responding to the problems.
- Numerous agencies and shelters for helping abused women and children are available. Call your local crisis line.
- Treatment steps for a victim: Get medical help for any injuries. Counseling is vital. The variety of treatment options will help a woman learn to cope, regain her self-confidence and the ability to function independently.
- Treatment for the abuser: Treatment is often resisted by an abuser. Educational and treatment groups have had some success for abusive men. Abusers must be confronted with the results of the behavior and learn that they will go to jail if they don't change.
- See the Resource section of this book for additional information or consult your local telephone directory.

MEDICATION—Usually not needed, but may be prescribed for anxiety or depression.

ACTIVITY—No restrictions.

DIET—No special diet.

CALL YOUR DOCTOR IF

You or a family member is a victim of domestic violence.

Face Lift & Blepharoplasty (Rhytidectomy)

 GENERAL INFORMATION

DEFINITION
- Face lift (rhytidectomy): Removal of excess skin, fat and tissue from the face in order to tighten sagging skin and eliminate wrinkles, jowls or a double chin.
- Blepharoplasty: Removal of excess fat and skin from around the eyelids to reduce puffiness, bags under the eyes and wrinkles.

REASONS FOR PROCEDURE
- Improved appearance of the face.
- Improved appearance and function of the eyelids.

RISK INCREASES WITH
- Obesity.
- Smoking.
- Stress.
- Poor nutrition.
- Recent illness.
- Alcoholism or chronic illness.
- Use of drugs such as antihypertensives, muscle relaxants, tranquilizers, sleep inducers, insulin, sedatives, beta-adrenergic blocker or cortisone.
- Use of mind-altering drugs, including narcotics, psychedelics, hallucinogens, marijuana, sedatives, hypnotics or cocaine.

DESCRIPTION OF PROCEDURE
- Laboratory blood and urine studies will be performed prior to surgery.
- Surgery is usually performed by a plastic and reconstructive surgeon, in a doctor's office, outpatient surgical facility or hospital.
- A local or a general anesthesia is administered.
- Incisions are made in areas where scarring will be minimal or less visible.
- Care is taken to clamp and tie tiny bleeding vessels during the procedure to prevent collection of scar tissue under the skin.
- Flaps of skin are cut away around the eyes and face. Excess tissue is removed from underlying areas, and excess skin is trimmed.
- The skin is closed with fine sutures, which can usually be removed about 1 week after surgery. Drains may be left in place for several days.
- Bandages and ice packs are applied to reduce swelling and bleeding.

PROBABLE OUTCOME—Expect complete healing and improved appearance without complications. Allow about 6 weeks for recovery from surgery.

POSSIBLE COMPLICATIONS
- Excessive bleeding or blood clot.
- Surgical-wound infection.
- Collection of serum under areas where skin has been removed.
- Abnormal scarring.
- Facial nerve damage.

 FOLLOW-UP CARE

GENERAL MEASURES
- Be sure you understand what results you can expect from surgery; ask your doctor to show you before-and-after photographs of some typical patients. Be realistic about your expectations.
- Hospital stay will usually be 0 to 3 days.
- If a wound bleeds during the first 24 hours after surgery, press a clean cloth or tissue to it for 10 minutes.
- Bathe and shower as usual. You may wash the wounds gently with mild unscented soap.
- Between baths, keep the wounds dry with a bandage for the first 2 or 3 days after surgery. If a bandage gets wet, change it promptly.
- Apply nonprescription antibiotic ointment to wounds before applying new bandages.
- Bruising and swelling are to be expected and may take 2 to 3 weeks to decrease. In most cases, it takes 3 to 6 months following a face lift for the surgery to produce its optimal effect.
- For most women, the benefits of a face lift will last anywhere from 6 to 10 years, after which time the effects of aging will again begin to show. The positive effects of a face lift can often be extended by avoiding excess exposure to the sun; limiting intake of alcohol, cigarettes and drugs; and by maintaining a constant weight.

MEDICATION
- Prescription pain relievers may be prescribed. Don't take them for longer than 4 to 7 days. Use only as much as you need.
- You may use nonprescription drugs, such as acetaminophen, for minor pain.
- Stool softeners to prevent constipation.
- Antibiotics to prevent or fight infection. Antibiotics may reduce the effectiveness of some oral contraceptives. If you are using oral contraceptives for birth control, discuss this with your doctor.

ACTIVITY
- To help recovery and aid your well-being, resume daily activities as soon as you are able.
- Avoid vigorous exercise for 6 weeks after surgery.
- Resume driving 3 days after returning home.

DIET—No special diet.

CALL YOUR DOCTOR IF

- Pain, swelling, redness, drainage or bleeding increases in the surgical area.
- You develop signs of infection: headache, muscle aches, dizziness or a general ill feeling and fever.
- You experience nausea or vomiting.
- New, unexplained symptoms develop. Drugs used in treatment may produce side effects.

Face Lift & Blepharoplasty (Rhytidectomy)

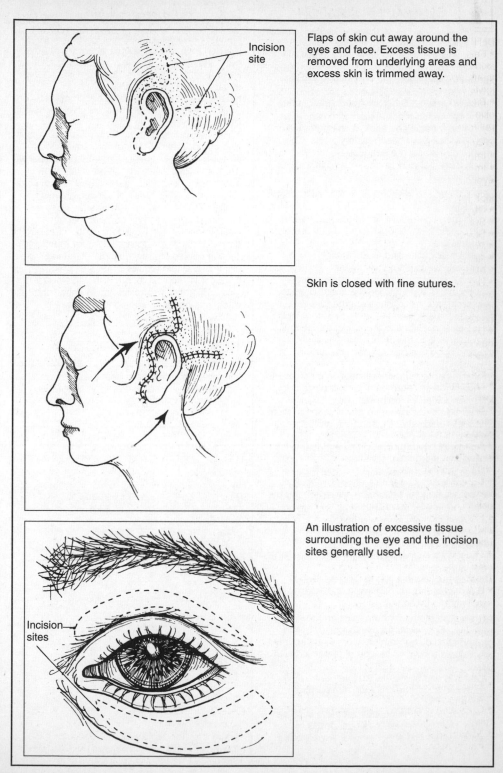

Incision site

Flaps of skin cut away around the eyes and face. Excess tissue is removed from underlying areas and excess skin is trimmed away.

Skin is closed with fine sutures.

An illustration of excessive tissue surrounding the eye and the incision sites generally used.

Incision sites

Health & Medical History

 GENERAL INFORMATION

DEFINITION—It is important to maintain a health and sickness history for yourself and for your children. This information can be invaluable for future reference. Any doctor you visit will ask about past medical experiences and about your health in general. Don't rely on memory. Write things down in a medical journal. It can be as simple as a spiral notebook, a computer file or specially designed health-history forms. The items listed below are suggestions for information that may be maintained in this personal medical record.

SOME ITEMS TO RECORD FOR YOU AND YOUR CHILDREN
• Birth date and details about the pregnancy, delivery and birth, and a record of any problems encountered.
• Serious illnesses and treatments.
• Chronic illnesses and treatments.
• Minor illnesses, problems or infections that recur such as ear infections, numerous colds, skin problems, headaches or others.
• Medications prescribed and any side effects or adverse reactions to them. List the generic name as well as the brand name of each medication; if unsure, ask your doctor or pharmacist.
• Information about nonprescription medications or supplements taken on a regular basis (e.g., vitamins, laxatives, antihistamines, aspirin) should be noted; also note any reaction to them and if the medications helped the problem being treated.
• Allergies to food or environmental agents.
• Immunizations.
• Medical tests and results. This can include such items as weight, height and blood pressure when taken in the doctor's office. Also include results of any eye exams and records of any corrective lenses prescribed.
• Operations and hospitalizations.
• Keep a record of your exercise habits.
• Note down any special weight loss diets tried and their results.
• Any significant weight changes that occur.
• Note dates and results of any self-testing performed, such as breast exam or skin exam.
• Sexual problems for both male and female partners. A nonmonogamous sexually active person should keep a history of sexual activity and should record what type of protection was used.
• Ongoing use of alcohol and amount consumed; cigarette smoking and number smoked.
• Make a note of emotional disorders such as stress, depression, feelings of sadness or other problems that can affect emotional well-being.

• Reproductive history (date of first menstrual period, length of menstrual cycles, contraceptive methods used and pregnancy history). Women who are going or have gone through menopause should be aware of any hormones they have used. You should also keep records of any uterine or breast evaluations (mammograms).
• Note any other facts about health matters, no matter how minor, that you think may be useful to the doctor.
• Medical history of parents, brothers, sisters and grandparents that includes any serious illnesses or other medical, mental or emotional problems. Especially important is information about asthma and allergies, breast and ovarian cancer, any other types of cancer, diabetes mellitus, glaucoma, Alzheimer's disease, alcoholism and carriers of recessive genes related to inherited disorders. Find out about the cause of death for deceased family members.
• Keep copies of prescriptions, immunization records and test results in the same file.
• Take this medical record with you when you visit a doctor. It will assist you in answering questions correctly and completely when a medical history is taken.

 CALL YOUR DOCTOR IF

You or a family member has questions or concerns about medical history information.

Hemorrhoids
(Piles)

 GENERAL INFORMATION

DEFINITION—Dilated (varicose) veins of the rectum or anus. Hemorrhoids may be located at the beginning of the anal canal (internal hemorrhoids) or at the anal opening (external hemorrhoids). Hemorrhoids may be present for years but go undetected until bleeding occurs.

SIGNS & SYMPTOMS
- Rectal bleeding. Bright-red blood may appear as streaks on toilet paper or adhering to fecal residue, or it may be a slow trickle for a short while following bowel movements. It often colors the toilet water.
- Pain, itching or mucus discharge after bowel movements.
- Constipation; bowel incontinence.
- A lump that can be felt in the anus.
- A sensation that the rectum has not emptied completely after a bowel movement (usually with large hemorrhoids only).
- Inflammation and swelling.
- Anal fissure.

CAUSES—Repeated pressure in the anal or rectal veins.

RISK INCREASES WITH
- Diet that lacks fiber.
- Prolonged sitting.
- Obesity.
- Pregnancy.
- Constipation.
- Loss of muscle tone in old age.
- Rectal surgery or episiotomy.
- Liver disease.
- Anal intercourse.
- Colon malignancy.
- Portal hypertension.

HOW TO PREVENT
- Don't try to hurry bowel movements, but do avoid straining and prolonged sitting on the toilet.
- Avoid prolonged sitting. If work or travel involves sitting for long periods, get up and move around periodically.
- Lose weight if you are overweight.
- Include plenty of fiber in your diet.
- Drink 8 to 10 glasses of water a day.
- Exercise regularly.

PROBABLE OUTCOME—Hemorrhoids usually clear up with proper care, but symptoms may come and go (may especially flare up after a bout of constipation). Stubborn cases may require surgery. Recurrence is common.

POSSIBLE COMPLICATIONS
- Iron-deficiency anemia if blood loss is significant (rare).
- Severe pain caused by a blood clot in a hemorrhoid.
- Infection or ulceration of a hemorrhoid.
- Incontinence.

HOW TO TREAT

GENERAL MEASURES
- Diagnosis may include an anoscopy (visual examination of the anus by means of a short tube called an anoscope, an optical instrument with lenses and a lighted tip) or proctoscopy (method of examining the rectum and lower part of the colon with a proctoscope, an optical instrument with a lighted tip).
- Treatment is aimed at easing the symptoms.
- Never strain to push stool out.
- When sitting on the toilet, place feet on a low footstool to aid bowel movement.
- Clean the anal area gently with soft, moist paper after each bowel movement.
- To relieve pain, sit in 8 to 10 inches of warm water for 10 to 20 minutes several times a day.
- To reduce pain and swelling of a blood clot or protruding hemorrhoid, stay in bed for 1 day and apply ice packs to the anal area.
- Surgery may be required in stubborn cases. Procedures include ligation (tying off the hemorrhoid with a rubber band to strangulate it); sclerotherapy (injection of a chemical to induce scarring); cryosurgery (freezing the hemorrhoid with liquid nitrogen); coagulation (by infrared light or laser); or hemorrhoidectomy (surgical removal of hemorroids).

MEDICATION
- For minor pain or itching, or to reduce swelling, you may use nonprescription drugs that are formulated to relieve symptoms of hemorrhoids. If these symptoms occur during pregnancy, ask your doctor which medications are appropriate to use.
- Use a stool softener, if a laxative is needed.

ACTIVITY—No restrictions. Bowel function often improves with good physical conditioning.

DIET
- To prevent constipation, eat a well-balanced diet that contains many high-fiber foods such as fresh fruit, bran muffins, whole-grain breads, beans, vegetables and whole-grain cereals.
- Drink 8 to 10 glasses of fluid daily.
- Weight loss diet if you are overweight.

CALL YOUR DOCTOR IF

- A hard lump develops where a hemorrhoid has been.
- Hemorrhoids cause severe pain that is not relieved by treatment measures listed above.
- Rectal bleeding is excessive (more than a trace or streak on toilet paper or stool). Rectal bleeding can be an early sign of cancer.

Hemorrhoid Removal (Hemorrhoidectomy)

 ## GENERAL INFORMATION

DEFINITION—Removal of hemorrhoids (varicose veins that occur inside or on the outside of the anus).

REASONS FOR PROCEDURE
• Relief of excessive itching, pain or bleeding.
• Relief of a painful thrombosed hemorrhoid (hemorrhoid containing a blood clot).

RISK INCREASES WITH
• Adults over 60.
• Obesity.
• Smoking.
• Poor nutrition.
• Excess alcohol consumption.
• Chronic illness.

DESCRIPTION OF PROCEDURE
• Laboratory blood studies will be performed prior to surgery.
• Surgery is usually performed by a proctologist, a colon-rectal surgeon or a general surgeon, in an outpatient facility or hospital.
• A general or local anesthetic is administered.
• The dilated veins from around the anus and inside the rectum are cut free and removed, with care taken to not damage the sphincter muscle. Sometimes anal muscles must be dilated vigorously to expose the hemorrhoids.
• The surgical area may be sewn closed or left open, and medicated gauze is used to cover it.

PROBABLE OUTCOME—Relief of symptoms of hemorrhoids. Allow about 3 weeks for recovery from surgery. Hemorrhoids may recur.

POSSIBLE COMPLICATIONS
• Excessive bleeding.
• Surgical-wound infection.
• Severe pain, especially with bowel movements.
• Recurrence of hemorrhoids.

 ## FOLLOW-UP CARE

GENERAL MEASURES
• Average hospital stay is 2 to 3 days.
• Warm baths every 4 hours or so relieve pain and help keep the rectal area clean. Sit in warm water for 10 to 20 minutes as often as it feels good.
• Avoid heavy lifting. If not possible, learn proper body mechanics to reduce strain contributing to recurrence.
• Don't strain with bowel movements or urination.

MEDICATION
• Pain relievers. Don't take prescription pain medication longer than 4 to 7 days. Use only as much as you need.
• Antibiotics to fight or prevent infection. Antibiotics may reduce the effectiveness of some oral contraceptives. If you are using oral contraceptives for birth control, discuss this with your doctor.
• Stool softeners or laxatives to prevent constipation.
• Analgesic ointment to relieve pain.
• Vitamins to encourage healing.

ACTIVITY
• Resume driving 1 week after returning home.
• Resume sexual relations as soon as you wish.

DIET—No special diet. Increase dietary fiber and fluid intake to prevent constipation. Straining during bowel movements can cause hemorrhoids to recur.

 ## CALL YOUR DOCTOR IF

• Pain, swelling, redness, drainage or bleeding increases in the surgical area.
• You develop signs of infection: headache, muscle aches, dizziness or a general ill feeling and fever.
• New, unexplained symptoms develop. Drugs used in treatment may produce side effects.

Hemorrhoid Removal
(Hemorrhoidectomy)

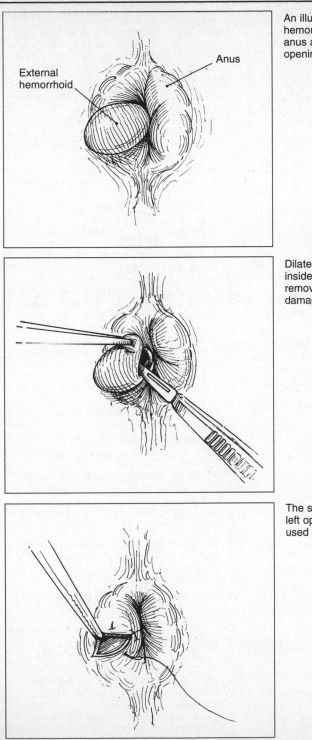

External hemorrhoid

Anus

An illustration of a typical external hemorrhoid arising from inside the anus and extending through the anal opening.

Dilated veins around the anus and inside the rectum are cut free and removed, with care taken not to damage the sphincter muscles.

The surgical area is sewn closed or left open and medicated gauze is used to cover.

Hepatitis, Viral

 GENERAL INFORMATION

DEFINITION—Inflammation of the liver caused by a virus. Hepatitis has several forms; the most common are type A and type B. Other types include hepatitis C, D, E and G.

SIGNS & SYMPTOMS
Early stages:
• Flu-like symptoms, such as fatigue, nausea, vomiting, diarrhea and loss of appetite. Fever may be present but is unusual with types B and C.
Several days later:
• Jaundice (yellow eyes and skin) caused by a build-up of bile in the blood.
• Dark urine from bile spilling over into the urine.
• Light, "clay-colored" or whitish stools.

CAUSES
• Types A and E: The virus usually enters the body through water or food, especially raw shellfish, that has been contaminated by sewage (fecal-oral contact).
• Type B: Usually transmitted sexually, through blood transfusions contaminated with the virus (rare in the U.S.) or from injections with nonsterile needles or syringes. An infected mother can pass it to her newborn. Can also be transmitted through body piercing or tattooing, and possibly through household contact such as shared towels, razors, eating utensils or toothbrushes. Some cases appear sporadically.
• Type C: Most commonly transmitted through intravenous drug use, blood transfusions (rare in the U.S.) and other exposures to contaminated blood or its products. In up to 40% of the cases, mode of transmission is unknown.
• Type D: Associated with an infection of hepatitis type B.
• Type G: Similar patterns to type C; usually blood-borne.

RISK INCREASES WITH
• Travel to areas with poor sanitation.
• Oral-anal sexual practices.
• Use of intravenous drugs; alcoholism.
• Blood transfusions (risk is low in the U.S. where blood products are tested for hepatitis).
• Health-care workers.
• Day-care centers or residential programs.
• Kidney-dialysis treatment.
• Poor nutrition.
• Illness that has lowered resistance.

HOW TO PREVENT
• Avoid risks listed above.
• If you are exposed to someone with hepatitis, seek medical advice about receiving gamma-globulin injections to prevent or decrease the risk of hepatitis.
• If you are in a high-risk group (such as hospital worker, dentist, dental worker), are sexually promiscuous or abuse intravenous drugs, obtain hepatitis vaccination (A and B are currently available; others are under study) and immune globulin in addition to the vaccination.
• Hepatitis B vaccination for all newborns.

PROBABLE OUTCOME—Jaundice and other symptoms usually peak and then gradually disappear over 3 to 16 weeks. Most people in good general health recover fully in 1 to 4 months. A small percentage proceed to chronic hepatitis. Recovery from viral hepatitis usually provides permanent immunity against it.

POSSIBLE COMPLICATIONS
• Liver failure; cirrhosis of the liver; liver cancer; even death.
• Chronic hepatitis. These patients are carriers and are potentially infectious to household and sexual contacts. These people may look and feel well and not realize they are infected.

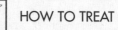 HOW TO TREAT

GENERAL MEASURES
• Diagnostic tests include laboratory blood tests to identify infection, liver-function studies and liver biopsy in severe or chronic cases.
• Most persons with hepatitis can be cared for at home without undue risk. Strict isolation is usually not necessary, but the ill person should have separate eating and drinking utensils, or should use disposable ones.
• If you have hepatitis or are caring for someone with it, wash your hands carefully and often, especially after bowel movements.
• If you are pregnant and a hepatitis B carrier, your child needs to be vaccinated and receive treatment (immune globulin) following birth to decrease the risk of transmission of the disease.

MEDICATION
• There are few specific medicines to treat hepatitis.
• An anti-inflammatory (cortisone) may be prescribed for severe cases to reduce liver inflammation and improve symptoms.
• Chronic hepatitis B or C may be treated with alpha-interferon.

ACTIVITY—Bed rest is recommended until jaundice disappears and appetite returns. People differ widely in the rate at which they can return to normal activity.

DIET—Small, well-balanced meals help aid recovery. Drink at least 8 glasses of water daily. Don't drink alcohol.

CALL YOUR DOCTOR IF

• You or a family member has symptoms of hepatitis or has been exposed to hepatitis.
• You experience increasing loss of appetite, excessive drowsiness, mental confusion, vomiting, diarrhea, abdominal pain, deepening jaundice, skin rash or itching.

Hyperthyroidism

GENERAL INFORMATION

DEFINITION—A clinical state resulting from overactivity of the thyroid, which causes an overproduction of thyroid hormone which, in turn, speeds the body's metabolic rate. The thyroid is a small, butterfly-shaped endocrine gland located in the neck. Virtually all metabolic processes in the body are affected by the thyroid hormone. The most common form of hyperthyroidism is called Graves' disease.

SIGNS & SYMPTOMS
• Hyperactivity.
• Feeling warm or hot all the time.
• Tremors.
• Increased sweating.
• Difficulty breathing.
• Itching skin.
• Pounding, rapid or irregular heartbeat.
• Weight loss, despite overeating. Older persons may gain weight.
• Marked anxiety and restlessness; nervousness.
• Sleeplessness.
• Fatigue and weakness.
• Tremors.
• Protruding eyes (exophthalmos) and double vision (sometimes).
• Diarrhea (sometimes).
• Hair loss (sometimes).
• Goiter (enlarged thyroid) (sometimes).

CAUSES
• Autoimmune disorder (body develops antibodies that stimulate excessive amounts of thyroid hormone).
• Thyroid nodules or tumors.
• Thyroiditis (inflammation of thyroid gland).

RISK INCREASES WITH
• Family history of hyperthyroidism.
• Stress.
• Female gender.
• Other autoimmune disorders.

HOW TO PREVENT—No specific preventive measures.

PROBABLE OUTCOME—Usually curable with medication or surgery. Allow 6 months of treatment for the condition to stabilize. Some forms may return to normal without treatment.

POSSIBLE COMPLICATIONS
• Misdiagnosis as a psychiatric anxiety reaction.
• Development of hypothyroidism (see Glossary) following treatment.
• Vision impairment.
• Congestive heart failure.
• "Thyroid storm," a life-threatening complication marked by a sudden worsening of all symptoms.

HOW TO TREAT

GENERAL MEASURES
• Since this condition develops gradually, symptoms may be difficult to recognize. If family and friends mention changes in your behavior or appearance, consult your doctor.
• Diagnostic tests may include laboratory blood studies to measure the levels of thyroid hormones (T3 and T4) and thyroid-stimulating hormones (TSH) in your body. Additional tests may include ECG (see Glossary) or radioactive studies such as I-131 uptake (see Glossary). Studies or treatment requiring radioactive isotopes are contraindicated in pregnancy.
• Appropriate treatment will depend on the level of thyroid overactivity and extent of thyroid enlargement, the causes, your age and how long surgery may be delayed (if you are a candidate for it).
• Medication may be prescribed that controls the problem in many patients.
• Your doctor may prescribe a concentrated liquid form of radioactive iodine, which will render your thyroid inactive. Radioactive iodine may not be used by pregnant or nursing women because it can destroy the thyroid of the fetus.
• Surgery (thyroidectomy), to remove part or all of the thyroid, may be performed if needed.
• Follow-up blood studies will usually be performed at regular intervals following treatment. Liver-function tests may also be performed.

MEDICATION
• Antithyroid drugs to depress thyroid activity.
• Beta-adrenergic blockers to decrease a rapid heartbeat.
• Radioactive iodine (radioiodine), which selectively destroys thyroid cells.
• If your thyroid is removed, or rendered underactive by treatment, you will need to take thyroid replacement hormones for the rest of your life.

ACTIVITY—Limit activity as much as possible until the disorder is controlled. Modify activities according to disease severity.

DIET
• Eat a diet high in protein to replace tissue lost from thyroid overactivity, and with sufficient calories to prevent weight loss.
• Weight loss diet if you are overweight.

CALL YOUR DOCTOR IF

• You or a family member has symptoms of hyperthyroidism.
• New, unexplained symptoms develop. Drugs used in treatment may produce side effects.
• You experience a sudden worsening of all symptoms. Get help immediately! This is an emergency!

Hypothyroidism

GENERAL INFORMATION

DEFINITION— A clinical state resulting from an underactive thyroid gland which causes an underproduction of thyroid hormone which, in turn, slows the body's metabolic rate. The thyroid is a small butterfly-shaped endocrine gland located in the neck. Virtually all metabolic processes in the body are affected by the thyroid hormone.

SIGNS & SYMPTOMS—It is unlikely one person will have all the following symptoms, but most will have several:
- Decreased tolerance for cold.
- Decreased sweating.
- Decreased appetite.
- Constipation.
- Chest pain.
- Coarse or slow-growing hair; hair loss on the head and eyebrows.
- Slow, rapid or irregular heartbeat.
- Weight gain or extreme thinness.
- Placidity or nervousness.
- Weakness; fatigue; lethargy.
- Insomnia.
- Mental impairment, including depression, psychosis or poor memory.
- Fluid retention, especially around the eyes.
- Dull facial expression and droopy eyelids; facial puffiness.
- Coarse skin; dry, brittle nails.
- Decreased tolerance for medication.
- Decreased sex drive; infertility.
- Menstrual disorders.
- Anemia.
- Numbness and tingling of the hands and feet.
- Deepened or hoarse voice.
- Hearing impairment.

CAUSES—Sometimes unknown. Following are the most common causes:
- Autoimmune disease, in which the body's immune system functions abnormally and attacks the thyroid gland.
- Radioactive iodine treatment.
- Surgery for hyperthyroidism.
- Iodine deficiency in the diet.
- Decreased activity of the pituitary gland, which secretes a thyroid-stimulating hormone.
- Use of drugs, such as lithium, that may depress thyroid function.

RISK INCREASES WITH
- Adults over 60.
- Females; more common in women than men.
- Obesity.
- Surgery for hyperthyroidism.
- X-ray treatments.

HOW TO PREVENT
- No known measures to prevent primary hypothyroidism.
- Take replacement thyroid for life after thyroid surgery or destruction of the thyroid gland by radiation treatment.

PROBABLE OUTCOME—Usually curable with careful thyroid replacement therapy. Relapses will occur if treatment is interrupted.

POSSIBLE COMPLICATIONS
- Myxedema coma, a life-threatening complication of hypothyroidism.
- Increased susceptibility to infection.
- Adrenal crisis with vigorous treatment of hypothyroidism.
- Infertility.
- Overtreatment over long periods can lead to bone demineralization.
- Treatment-induced congestive heart failure in women with coronary artery disease.

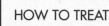

HOW TO TREAT

GENERAL MEASURES
- Diagnostic laboratory blood studies will be performed to measure the levels of thyroid stimulating hormones (TSH) in your body. Lab studies can confirm the diagnosis of hypothyroidism, but they cannot indicate how much replacement therapy is needed.
- Treatment will consist of thyroid replacement medication. The goal of treatment is to provide the body with enough thyroid substance for efficient body function. Medical evaluation may be necessary for several months to establish the correct dose of thyroid replacement.
- Blood serum levels of TSH should be checked regularly during treatment in order to avoid hyperthyroidism (see Glossary).
- You may require hospitalization if complicating emergencies, such as myxedema coma (see Glossary), occur.

MEDICATION—Your doctor will prescribe thyroid replacement hormones, usually levothyroxine (Synthroid), which is a synthetic form of the thyroid hormone thyroxine. Dosage requirements will depend on age, weight, sex, capacity of thyroid function, other drugs you take and intestinal function. Dosages may need to be adjusted until an optimum level is achieved.

ACTIVITY—No restrictions. Stay as active as possible.

DIET—No special diet for hypothyroidism. Avoid constipation by eating a high-fiber diet. Weight loss diet recommended if you are overweight.

CALL YOUR DOCTOR IF

- You have symptoms of hypothyroidism.
- Symptoms don't improve within 3 weeks after treatment begins.
- New, unexplained symptoms develop. Drugs used in treatment may produce side effects.

Insomnia
(Sleep Disorders)

 GENERAL INFORMATION

DEFINITION—Sleep disturbance that includes difficulty falling asleep or remaining asleep, intermittent wakefulness, early morning awakening or a combination of these. Insomnia affects all age groups but is more common in the elderly. Insomnia may be transient, due to a life crisis or lifestyle change, or chronic, due to medical or psychological problems or drug intake.

SIGNS & SYMPTOMS
• Restlessness ("tossing and turning") when trying to fall asleep.
• Brief sleep followed by wakefulness.
• Normal sleep until very early in the morning (3 a.m. or 4 a.m.), then wakefulness (often with frightening thoughts).
• Periods of sleeplessness, alternating with periods of excessive sleep or sleepiness at inconvenient times.

CAUSES
• Depression. This is usually characterized by early morning wakefulness.
• Overactivity of the thyroid gland.
• Anxiety caused by stress.
• Daytime napping; erratic nighttime sleep patterns.
• Noisy environment (including a snoring partner).
• Allergies and early morning wheezing.
• Heart or lung conditions that cause shortness of breath when lying down.
• Painful disorders, such as fibromyalgia or arthritis.
• Urinary or gastrointestinal problems that require urination or bowel movements during the night.
• Consumption of stimulants, such as coffee, tea or cola drinks.
• Use of some medications, including dextroamphetamines, cortisone drugs or decongestants.
• Erratic work hours.
• New environment or location.
• Jet lag after travel.
• Lack of physical exercise.
• Alcoholism.
• Sleep apnea (see Glossary).
• Drug abuse, including overuse of sleep-inducing drugs.
• Withdrawal from addictive substances.

RISK INCREASES WITH
• Stress.
• Obesity.
• Age over 50.
• Smoking.

HOW TO PREVENT
• Establish a lifestyle that fosters healthy sleep patterns (see General Measures). If unable to sleep, get up and do something. Avoid lengthy daytime napping.
• Avoidance of causes when possible.

PROBABLE OUTCOME—Most persons can establish good sleep patterns if the underlying cause of insomnia is treated or eliminated.

POSSIBLE COMPLICATIONS
• Transient insomnia becomes chronic.
• Increased daytime sleepiness that can affect all aspects of your life.

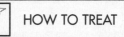 HOW TO TREAT

GENERAL MEASURES
• Seek ways to minimize stress. Learn and practice relaxation techniques.
• Don't use stimulants or drink alcohol for several hours before bedtime.
• Treat any underlying drug use or medical cause.
• Relax in a warm bath before bedtime.
• Don't turn your bedroom into an office or a den. Create a comfortable, restful sleep setting.
• Turn off your mind. Focus on peaceful and relaxing thoughts. Play soft music or relaxation tapes.
• Set a rigid sleep schedule.
• Use mechanical aids such as ear plugs, eye shades or blackout shades on windows.
• Seek counseling or psychotherapy if the cause is psychological.

MEDICATION
• Sleep-inducing drugs may be prescribed for a short time if temporary insomnia is interfering with your daily activities, you have a medical disorder that regularly disturbs sleep or you need to establish regular sleep patterns.
• Long-term use of sleep inducers may be counter-productive or addictive. Don't use sleeping pills given to you by friends.

ACTIVITY
• Exercise regularly to create healthy fatigue, but don't exercise less than 2 hours before going to bed.
• Have sexual relations, if they are fulfilling and satisfying, before going to sleep.

DIET—No special diet, but don't eat heavy late-night snacks or meals. Drinking a glass of warm milk or eating a light snack before bedtime helps some people.

 CALL YOUR DOCTOR IF

• You or a family member has insomnia.
• New, unexplained symptoms develop. Drugs used in treatment may produce side effects.

Liposuction
(Suction Lipectomy)

 GENERAL INFORMATION

DEFINITION—A surgical technique using suction equipment to permanently remove fat deposits, usually from the thighs, hips, buttocks, abdomen or chin.

REASONS FOR PROCEDURE—Cosmetic improvement of fat deposits that are resistant to diet and/or exercise.

RISK INCREASES WITH
- Extreme obesity.
- Smoking.
- Chronic illness or disease, such as diabetes.
- Excess alcohol consumption.
- History of phlebitis.
- Use of mind-altering drugs, including narcotics, psychedelics, hallucinogens, marijuana, sedatives, hypnotics or cocaine.

DESCRIPTION OF PROCEDURE
- Laboratory blood and urine studies will be performed prior to surgery.
- Surgery is usually performed by a plastic surgeon, in a hospital or outpatient surgical facility.
- Local anesthesia and sedation are often used when liposuction is to be performed on small areas of fat.
- General anesthesia, by injection and inhalation with an airway tube placed in the windpipe, is usually used for larger areas of fat.
- The plastic surgeon marks the areas where fat is to be removed.
- Incisions (usually about 1 inch each) are made in suction areas.
- A suction tube, with one end attached to suction equipment, is pushed through the incision into the excess fat and moved back and forth repeatedly (20 to 30 times at each site) until the desired amount of fat has been removed.
- Each incision is stapled or stitched shut, and a pressure dressing is placed over the wounds.
- Drains may be left in place under the skin for several days.

PROBABLE OUTCOME
- Expect complete healing and improved appearance without complications.
- There may be some discomfort following the procedure.
- Swelling and bruising may last for several weeks, depending on the areas and amount of fat removal.

POSSIBLE COMPLICATIONS
- Phlebitis (see Glossary).
- Surgical-wound infection.
- Excess bleeding; anemia.
- Excessive scarring (keloid).

 HOW TO TREAT

GENERAL MEASURES
- Be sure you understand what type of results you can expect from your surgery. Ask your doctor to show you before-and-after photographs of typical patients. Following liposuction, there may be some rippling or sagging of the skin, or an uneven effect. Be realistic about your expectations.
- Following surgery, you should not smoke and should avoid exposure to second-hand smoke to minimize the chances of problems in healing.
- A hard ridge should form along the incision. As it heals, the ridge will gradually recede.
- Don't be concerned about small amounts of oozing at the surgical sites.
- Bathe and shower as usual. You may wash the incision gently with mild unscented soap.
- Use an electric heating pad, a heat lamp or a warm compress to relieve incisional pain.
- It may take several weeks to several months for tenderness to subside.
- Allow time for healing and for appearance to improve.

MEDICATION
- Prescription pain medicine should generally be taken for no longer than 4 to 7 days. Use only as much as you need.
- Antibiotics to fight or prevent infection. Antibiotics may reduce the effectiveness of some oral contraceptives.
- You may use nonprescription drugs, such as acetaminophen, for minor pain.
- Avoid aspirin.

ACTIVITY
- Resume driving 2 weeks after surgery.
- Avoid heavy lifting for 6 weeks after surgery. Learn proper body mechanics to reduce strain.
- Don't strain with bowel movements or urination.

DIET
- No special diet required.
- Vitamin or mineral supplements (sometimes).

 CALL YOUR DOCTOR IF

- Pain, swelling, redness, drainage or bleeding occurs in the surgical area.
- Your temperature rises to 101F (38.3C).
- You develop signs of infection: headache, muscle aches, dizziness or a general ill feeling and fever.
- You become constipated.
- Leg becomes swollen or painful.
- New, unexplained symptoms develop. Drugs used in treatment may produce side effects.

Liposuction
(Suction Lipectomy)

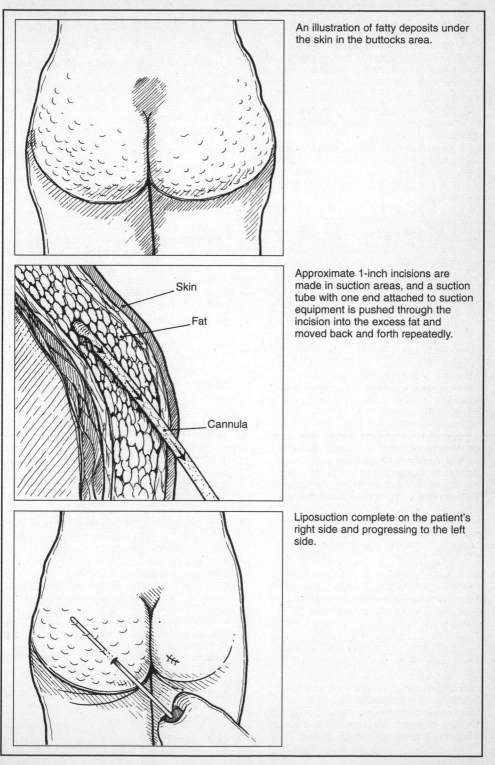

An illustration of fatty deposits under the skin in the buttocks area.

Approximate 1-inch incisions are made in suction areas, and a suction tube with one end attached to suction equipment is pushed through the incision into the excess fat and moved back and forth repeatedly.

Skin

Fat

Cannula

Liposuction complete on the patient's right side and progressing to the left side.

Living Longer & Healthier

 GENERAL INFORMATION

Simple as they seem, these suggestions require accepting, reviewing and following—if you desire to maintain optimum health and stay at your highest level of physical fitness, mental alertness and creativity.

HEALTHFUL EATING
- Regular meals keep the metabolic and digestive systems functioning at their most efficient levels.
- Don't skip breakfast. Failing to eat because "you don't have time" can cause low energy levels and can contribute to poor health.
- Limit your intake of fat, caffeine, salt and refined sugar.
- If you get hungry between meals, eat fruit, raw vegetables or whole-grain snacks.
- Drink at least 8 eight-ounce glasses of water a day.

EXERCISE REGULARLY
- Exercise that you enjoy is most likely to be exercise that is successful and that you will continue. Activities such as gardening, housework and, particularly, walking count.
- Regular exercise increases your energy levels, helps to fight stress, boosts overall health, aids in fighting off a variety of illnesses and disorders and promotes weight loss.

CONTROL YOUR WEIGHT
- Even small amounts of excess weight can possibly shorten your life or put you at risk for illness.
- Extreme obesity is associated with many physical and mental disorders. If you need to reduce your weight, do so through a healthy, well-balanced weight reduction plan. Crash dieting or ill-advised reduction of calories per day can lead to poor health. Obtain medical advice before embarking on any weight loss diet.
- If your weight is ideal, work to keep it that way.

DRINK ALCOHOL MODERATELY OR NOT AT ALL
—Alcohol abuse can cause serious diseases, reduce your life span and make your life miserable. Moderate consumption can be defined as drinking no more than 3 ounces of alcohol in any form on any day.

GET ENOUGH SLEEP
- Get the right amount of sleep (average 7 to 8 hours) each night.
- Avoid taking business or personal worries to bed with you.
- Avoid getting caught up in suspenseful reading or television while relaxing in bed.
- If you toss and turn on occasion and can't get to sleep, go to another room and do something productive until you feel ready to sleep.

MANAGE THE STRESS AND ANXIETY IN YOUR LIFE
- Learn and practice relaxation techniques.
- Be realistic so that you don't overreact to situations or circumstances. Remember, almost nothing is hopeless.
- Exercise regularly and eat a well-balanced, nutritional diet.
- Write about your concerns and feelings in a journal.

DON'T SMOKE
- There is overwhelming evidence that smoking damages the human body and shortens life. Cigarette smoking is a risk factor for many illnesses, particularly lung cancer, chronic lung disease, hardening of the arteries, heart attack and damage to unborn children of pregnant women who smoke.
- Anyone who smokes is at greater risk of problems with anesthesia during surgery.
- Avoid second-hand smoke.

DON'T ABUSE DRUGS
- Evidence is mounting about the cumulative ill effects of drug abuse.
- Common sense dictates avoiding drugs if you want to stay mentally and physically healthy.

STAY INVOLVED
- Communicate and visit with friends and family frequently. Take the initiative. Don't wait for them to call you.
- Stay active through work, recreation, church, volunteer and community activities.

MEDICAL HELP
- Get regular medical and dental checkups.
- See a doctor or dentist when you detect a problem. Don't put it off.
- Wear a medical identification bracelet or neck tag if you have any chronic disorder, have known allergies to medications or take medications that emergency personnel would need to know about.

SAFETY
- Use seat belts when you drive or ride in any vehicle. Never drive or operate heavy machinery while under the influence of alcohol or drugs, and never ride in a vehicle with a driver who is under the influence.
- Practice good safety measures at home to avoid accidents such as falls and to prevent fires.
- Avoid overexposure to sun, heat or cold. Use sunscreen and wear sunglasses when outdoors.

 CALL YOUR DOCTOR IF

You want additional information about making lifestyle changes.

Low Grade Depression (Dysthymia)

GENERAL INFORMATION

DEFINITION—A chronic depressive mood with symptoms that are milder, but longer lasting, than those of a major depressive episode. The onset of dysthymia is often unnoticed, and many people are not aware of the change in their lives. Symptoms may begin in childhood or in adolescence and continue over years or decades.

SIGNS & SYMPTOMS—Dysthymia may be diagnosed if several of the following signs and symptoms have been consistently present for two years or more (one year for children or teens), generally with no more than two months of that time symptom-free:
- Poor appetite or eating too much.
- Sleep problems (too much or too little sleep).
- Lack of energy; feeling tired all the time.
- Preoccupation with failure, inadequacy and negative thoughts (hopelessness).
- Feelings of self-pity; pessimistic attitude.
- Lack of productivity at home and work.
- Trouble with concentration and decision-making.
- Lack of interest or enjoyment in pleasurable activities, social activities or sex.
- Irritability.
- Crying for no reason.
- Overcritical or complaining.
- Skepticism.
- Psychosomatic illnesses (see Glossary).

CAUSES—Probably due to a combination of genetic factors, developmental factors and psychosocial factors (e.g., job loss, divorce).

RISK INCREASES WITH
- Family history of depressive illnesses.
- History of sexual or physical abuse.
- Discord in marriage, family, work or other personal relationships.
- Alcohol or drug abuse.

HOW TO PREVENT
No specific preventive measures. Anticipate and prepare for major life changes when possible.

PROBABLE OUTCOME—The majority of people are helped with treatment. It may take several months before symptoms show improvement. Sometimes, it is not until a woman has been treated and is feeling better that she realizes just how depressed she was before treatment.

POSSIBLE COMPLICATIONS
- Chronic recurrence; major depression.
- Alcohol abuse or dependency.

HOW TO TREAT

GENERAL MEASURES
- Diagnosis is usually based on your own observation of symptoms, a medical history and physical examination by your doctor.
- Treatment includes psychotherapy or counseling (may be combined with antidepressant medications). Several techniques are effective in treating dysthymia, such as cognitive or behavior therapy (focuses on changing negative thought patterns into positive ones), interpersonal therapy (focuses on building better relationships) and cultural analysis (deals with the role of society in contributing to low self-esteem and powerless feelings).
- Vocational counseling, to be sure your work suits your temperament, is helpful for some patients.
- Joining a support group can help by providing a forum for sharing problems and fostering friendships.
- Make an effort to attend social activities such as concerts, parties, plays, athletic events and movies. Keep in touch with friends and loved ones.
- Avoid alcohol. If you need help abstaining from alcohol, ask your doctor or contact an Alcoholics Anonymous group in your community.
- Reduce emotional stress in your life. Learn techniques to cope with stress.
- See the Resource section of this book for additional information.

MEDICATION—Your doctor may prescribe antidepressants, which you may need to take for several months or several years. If one medication doesn't work, it is possible that another will.

ACTIVITY—No restrictions. A regular physical exercise program is recommended and can help relieve depression.

DIET—Eat a nutritionally balanced diet to help maintain optimum health.

CALL YOUR DOCTOR IF

- You or a family member has symptoms of dysthymia.
- Symptoms worsen, recur or don't improve despite treatment.
- You have thoughts of death or suicide.
- New, unexplained symptoms develop. Drugs used in treatment may produce side effects.

Lymphedema

GENERAL INFORMATION

DEFINITION—An accumulation of lymphatic fluid in the interstitial tissue that causes swelling, most often in the arm(s) or leg(s) and, occasionally, in other parts of the body. Lymphedema can develop when lymphatic vessels are missing or impaired (primary), or when lymph vessels are damaged or lymph nodes are removed (secondary). In women who undergo excison of lymph nodes and/or radiation for breast cancer, approximately 5% will be affected with lymphedema within 1 year; 30% within 10 years; and 65% within 20 years. It is estimated that over 2 million people in the U.S. have lymphedema.

SIGNS & SYMPTOMS—Lymphedema can develop in any part of the body. Symptoms can include:
Stage one:
• A sensation of fullness, heaviness or warmth in the affected limb(s).
• Palpable swelling.
• Tight skin in the affected area.
• Difficulty fitting clothing onto one specific area of the body.
• Increased tightness of wristwatch, rings or bracelets.
• Discoloration or blistering of the skin.
Stage two:
• Increased and persistent swelling.
• Hardening of tissue as a result of fibrosis.
• Decreased flexibilty and mobility in the affected area.
Stage three:
• Elephantiasis: The affected limb reaches grotesque proportions and enormous weight. There may be actual leakage of lymphatic fluid through the skin.

CAUSES

Primary lymphedema: Congenital and can be present at birth, or can develop at puberty or in adulthood. Causes are unknown, although it is often associated with arterial-venous abnormalities, such as hemangioma (see Glossary) or port wine stain.
Secondary (or acquired) lymphedema can develop as a result of:
• Surgery, especially for breast, gynecological, head, neck, bladder or colon cancer, all of which may require removal or dissection of lymph nodes. Lymphedema may develop immediately following surgery or as long as 20 or 30 years later.
• Radiation therapy.
• Lymphangitis (infection or inflammation of the lymphatic vessels).
• Severe traumatic injury to the lymphatic system.
• Use of the drug tamoxifen (rarely).

• Mosquito bites can cause a form of secondary lymphedema called filariasis (extremely rare in developed countries).

RISK INCREASES WITH
• Aircraft flight at any point following surgery or radiation for cancer.
• Chemotherapy administered to the same side of the body as cancer surgery was previously performed on.
• Any injury, however slight, to the limb(s) on the side of the body where surgery requiring removal or dissection of lymph nodes was previously performed.

HOW TO PREVENT—No specific measures are known to prevent lymphedema. Following the steps outlined in this discussion may help to lessen the chances of developing lymphedema following radiation or surgery for cancer.

PROBABLE OUTCOME—There is presently no known cure for lymphedema. However, by following the instructions listed under General Measures, Activity, and Diet, and with early diagnosis and treatment, prognosis and general outlook may be greatly improved.

POSSIBLE COMPLICATIONS
• Impaired quality of life as a result of lymphedema.
• Lymphangitis (infection in the lymphatic fluid), which can further damage the lymphatic system. Without treatment, lymphangitis may be life-threatening.
• Lymphangiosarcoma, a form of cancer that is almost always fatal (this is a rare complication).

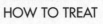

HOW TO TREAT

GENERAL MEASURES
• Following radiation and/or cancer surgery that involves lymph node dissection or removal:
Keep the "at risk" limb(s) spotlessly clean. Use lotion (e.g., Eucerin or Nivea) after bathing. When drying the limb, be gentle but thorough. Make sure it is dry between the fingers and toes, and in any creases.
When manicuring your nails, do not trim the cuticles.
Use an electric razor when shaving an "at risk" leg or under the arm on the affected side.
Avoid extreme temperature changes when bathing or washing dishes. Do not use saunas or hot tubs. Keep the limb protected from the sun.
Wear gloves when doing housework, gardening or any other type of work that could result in even minor injury to an "at risk" arm.
Wear closed-toed shoes at all times if a leg is "at risk."
Do not allow any injections, blood tests or blood pressure checks on the "at risk" arm.

Lymphedema (cont.)

Do not ignore any increase in swelling, however slight, or any redness or rash in the arm, hand, fingers or chest wall (or the toes, foot, ankle, leg, genitals or abdomen if applicable) on the affected side. Call your doctor immediately.

Avoid any type of trauma to the "at risk" limb, including cuts, insect bites, sports injuries, bruising, cat scratches, sunburn or other burns.

Do not wear tight jewelry or elastic bands around an affected arm, or on the fingers on the affected side.

• When traveling by air, patients with lymphedema must wear a compression stocking on the affected limb. Long flights may require the use of additional bandages.

• Depending on the severity of the lymphedema and the presence of current infection, the recommended treatment plan will usually be based on complex decongestive physiotherapy (CPD) methods which consist of manual lymphatic drainage (MLD); bandaging; proper skin care, diet and exercise and the use of compression garments including sleeves and devices such as CircAid leggings, a Legacy Sleeve or a Reid Sleeve. Self-treatment methods can be learned at an increasing number of specialized treatment centers throughout the U.S.

• Because the risks of developing lymphedema and its complications are life-long, these are measures that will need to be followed for the remainder of your life.

MEDICATION—Antibiotics will be prescribed if infection develops. Because of the high risk of infection in the limb(s) affected by lymphedema, it is advisable to carry antibiotics, or a prescription for antibiotics, whenever you travel.

ACTIVITY
• Do not smoke.
• Exercise is important, but do not overtire a limb at risk. Consult with your doctor about an appropriate exercise routine.
• Avoid heavy lifting or vigorous, repetitive movements with the arm and shoulder (or the leg in the case of groin surgery or radiation) on the affected side.

DIET
• Maintain your ideal weight. If overweight, consult your doctor about a weight loss diet.
• Eat a well-balanced, low-sodium, low-fat, high-fiber diet. Your diet should contain protein that is easily digested, such as chicken, fish or tofu.
• Avoid alcoholic beverages.

 CALL YOUR DOCTOR IF

• You or a family member has symptoms of lymphedema.
• Symptoms worsen, recur or don't improve despite treatment.
• You develop signs of infection: headache, muscle aches, dizziness, a general ill feeling, fever, redness, increased swelling, or a feeling of heat in the affected area of the body.
• New, unexplained symptoms develop. Drugs used in treatment may produce side effects.

Obesity

GENERAL INFORMATION

DEFINITION—A condition of excess body weight. Obesity may be defined as over 25% body fat in females and over 20% body fat in males. The concept that obesity is a will-power or self-discipline problem is outmoded. However, there is no clear understanding of the biochemical defects that cause it.

SIGNS & SYMPTOMS
- Excessive body weight and fat composition.
- Emotional problems.
- Poor exercise tolerance. Excess weight increases the heart's work.

CAUSES
- Genetic factors; parental obesity.
- Environmental factors: Diet and eating habits; levels of activity; emotional and physical stress; other emotional problems; drugs; cultural.
- Metabolic and endocrine disorders.
- Other factors not fully understood as yet include developmental factors and physiologic regulation that involves the "set point" theory (it helps explain the difficulty obese people have in losing weight and maintaining weight loss).
- Use of corticosteroid drugs.

RISK INCREASES WITH
- Factors listed under Causes.
- Pregnancy; puberty.
- Sedentary lifestyle.
- High-fat diet.

HOW TO PREVENT—Life-long adherence to a program consisting of proper diet, nutrition and exercise, and behavior and lifestyle modification as needed.

PROBABLE OUTCOME—Obesity can be controlled if motivation stays high. Long-term management of weight loss can be extremely difficult.

POSSIBLE COMPLICATIONS
- Obesity may contribute to the development of diabetes mellitus, high blood pressure, sleep apnea (see Glossary), heart disease and gallbladder disease. It complicates treatment and decreases survival chances of patients with stroke, kidney disease and other disorders.
- Psychosocial complications (poor self-image, difficulty in getting jobs, lack of social contacts with the opposite sex).

HOW TO TREAT

GENERAL MEASURES
- Medical assessment to determine the degree of health risk. The most accurate methods of determining body composition are underwater weighing and the skinfold measurements of multiple sites. Also used are body mass index (BMI) and waist to hip ratio (WHR).
- Many commercial and community programs are available that provide help in losing weight. Choose a program whose diet plans meet the RDA guidelines for nutrients, provide exercise and behavior counseling and include long-term maintenance support.
- Keep diaries for food intake, exercise activities and behavior changes. Review them with your weight loss advisor weekly.
- Several techniques exist for behavior modification. Determine the technique that best fits your needs (e.g., assertiveness, rewards, cognitive, substitution, imagery and others).
- Surgical procedures to reduce weight, such as bypassing part of the intestine or stomach, cutting or suctioning away fat or wiring the jaw shut, are desperate measures. They are used only in extreme circumstances.

MEDICATION
- Drug therapy as an aid to weight loss may or may not be helpful. Drugs for obesity may be recommended for you on a trial basis to see if they are of benefit to you. The effectiveness of many appetite suppressants diminishes after a few weeks and there are side effects to these drugs. Amphetamine compounds are not recommended for treating obesity.
- Experimental therapy for weight loss with medications is ongoing and new regimens may become available that are effective and have fewer side effects.

ACTIVITY
- Increase your current level of activity. Daily exercise (e.g., bicycle riding, walking, swimming) helps you lose weight, feel better and control appetite.
- 30 minutes of activity, 5 times a week should be the goal. Keep an activity diary to monitor your progress.

DIET
- Many different diet plans are available to choose from. Diets that are not nutritionally balanced can cause more problems than the obesity. Crash diets and fad diets don't produce long-term results. Schemes that promise easy weight loss are usually unsuccessful.
- During your diet and exercise program, there may be periods when you don't lose weight. This is normal; don't stop the program. Weight loss will begin again in a week or two.
- A realistic weight loss is 1 to 2-1/2 pounds a week. This may seem slow, but 1 pound of fat lost per week totals 52 pounds in 1 year.
- Keep a daily food diary to record everything you eat.

CALL YOUR DOCTOR IF

- You or a family member wants help with weight loss.
- Weight increases, despite measures taken to lose weight.

Osteoporosis

♀ GENERAL INFORMATION

DEFINITION—Loss of normal bone density, mass and strength, leading to increased thinning of bones and vulnerability to fracture. It most often affects women after menopause. Twenty million American women may have osteoporosis or be at risk for it.

SIGNS & SYMPTOMS
Early symptoms:
• Backache.
• No symptoms (often).
Late symptoms:
• Sudden back pain with a cracking sound indicating fracture.
• Deformed spinal column with humps.
• Loss of height.
• Fractures, especially of the spine, hip or arm, which occur with minor injury.

CAUSES—Loss of bone structure and strength. Factors include:
• Insufficient calcium intake.
• Excessive protein or phosphate intake.
• Low estrogen levels after menopause.
• Decreased activity with increased age.
• Smoking; heavy caffeine intake.
• Use of steroid (cortisone) drugs.
• Prolonged disease, including alcoholism.
• Vitamin deficiency (especially of vitamin D).
• Hyperthyroidism.
• Cancer.
• Genetic predisposition (female family members afflicted with osteoporosis).

RISK INCREASES WITH
• Surgery to remove the ovaries.
• Radiation treatment for ovarian cancer.
• Poor nutrition, especially inadequate calcium.
• Body type. Thin women with a small frame are more susceptible.
• Fair complexion.
• Family history of osteoporosis.
• Smoking.
• Heavy drinking of alcohol.
• Long-term use of cortisone drugs.
• Use of thyroid medications.

HOW TO PREVENT
• Hormonal replacement therapy starting at menopause.
• Ensure an adequate calcium intake (up to 1500 mg a day) with milk and milk products or calcium supplements.
• Regular exercise, such as brisk walking, which is weight-bearing and is better for preventing osteoporosis than swimming (nonweight-bearing).
• Seek medical advice about taking estrogen, calcium and fluoride after menopause begins or the ovaries have been removed.
• Avoid risk factors when possible.

PROBABLE OUTCOME—Diet, calcium and fluoride supplements, vitamin D, exercise and estrogen can halt and may reverse bone deterioration. Fractures usually heal with standard treatment.

POSSIBLE COMPLICATIONS
• Falls that cause bone fractures, especially of the hip or spine. Sometimes a bone will break or collapse without injury or fall.
• Severe, disabling pain.
• Permanent disability, or even death, as a result of bone fractures.

⚕ HOW TO TREAT

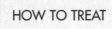

GENERAL MEASURES
• Medical tests include bone x-rays and bone-density studies.
• Treatment goals are directed to relieving pain and preventing any fractures and, sometimes, rebuilding bone.
• Avoid all circumstances which may lead to injury. Stay off icy streets and wet or waxed floors. Hold banisters when using stairs, and make sure banisters are sturdy.
• If estrogen is prescribed, get regular medical pelvic exams, Pap smears and mammograms. Examine your breasts for lumps once a month. Report any vaginal bleeding or discharge.
• Use heat or ice in any form to ease pain.
• Sleep on a firm mattress.
• Use a back brace, if prescribed.
• Use correct posture when lifting.
• Avoid mind-altering medications, such as sedatives or tranquilizers, which may cause falls and fractures.
• See the Resource section of this book for additional information.

MEDICATION
• For minor pain, you may use nonprescription drugs such as acetaminophen.
• Calcium, calcitonin (a hormone produced by the thyroid) or vitamin D supplements, hormone replacement therapy (HRT) or fluoride may be prescribed.
• Other medications that can slow bone loss or increase bone growth may also be prescribed.

ACTIVITY—Stay active, but avoid the risk of falls. Exercise is important, especially weight-bearing exercise, such as walking or running, to maintain bone strength.

DIET—Eat a well-balanced diet high in calcium and vitamin D. If you are overweight, initiate a weight loss plan.

☎ CALL YOUR DOCTOR IF

• You or a family member has symptoms of osteoporosis.
• Pain develops, especially after injury.
• New, unexplained symptoms develop. Drugs used in treatment may produce side effects.

Otoplasty
(Ear Plastic Surgery)

 GENERAL INFORMATION

DEFINITION—Cosmetic or reconstructive surgery on the outer ear.

REASONS FOR PROCEDURE
• Improve appearance of the outer ear (usually to flatten protruding ears).
• To construct or repair a missing or badly damaged ear.

RISK INCREASES WITH—Previous severe ear injury such as burn or extensive laceration.

DESCRIPTION OF PROCEDURE
• Laboratory blood and urine studies will usually be performed prior to surgery.
• Surgery is performed by a plastic or reconstructive surgeon or by an ear, nose and throat specialist, in a hospital or outpatient facility. Occasionally, surgery may be performed in a doctor's office.
• A local anesthetic is usually used. However, for more extensive surgery, or for a patient who may have trouble lying still for the procedure, a general anesthetic may be used.
To flatten protruding ears (several procedures are available; one is described here):
• A flap of skin is removed from the back of each ear.
• The underlying cartilage is remolded and the two edges of the wound stitched together. This brings the ear closer to the head.
• Bulky dressings are applied to the ear and left for a few days. They are replaced by a headband that is worn for several weeks. Stitches are removed about a week after surgery.
For a missing or badly damaged ear:
• The procedure is extensive and complex and normally involves more than one operation with long intervals of healing in between.
• A piece of rib cartilage is removed and sculptured to resemble a normal ear.
• The cartilage is transferred to a pocket of skin at the site where the ear will be located. Sometimes a skin graft is necessary.
• Dressings are applied to the ear and left on for 10-14 days until healing is completed and the stitches are removed.
• Hearing in the reconstructed ear may not be normal. When the hearing is normal in the other ear, there is usually no attempt made to improve the hearing in the reconstructed ear.

PROBABLE OUTCOME—Expect complete healing without complications. Allow about 2 weeks for recovery from surgery.

POSSIBLE COMPLICATIONS
• Sensitivity to cold weather, especially in the first year following surgery.
• Excessive bleeding (rare).
• Excessive scarring (keloid).
• Skin graft failure.
• Surgical-wound infection (rare).

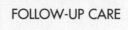 FOLLOW-UP CARE

GENERAL MEASURES
• Be sure you understand what results you can expect from your surgery. Ask your surgeon to show you before-and-after photographs of typical patients. Be realistic about your expectations.
• An overnight stay in the hospital may be required.
• A hard ridge should form along the incision. As it heals, the ridge will gradually recede. The scar will usually be hidden in the crease between the ear and the scalp.
• Bathe and shower as usual. Keep the dressings dry by wearing a shower cap.
• While resting or sleeping, keep the head elevated on 2 pillows to provide greater comfort.

MEDICATION
• Your doctor may prescribe pain relievers. Don't take prescription pain medication longer than 4 to 7 days. Use only as much as you need.
• Antibiotics to fight or prevent infection. Antibiotics may reduce the effectiveness of some oral contraceptives. If you are using oral contraceptives for birth control, discuss this with your doctor.
• You may use nonprescription drugs, such as acetaminophen, for minor pain. Avoid aspirin.

ACTIVITY
• Resume work and everyday activity as soon as possible, usually within 5 days.
• Resume mild exercise 2 to 3 weeks after surgery.
• Avoid vigorous exercise, swimming or contact sports for 6 weeks after surgery.

DIET—No special diet. Eat soft foods if chewing causes discomfort.

CALL YOUR DOCTOR IF

• You experience nausea or vomiting.
• Pain, swelling, redness, drainage or bleeding increases in the surgical area.
• You develop signs of infection: headache, muscle aches, dizziness, general ill feeling or fever.
• New, unexplained symptoms develop. Drugs used in treatment may produce side effects.

Otoplasty
(Ear Plastic Surgery)

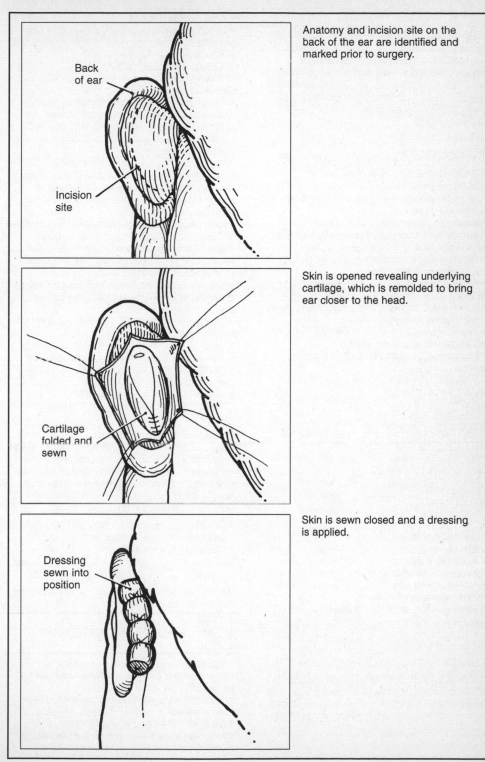

Anatomy and incision site on the back of the ear are identified and marked prior to surgery.

Back of ear

Incision site

Skin is opened revealing underlying cartilage, which is remolded to bring ear closer to the head.

Cartilage folded and sewn

Skin is sewn closed and a dressing is applied.

Dressing sewn into position

Panic Disorder

GENERAL INFORMATION

DEFINITION—A severe, spontaneous form of anxiety that is recurrent, unexplained and unpredictable. Most attacks last 2 to 10 minutes, but some may extend over an hour or two. This type of anxiety occurs with attack-like symptoms (often during sleep), while chronic anxiety (generalized anxiety) is a persistent state of anxiety.

SIGNS & SYMPTOMS
Physical symptoms:
- Palpitations, rapid heartbeat, chest pains.
- Shortness of breath, choking feeling, hyperventilation.
- Numbness and tingling around the mouth, hands and feet.
- Weakness or faintness; dizziness.
- Muscle spasm or contractions in the hands and feet.
- Fainting (occasionally).
- Sweating and trembling.
- Feeling of "butterflies in the stomach."

Emotional symptoms:
- Intense fear of losing one's sense of reason (fear of going crazy).
- Fear of dying.
- Sense of terror, doom or dread.
- Feelings of unreality, loss of contact with people and objects.

CAUSES
- Most often an unresolved emotional conflict or unrecognized conflict. The physical symptoms are a result of the autonomic nervous system being set in motion by the arousal of frightening fantasies, impulses and emotions.
- A variety of disorders can simulate panic attacks (heart rhythm problems, angina, respiratory illness, asthma, obstructive pulmonary disease, endocrine disorders, seizure disorders, stimulating drugs and withdrawal from certain drugs).

RISK INCREASES WITH
- Stress.
- Feelings of guilt.
- Fatigue or overwork.
- Illness.
- Alcohol and/or drug abuse.
- Family history of panic disorder.

HOW TO PREVENT—There are no specific measures to prevent a first panic attack; once diagnosed, therapy helps prevent additional episodes.

PROBABLE OUTCOME—For many, this disorder may run a limited course with a few attacks and long periods of remission. For others, treatment with psychotherapy and/or medication is effective.

POSSIBLE COMPLICATIONS
- Chronic anxiety.
- Phobias, including agoraphobia, a fear of being alone or in public places.
- Chronic depression.
- Drug dependency.

HOW TO TREAT

GENERAL MEASURES
- Diagnosis is usually determined by patient history and interviews and a description of behavior by the patient, family and friends. Laboratory blood studies may be done to rule out other disorders.
- Treatment involves psychotherapy or counseling and/or medications. Psychotherapy may involve cognitive therapy (learning to recognize thoughts and emotions which may underlie the panic attacks) or behavior therapy (using desensitization and relaxation techniques to control the body's response to anxiety).
- Talk to a friend or family member about your feelings. This can sometimes help to defuse your anxious thoughts.
- Keep a journal or diary about your anxious thoughts or emotions. Consider the causes and possible solutions.
- Join a self-help group. Call your local mental health society for referrals.
- Learn relaxation techniques. Meditation, a specific form of relaxation, may be effective.
- For hyperventilation symptoms, cover the mouth and nose with a small paper bag and breathe into it for several minutes.
- See the Resource section of this book for additional information.

MEDICATION—An antidepressant, benzodiazepine, or beta-blocking agent may be prescribed but may take 2 to 3 weeks to have an effect. The medicine is usually slowly reduced or discontinued after 6 months to a year to determine if the panic attacks return. If not, the medicine can be discontinued.

ACTIVITY
- Get regular physical exercise.
- Get adequate rest at night.

DIET—Consider giving up caffeine (coffee, tea, soft drinks, chocolate). You may experience caffeine withdrawal symptoms of headache or tiredness, but they stop in a few days.

CALL YOUR DOCTOR IF

- You or a family member has symptoms of panic disorder that don't diminish with self-treatment.
- Treatment program fails to produce an effect after 8 weeks.
- New, unexplained symptoms develop. Drugs used in treatment may produce side effects.

Phobias

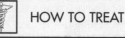

GENERAL INFORMATION

DEFINITION—A type of anxiety involving persistent, irrational or an exaggerated fear of a particular object, situation, activity, setting or even a bodily function (all of which are not basically dangerous nor an appropriate source for anxiety). Most people with phobias recognize that the fear is inappropriate to the situation. Phobias are classified as:
• Social (fear of embarrassment or humiliation in social situations such as public speaking and/or performing, or using public bathrooms).
• Agoraphobia (fear of being alone or fear of public places).
• Simple (fear of a particular stimulus such as animals, insects, flying, heights [acrophobia], closed places [claustrophobia], etc.).

SIGNS & SYMPTOMS—Anxiety symptoms occur when exposed to, or thinking of, the phobic stimulus:
• Palpitations.
• Sweating.
• Tremors.
• Flushing.
• Nausea.
• Experiencing negative thoughts and scary images.

CAUSES—Exact cause is unknown. Possibly a learned response (conditioning) such as being raised by someone with a similar fear or having an early frightening experience that has become associated with the object or situation. Other theories focus on the phobia as having a symbolic meaning.

RISK INCREASES WITH
• Family history of anxiety.
• Separation anxiety in childhood.
• Presence of another psychiatric disorder.
• Introverted, dependent or perfectionist type individuals.

HOW TO PREVENT—No specific measure to prevent the phobia. Techniques are available to prevent or control the reaction.

PROBABLE OUTCOME
• Simple phobias—some spontaneously stop as a person ages; others don't cause any impairment if the object can be avoided (such as fear of snakes). For some phobias, the people struggle through their fearful situations (such as flying); others can be cured with treatment, but the phobia may later recur.
• Social phobias—may be overcome with treatment; medication is often helpful.
• Agoraphobia—often associated with panic disorder. Without treatment, the person becomes more and more homebound. Treatment with medication and/or therapy is often effective.

POSSIBLE COMPLICATIONS
• Lifestyle constrictions brought on by avoidance of the phobic stimulus. Agoraphobia in particular restricts an individual's activities and is severely disabling.
• Dependence on drugs or alcohol to overcome anxiety.

HOW TO TREAT

GENERAL MEASURES
• Diagnosis involves a medical and social history and physical examination (sometimes).
• Psychotherapy or counseling for severe phobias and for phobias that are lifestyle restricting. Several different types of therapy are used such as desensitization or flooding.
• Fear-of-flying clinics are available in many communities.
• If you feel your fear taking hold:
  Shift your thoughts from negative—"the dog will bite"—to thoughts that are positive and real—"the dog is on a leash."
  Do something manageable—count backward from 1000, read a book, talk aloud, take deep measured breaths.
  Shift your thoughts to pleasant ones.
  Practice relaxation techniques.
• Join a support group if available.
• See the Resource section of this book for additional information.

MEDICATION—Medications may be prescribed for a short period of time during therapy.

ACTIVITY—No restrictions.

DIET—No special diet. Avoiding caffeine (coffee, tea, sodas and chocolate), nicotine and drugs that contain stimulants (e.g., ephedrine, epinephrine, phenylephrine, xanthine and pseudoephedrine) may help.

CALL YOUR DOCTOR IF

• You or a family member feels any phobia is restricting or disrupting your life.
• Symptoms of the phobia return after treatment.
• New, unexplained symptoms develop. Drugs used in treatment may produce side effects.

Recto-Vaginal-Fistula Repair

GENERAL INFORMATION

DEFINITION—Repair of a fistula (an abnormal tract) between the rectum and vagina that usually results from tearing during childbirth, surgical procedures, cervical cancer, radiation therapy or inflammatory bowel disease.

REASONS FOR PROCEDURE
- Prevention of fecal matter from contaminating the vagina or urinary tract.
- Discomfort and embarrassment caused by feces and rectal gas passing through the vagina.

RISK INCREASES WITH
- Obesity; smoking.
- Poor nutrition; alcoholism.
- Recent or chronic illness.
- Use of drugs such as antihypertensives, muscle relaxants, tranquilizers, sleep inducers, insulin, sedatives, beta-adrenergic blockers or cortisone.

DESCRIPTION OF PROCEDURE
- Laboratory blood and urine studies and x-rays of lower gastrointestinal tract and kidneys will often be performed prior to surgery.
- Surgery is performed in a hospital, usually by an obstetrician-gynecologist, a proctologist or a general surgeon.
- General anesthesia is administered by injection and inhalation with an airway tube place in the windpipe.
- An incision is made in the perineum.
- Scar tissue and the fistula between the vagina and rectum are cut free and removed.
- The openings into the rectum and vagina are closed with sutures that will be absorbed by the body.
- With some fistulas, a temporary colostomy (see Glossary) may be necessary for 2 to 3 months.
- The skin is closed with sutures, which usually may be removed about 1 week after surgery.

PROBABLE OUTCOME—Expect complete healing without complications. Allow about 6 weeks for recovery from surgery.

POSSIBLE COMPLICATIONS
- Excessive bleeding.
- Surgical-wound infection.
- Failure to heal completely.

FOLLOW-UP CARE

GENERAL MEASURES
- Hospital stay will usually last 5 to 7 days.
- Take hot baths several times a day to relieve discomfort.
- Bathe after bowel movements to prevent infection.
- Use sanitary pads instead of tampons during menstrual periods for 6 months.

MEDICATION
- Prescription pain medication should generally be taken for no longer than 4 to 7 days. Use only as much as you need.
- Stool softeners to prevent constipation.
- Antibiotics to fight or prevent infection. Antibiotics may reduce the effectiveness of some oral contraceptives. If you are currently using oral contraceptives for birth control, discuss this with your doctor.
- You may use nonprescription drugs, such as acetaminophen, for minor pain. Avoid aspirin.

ACTIVITY
- To help recovery and aid your well-being, resume daily activities, including work, as soon as you are able.
- Avoid vigorous exercise for 6 weeks after surgery. Resume sexual relations when your doctor determines that healing is complete.
- Resume driving 1 week after returning home.

DIET—Clear liquid diet until the gastrointestinal tract functions again. Then eat a well-balanced diet to promote healing.

CALL YOUR DOCTOR IF

- Pain, swelling, redness, drainage or bleeding increases in the surgical area.
- You develop signs of infection: headache, muscle aches, dizziness or a general ill feeling and fever.
- You experience nausea, vomiting, constipation or diarrhea.
- New, unexplained symptoms develop. Drugs used in treatment may produce side effects.

Recto-Vaginal-Fistula Repair

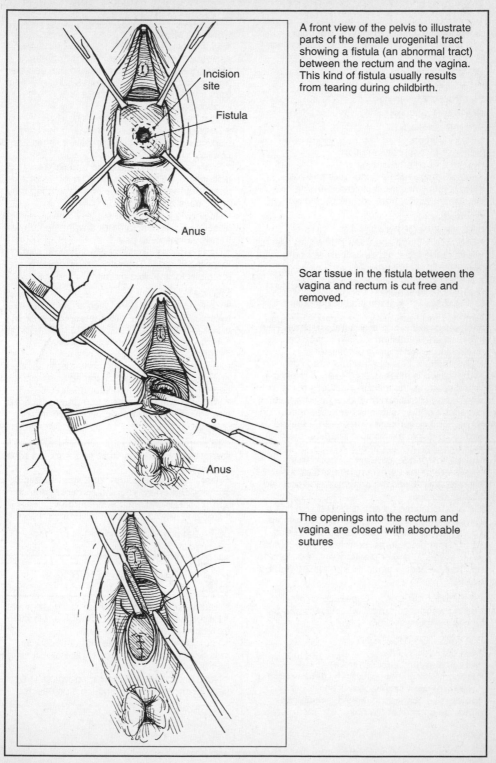

A front view of the pelvis to illustrate parts of the female urogenital tract showing a fistula (an abnormal tract) between the rectum and the vagina. This kind of fistula usually results from tearing during childbirth.

Scar tissue in the fistula between the vagina and rectum is cut free and removed.

The openings into the rectum and vagina are closed with absorbable sutures

Rhinoplasty & Septoplasty

 GENERAL INFORMATION

DEFINITION—Reconstruction of the nose (rhinoplasty) and removal of deformities of the septum (septoplasty).

REASONS FOR PROCEDURE
- Opening of blocked nasal passages.
- Improved appearance.

RISK INCREASES WITH
- Obesity; smoking.
- Poor nutrition.
- Excess alcohol consumption.
- Recent or chronic illness.
- Use of drugs such as antihypertensives, muscle relaxants, tranquilizers, sleeping pills, insulin, sedatives, beta-adrenergic blockers or cortisone.

DESCRIPTION OF PROCEDURE
- Laboratory blood and urine studies, as well as x-rays of the facial bones, will usually be performed prior to surgery.
- Surgery is performed by a plastic and reconstructive surgeon or an ear, nose and throat specialist, in a hospital or outpatient facility.
- A local anesthetic or a general anesthesia by injection and inhalation with an airway tube placed in the windpipe is administered.
- The nostril is held open with a speculum.
- An incision is made in the nose. To minimize visual scarring, the incison is usually made from within the nostrils; external cuts may be made if the shape of the nostrils is being changed.
- The bone or cartilage is fractured, trimmed and molded into the desired shape. If the goal is to increase the length of the nose, or to elevate the bridge, cartilage or bone from elsewhere in the body may be used as an implant. A synthetic material may also be used for the implant.
- The mucous membrane is closed with fine sutures, which usually can be removed about 10 days after surgery. Bandages are applied.
- For some procedures, petroleum-jelly-coated packing gauze and/or plastic splints are used to hold the septum in place during healing (up to 2 weeks).

PROBABLE OUTCOME—Expect complete healing without complications. Allow about 3 weeks for recovery from surgery.

POSSIBLE COMPLICATIONS
- Excessive bleeding.
- Surgical-wound infection (rare).
- Discomfort and pain caused by gauze packing.
- Recurrence of airway obstruction.
- Excessive scar tissue (keloid), which can affect the contour of the nose.

 FOLLOW-UP CARE

GENERAL MEASURES
- If surgery is being done for cosmetic reasons, ask your doctor to provide before-and-after photographs of typical patients so that you may have some idea of what results you can expect from surgery. Be realistic about your expectations.
- Hospital stay is usually 0 to 1 day.
- Swelling and discoloration around the eyes (raccoon eyes) will usually diminish within 2 to 3 weeks.
- Apply ice packs to the nose to relieve discomfort. Do this for 10 to 20 minutes at a time, and repeat 4 to 8 times a day during the first 2 days after surgery.
- Beginning 2 days after surgery, use an electric heating pad, a heat lamp or a warm compress to relieve incisional pain.
- Don't blow your nose at all in the first week following surgery. Then don't blow your nose forcefully for the next month.

MEDICATION
- Prescription pain medication should not be taken for longer than 4 to 7 days. Use only as much as you need.
- Antibiotics to fight infection or prevent infection. Antibiotics may reduce the effectiveness of some oral contraceptives. If you are currently using oral contraceptives for birth control, discuss this with your doctor.
- You may use nonprescription drugs, such as acetaminophen, for minor pain. Avoid aspirin.

ACTIVITY
- To help recovery and aid your well-being, resume daily activities, including work, as soon as you are able.
- Avoid vigorous exercise for 3 weeks after surgery. Generally, you should avoid contact sports for 6 months following surgery.
- Resume driving 1 week after returning home.

DIET—Eat a well-balanced diet to promote healing.

 CALL YOUR DOCTOR IF

- Nausea or vomiting occur following surgery.
- Pain, swelling, redness, drainage or bleeding increases in the surgical area.
- You develop signs of infection: headache, muscle aches, dizziness or a general ill feeling and fever.
- New, unexplained symptoms develop. Drugs used in treatment may produce side effects.

Rhinoplasty & Septoplasty

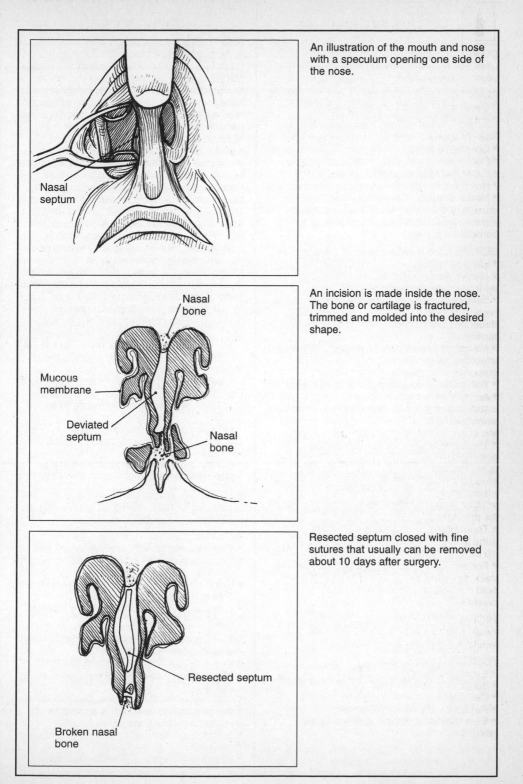

An illustration of the mouth and nose with a speculum opening one side of the nose.

Nasal septum

An incision is made inside the nose. The bone or cartilage is fractured, trimmed and molded into the desired shape.

Nasal bone

Mucous membrane

Deviated septum

Nasal bone

Resected septum closed with fine sutures that usually can be removed about 10 days after surgery.

Resected septum

Broken nasal bone

Seasonal Affective Disorder (SAD)

GENERAL INFORMATION

DEFINITION—A seasonal disruption of mood that occurs during the winter months and ceases with the advent of spring. Symptoms usually begin in September, when days begin to shorten, and last through the winter and into March, when the days begin to lengthen again. Light plays a large part in its origin, as well as in its treatment. It can affect both adults and children but is most common in women; approximately 80% of people with seasonal affective disorder (SAD) are women. In rare instances, the symptoms of SAD occur in the summer months and may be caused by an intolerance to heat.

SIGNS & SYMPTOMS—Usually experienced at the start of winter:
• Depression.
• Fatigue; sluggishness; lethargy.
• Increased appetite (especially for sweets and carbohydrates).
• Weight gain.
• Irritability.
• Increased need for sleep.
• Feeling less cheerful.
• Poor concentration.
• Decreased interest in work, social activities or sex.
• Difficulty coping with life as a result of these changes.

CAUSES—It is believed that the cause of SAD is related to the effects of light on melatonin. Melatonin is a hormone produced by the pineal gland, which is thought to be involved in the regulation of our sleep-wake cycles. Very little melatonin is secreted in light (daytime); the peak production is usually at night, between 2 and 3 a.m. Winter months (with their longer nights) stimulate extra production of melatonin, so the level in the body is increased, and this may interfere with a person's sleep. The average nighttime illumination in homes or offices is not adequate to counteract this effect.

RISK INCREASES WITH
• Geographical location; the farther a woman lives from the equator, the more likely she is to develop SAD.
• Other depressive illness.

HOW TO PREVENT—No specific preventive measures. Increased lighting may have some effect.

PROBABLE OUTCOME—With correct diagnosis and treatment, symptoms can usually be minimized.

POSSIBLE COMPLICATIONS—Continuation of the symptoms and lifestyle disruptions.

HOW TO TREAT

GENERAL MEASURES
• Laboratory blood studies may be done to rule out other medical disorders. Diagnosis usually requires a three-year mood disturbance pattern, with the onset occurring in the autumn, and a remission in the spring.
• Mild symptoms may be resolved with simple measures: keep drapes and blinds open in your house; sit near windows and gaze outside frequently; turn on bright lights on cloudy days; keep a diary or journal of your moods so that any changes or patterns can be evaluated; don't isolate yourself (visit friends, see shows, etc.). Read suggestions in Activity section.
• Other therapies usually involve extending the day artificially in various ways with light therapy (phototherapy). Duration and intensities of the therapy may vary for individuals and they need to be adjusted to fit your personal needs. Even though these light sources are commercially available, it is recommended that they not be used without medical advice. Examples include:
  Sitting in a very bright light (equivalent to 10 100 watt bulbs or more) for an hour in the morning and evening.
  Installing a computerized system of lighting in your bedroom that creates an artificial dawn. The light goes from very dim to bright like a sunrise.
• For some patients, the light therapy is unsuccessful and other forms of treatment, such as drugs or psychotherapy, may be required.
• See the Resource section of this book for additional information.

MEDICATION—Antidepressants may be prescribed for patients who do not respond to other forms of therapy.

ACTIVITY
• Stay as active as your energy permits. Physical activity is usually therapeutic for mood disorders.
• Get outside as much as possible, especially in the early morning light.
• Try to take a vacation in the winter months instead of in the summer.

DIET—Eat a nutritionally balanced diet to help maintain optimum health.

CALL YOUR DOCTOR IF

• You or a family member has symptoms of seasonal affective disorder.
• Symptoms worsen or don't improve despite treatment.
• You have thoughts of death or suicide.

Smoking

👤 GENERAL INFORMATION

DEFINITION—Cigarette smoking is an addiction disorder and the cause of many serious health problems. Among the thousands of chemicals in cigarette smoke are three substances which are known to be dangerous to the smoker, as well as to those who breathe in the second-hand smoke. The three are tar, nicotine and carbon monoxide (a poisonous gas). Tar condenses into a sticky substance in the lungs, nicotine is the addictive component of tobacco smoke and carbon monoxide decreases the oxygen carried by the red blood cells throughout the body. There is overwhelming evidence that anyone who smokes should make every attempt to quit.

SIGNS & SYMPTOMS—Any amount of cigarette smoking. The more one smokes, the greater the health risks. There is no safe level of exposure; someone who smokes occasionally (1 to 4 cigarettes a day) is still at greater risk for health problems than nonsmokers. An average smoker smokes 15 to 20 cigarettes a day.

CAUSES—Tobacco use usually begins as a social behavior and becomes an addiction that results in significant physical consequences.

RISK INCREASES WITH
• Addictive personality traits such as sensation-seeking, impulsiveness, difficulty in delaying gratification, rebelliousness, weak commitment to social goals, sense of alienation or low tolerance for stress. Other characteristics are low self-esteem, anxiety and depression.
• Lower education.
• Lower socioeconomic group.
• Ages 25 to 44 have highest smoking rates.
• Blue collar occupation group.

HOW TO PREVENT
• Education about health risks.
• Smoking restrictions in the workplace and other public facilities.

PROBABLE OUTCOME—For discontinuing smoking:
• It is never too late to quit. Discontinuing smoking can reverse the majority of health risks; some within 1 year, others within 10 to 15 years.
• Smoking cessation helps improve quality of life: Food tastes better; coughing is decreased; stamina is increased; mental health is improved.

POSSIBLE COMPLICATIONS—For continued smoking:
• Cancer of the lung, esophagus, pancreas, bladder, mouth, larynx or cervix.
• Heart and cardiovascular disease including heart attacks; coronary artery disease; hypertension; stroke. Use of oral contraceptives compounds the risk of cardiovascular disease.
• Chronic obstructive pulmonary disease.
• More prominent skin wrinkling.
• Infertility; numerous risks of complications in pregnancy; threats to the health of a newborn.
• Earlier menopause and possible osteoporosis.
• Harmful effects of second-hand smoke on family and friends.
• Death from disease or residential fire.

⚕ HOW TO TREAT

GENERAL MEASURES
• The majority of smokers who quit do so on their own; others are helped by a variety of methods. No one way works for everyone.
• Self-help steps for quitting:
1) Analyze your smoking habits by determining when and why you smoke. 2) Make up your mind to quit and do it. 3) Use any kind of substitute (gum, hard candy). 4) Temporarily give up those activities that you associate with smoking. 5) Reward yourself for not smoking. 6) During the first few weeks, eat plenty of low-calorie snacks and drink lots of water.
• Join a support group or a formal smoking cessation program.
• Try out other ideas such as hypnosis or acupuncture.
• Concerns about quitting: 1) Weight gain—average amount is 5 to 8 pounds over 5 years; for some, there is no weight gain. 2) Stress—get counseling or help with stress management. 3) Withdrawal—physical symptoms subside in about 10 to 14 days; psychological symptoms may persist for months or longer. 4) Fear of failure—relapse is common; if it happens, try again immediately. Many people have had to try more than once and by more than one method.

MEDICATION—Stop-smoking aids include nicotine gum, transdermal nicotine patches and a nasal spray. The idea of this therapy is to provide nicotine in a form other than a cigarette, so as to minimize the symptoms of withdrawal while being weaned from smoking. There are side effects associated with these aids, so be sure you discuss the risks and benefits with the doctor. Aids are to be used in conjunction with counseling or a smoking-cessation program.

ACTIVITY—Establish a regular exercise routine to help control weight, combat restlessness and make you feel better mentally and physically. Lung capacity improves when smoking is discontinued, so there is less shortness of breath when engaging in physical activities.

DIET—There is no special diet associated with smoking cessation. Metabolism rate tends to slow after quitting and a weight gain may occur. Low calorie snacks are recommended to replace the oral sensation of smoking.

📞 CALL YOUR DOCTOR IF

You or a family member is a cigarette smoker and wants help quitting.

Stress

GENERAL INFORMATION

DEFINITION—Changes and demands in your life can result in stress, which is the physical, mental and emotional reactions you experience. The life changes can be either large or small, and each person will respond to these changes somewhat differently. Some people are more susceptible to stress than others. Positive stress can be a motivator, while negative stress occurs when these changes and demands are overwhelming to you. Stress can affect any body system and aggravate any chronic disease.

SIGNS & SYMPTOMS
• Physical symptoms include muscle tension, headache, chest pain, upset stomach, diarrhea or constipation, racing heartbeat, cold, clammy hands, fatigue, sweating, rashes, dizziness, rapid breathing, shaking, tics, jumpiness, poor or excessive appetite, weakness and tiredness.
• Emotional reactions include anger, low self-esteem, depression, apathy, irritability, guilt, worry, fear, difficulty concentrating, agitation, anxiety, phobias and panic.
• Behavioral reactions may cause alcohol or drug abuse, increased smoking, memory loss, sleep disorders, overeating or confusion.

CAUSES—In a stressful situation, the body responds by increasing the production of certain hormones, which causes changes in the heart rate, blood pressure and metabolism.

RISK INCREASES WITH
• Recent death of a family member or friend.
• Loss of anything valuable to you.
• Injuries or severe illnesses.
• Getting fired or changing jobs.
• Recent move to a new city or state.
• Sexual difficulties between you and your partner.
• Business or financial reversal, or taking on a large debt, such as purchasing a new home.
• Regular conflict between you and a spouse or family member, friend or business associate.
• Constant fatigue brought about by inadequate rest, sleep or recreation.
• Demands on your time and energy by other family members, leaving little time for self-care.

HOW TO PREVENT
• To help prevent stress, try to take charge of those aspects of your life that you can manage.
• Since stress cannot always be prevented, learn coping techniques to protect your mental and physical health. Educate yourself about stress, its causes, effects and self-treatment techniques.

PROBABLE OUTCOME—Usually resolved with time, self-treatment or professional therapy.

POSSIBLE COMPLICATIONS
Chronic stress can play a role in many health problems including accidents, asthma, cancer, colds, colitis, diabetes mellitus, fatigue, muscle aches, endocrine disorders, headaches, heart disease, digestive and skin problems, ulcers, hypertension, insomnia and sexual dysfunction.

HOW TO TREAT

GENERAL MEASURES
• Diagnosis is usually by your own or others' observation of symptoms. Sometimes medical tests may be necessary to rule out medical disorders that could be the cause of the symptoms. Patients often don't recognize that they are stressed.
• Psychotherapy or counseling may be helpful.
• Learn a meditation or relaxation technique and practice it regularly, daily if possible.
• Rearrange daily schedules to make them less stressful.
• If possible, get help with physical responsibilities and decrease the burden of other responsibilities when you can. Determine what is important and what can be postponed, left undone or passed on to others.
• Take a short time away from any stressful situation you encounter during a day.
• Learn and practice a muscle-tensing and muscle-relaxing technique. Take warm baths.
• Make a list of what needs to be done each day and then cross the items off as you complete them; this will bring a feeling of accomplishment.
• Take time for some form of enjoyable recreation for yourself.
• Try to increase self-esteem by finding ways to validate your worth and your needs.
• Avoid taking your problems home or to bed with you. At the end of the day, spend a few minutes reviewing your entire day, event by event, as if you're replaying a tape. Release all negative emotions you have harbored, and relish all good energy or emotion. Reach a decision about unfinished events, and release mental or muscular tension. Now you're ready for a relaxing and emotionally healing sleep.
• Join a support group in your community.

MEDICATION—Usually not necessary, unless symptoms are severe.

ACTIVITY—Adopt an exercise program. People in good physical condition are less likely to suffer the negative effects of stress.

DIET—Eat a normal, well-balanced diet. Don't skip meals. Vitamin supplements may be recommended.

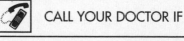

CALL YOUR DOCTOR IF

You or a family member is concerned about stress.

Substance Abuse & Addiction

 ## GENERAL INFORMATION

DEFINITION—Preoccupation with mood-altering substances (drugs, alcohol, nicotine), loss of self-control and a compulsion to continue despite adverse personal and social consequences.

SIGNS & SYMPTOMS—Depends on the substance of abuse. Most produce:
- A temporary pleasant mood.
- Relief from anxiety.
- False feelings of self-confidence.
- Increased sensitivity to sights and sounds (including hallucinations).
- Altered activity levels (either stupor and sleeplike states or frenzies).
- Unpleasant or painful symptoms when the abused substance is withdrawn.

CAUSES—Substances of abuse may produce addiction or dependence. The most common substances of abuse include:
- Nicotine.
- Alcohol.
- Marijuana.
- Amphetamines, including diet pills.
- Barbiturates, including sleeping pills.
- Cocaine.
- Opiates, including codeine, heroin, methadone, morphine and opium.
- Prescription medications containing narcotics (e.g., Demerol, Percocet and Percodan); tranquilizers such as Valium and Xanax.
- Psychedelic or hallucinogenic drugs, including PCP (or "angel dust"), mescaline and LSD.
- Volatile substances that are inhaled, such as glue, solvents and paints.

RISK INCREASES WITH
- Illness that requires prescription pain relievers or tranquilizers.
- Family history of drug abuse.
- Genetic factors. Some persons may be more susceptible to addiction than others.
- Excess alcohol consumption.
- Fatigue or overwork.
- Poverty.
- Psychological problems, including depression, dependency or poor self-esteem.

HOW TO PREVENT
- Don't socialize with persons who use and abuse drugs, alcohol or nicotine.
- Seek counseling for mental health problems, such as depression or chronic anxiety, before they lead to drug or alcohol problems.
- Pursue wholesome interests and activities.
- After surgery, illness or injury, stop taking prescription pain relievers or tranquilizers as soon as possible. Don't use more than you need.

PROBABLE OUTCOME—Curable with strong motivation, good medical care and support from family and friends.

POSSIBLE COMPLICATIONS
- Sexually transmitted diseases in addicts who share needles or practice careless sexual behavior while under the influence of drugs.
- Severe infections from intravenous injections with nonsterile needles.
- Malnutrition.
- Accidental injury to oneself or others while in a drug-induced state.
- Loss of job or family.
- Irreversible damage to body organs.
- Birth defects, premature birth, increased risk of fetal or newborn death, and withdrawal in newborns of mothers who used drugs or alcohol during pregnancy.
- Death caused by overdose.

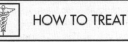 ## HOW TO TREAT

GENERAL MEASURES
- Diagnosis is made by your own and other's observations of symptoms.
- Recovery begins with admitting that you have a problem and seeking professional help.
- Your doctor may perform a medical history and physical examination; laboratory blood and urine studies may also be done.
- Treatment consists of psychotherapy or counseling, either on an outpatient basis or as a patient in a specialized treatment center.
- Hospitalization may be required for drug withdrawal symptoms.
- Be open and honest with your family and good friends, and ask for their help. Avoid friends who tempt you to resume your habit.
- Join self-help groups such as Narcotics Anonymous or Alcoholics Anonymous.
- See the Resource section of this book for additional information.

MEDICATION
- Disulfiram for alcoholism. This drug produces severe illness when alcohol is consumed.
- Naltrexone, which blocks the effect of opiates.
- Methadone for narcotic abuse. This drug is a less potent narcotic that is used to decrease the severity of physical withdrawal symptoms and allow a return to a normal life.

ACTIVITY—No restrictions. Exercise regularly.

DIET—Eat a normal, well-balanced diet that is high in protein. Vitamin supplements may be necessary if you suffer from malnutrition.

 ## CALL YOUR DOCTOR IF

- You abuse or are addicted to alcohol, cigarettes or drugs, and want help.
- New, unexplained symptoms develop. Drugs used in treatment may produce side effects.
- Coma or seizures occur. Get help immediately! This is an emergency!

Tummy Tuck (Abdominoplasty)

 GENERAL INFORMATION

DEFINITION—Removal of excess skin and fat from the abdomen.

REASONS FOR PROCEDURE—Improved appearance.

RISK INCREASES WITH
- Stress; smoking; alcoholism.
- Poor nutrition.
- Previous abdominal surgery.
- Recent or chronic illness.
- Use of drugs such as antihypertensives, muscle relaxants, tranquilizers, sleep inducers, insulin, sedatives, beta-adrenergic blockers or cortisone.

DESCRIPTION OF PROCEDURE
- Laboratory blood and urine studies will be performed prior to surgery.
- Surgery is usually performed in a hospital, by a plastic and reconstructive surgeon.
- General anesthesia is administered by injection and inhalation with an airway tube placed in the windpipe.
- A large, elliptical incision, usually running from hip to hip just above the pubic area, is made in the abdomen. Another incision is usually made around the navel so that it can be moved to a new position after the excess skin has been removed.
- Excessive skin and the underlying apron of excess fat are cut free and removed. Liposuction may also be performed to remove some of the excess fat.
- The navel is reattached in its new location.
- Drains are left under the operative site to prevent accumulation of blood and fluid from tissue drainage.
- Both edges of the skin are gently stretched and carefully sewn together with sutures.
- Bandages and a firm, elastic dressing similar to a girdle may be placed over your abdomen and buttocks to help hold the stitches together while healing takes place.
- Sutures can usually be removed in 10 to 14 days.

PROBABLE OUTCOME—Expect complete healing and improved appearance without complications. Allow about 10 weeks for recovery from surgery. Excess abdominal fat may return if caloric intake is not controlled.

POSSIBLE COMPLICATIONS
- Wide or excessive (keloid) scars.
- Excessive bleeding.
- Surgical-wound infection.
- Blood or serum collection beneath the flap where fat was removed.
- Necrosis (see Glossary) of surgical flaps.
- Wound breaking open.

 FOLLOW-UP CARE

GENERAL MEASURES
- Ask your surgeon to show you before-and-after photographs of typical patients so that you will have some idea of what type of results you can expect from this surgery. Be realistic about your expectations.
- Hospital stay is usually 2 to 5 days.
- Abdominoplasty is an extensive procedure, and you will probably experience at least moderate pain and discomfort following the surgery. Usually, pain can be relieved with the use of prescription or nonprescription pain relievers.
- A hard ridge should form along the incision. As it heals, the ridge will gradually recede.
- Use an electric heating pad, a heat lamp or a warm compress to relieve incisional pain.
- Bathe and shower as usual. You may wash the incision gently with mild unscented soap.
- Between showers, keep the wound dry with a bandage for the first 2 or 3 days after surgery. If a bandage gets wet, change it promptly.
- Apply nonprescription antibiotic ointment to the wound before applying new bandages.

MEDICATION
- Prescription pain medication should generally be taken for no longer than 4 to 7 days. Use only as much as you need.
- Stool softeners to prevent constipation.
- Antibiotics to fight or prevent infection. Antibiotics may reduce the effectiveness of some oral contraceptives.
- You may use nonprescription drugs, such as acetaminophen, for minor pain. Avoid aspirin.

ACTIVITY
- To help recovery and aid your well-being, resume daily activities, including work, as soon as you are able.
- Resume sexual relations when able.
- Exercise will help maintain improved appearance. Consult your doctor about an exercise program after recovery.

DIET—No special diet, but diet must be controlled to maintain improved appearance.

 CALL YOUR DOCTOR IF

- Pain, swelling, redness, drainage or bleeding increases in the surgical area.
- You develop signs of infection: headache, muscle aches, dizziness or a general ill feeling and fever.
- You experience nausea, vomiting, constipation or abdominal swelling.
- New, unexplained symptoms develop. Drugs used in treatment may produce side effects.

Tummy Tuck
(Abdominoplasty)

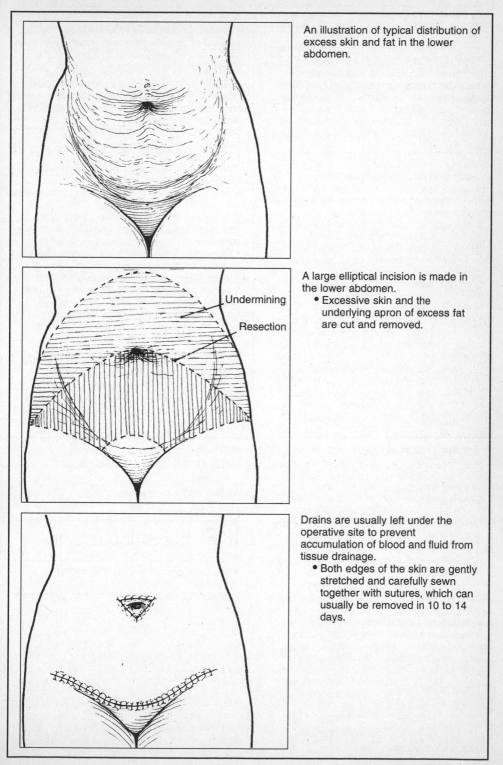

An illustration of typical distribution of excess skin and fat in the lower abdomen.

A large elliptical incision is made in the lower abdomen.
- Excessive skin and the underlying apron of excess fat are cut and removed.

Undermining

Resection

Drains are usually left under the operative site to prevent accumulation of blood and fluid from tissue drainage.
- Both edges of the skin are gently stretched and carefully sewn together with sutures, which can usually be removed in 10 to 14 days.

Ultrasound Scanning

GENERAL INFORMATION

DEFINITION—A noninvasive diagnostic technique that produces an image on a screen (sonogram) by passing high frequency soundwaves into the body. The reflected echoes are detected and analyzed to establish the picture of internal organs or a fetus in the uterus. Ultrasound can be used to examine most parts of the body except those surrounded by bone (the brain) or that contain gas (lungs or intestines).

REASONS FOR PROCEDURE—In obstetric and gynecological diagnostic situations:
• To detect foreign bodies and distinguish between cystic and solid masses (tumors) in the uterus, fallopian tubes and ovaries.
• To evaluate fetal viability, position, gestational age and growth rate (often recommended between 12th and 20th weeks of pregnancy).
• To determine the location of the placenta.
• Suspected ectopic pregnancy.
• To guide amniocentesis by determining placental location and fetal placement.
• To detect multiple pregnancies.
• Can be used to evaluate fetal anatomy for a wide variety of birth defects (when performed by specially trained and experienced ultrasound operators).
• Used to evaluate fetal well-being with an examination called a biophysical profile (BPP). It assesses fetal breathing movement, heart rate, limb movement, trunk attitude and movement and amount of amniotic fluid.

RISK INCREASES WITH—None expected.

DESCRIPTION OF PROCEDURE
• The procedure is usually done in the doctor's office. No anesthetic is required unless it is associated with other testing, such as amniocentesis.
• In early pregnancy testing, a woman is often advised to drink several glasses of fluid and not to empty the bladder for a few hours prior to the test. A full bladder can help improve the view of the uterus when the ultrasound is done through the abdomen.
• Clothing over the area to be scanned is removed, and oil or jelly is applied to the skin to achieve good contact.
• A transducer (an instrument that converts an electrical current into sound waves) is passed back and forth over the skin and the images appear on a black and white video screen.
• In some cases, the transducer may be placed inside the vagina to allow certain enhanced details to be seen. The vaginal procedure allows better visualization of the pelvis. In this case, a full bladder is not necessary.
• The technique produces no detectable sensation or pain.

PROBABLE OUTCOME
• The ultrasound reveals no abnormalities or problems.
• To date, there are no significant aftereffects, either short-term or long-term, which have been associated with ultrasound to a patient or a fetus.

POSSIBLE COMPLICATIONS—None expected. However, the ultrasound results may be considered abnormal and further testing may be necessary.

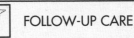

FOLLOW-UP CARE

GENERAL MEASURES
• You may empty your bladder immediately after the test.
• Results of the procedure will be explained to you by the doctor. Further diagnostic tests may be indicated.
• Most often, the results show a normal uterus and ovaries and no other visible masses. If done in pregnancy, the gestational sac and fetus usually show normal size and development.
• If testing is to determine the difference between cystic and solid masses, the solid masses will appear more dense on the sonogram.
• Results may indicate inappropriate fetal size, which can indicate a miscalculation of conception or delivery date. Abnormal echo patterns may indicate foreign bodies, such as an intrauterine device (IUD); multiple pregnancy; problems with placental placement; fetal abnormalities and breech or shoulder presentation.

MEDICATION—Medicine is usually not necessary.

ACTIVITY—No restrictions.

DIET—No special diet.

CALL YOUR DOCTOR IF

• You have concerns about the testing procedure.
• Results of the test are not clearly understood.

Ultrasound Scanning

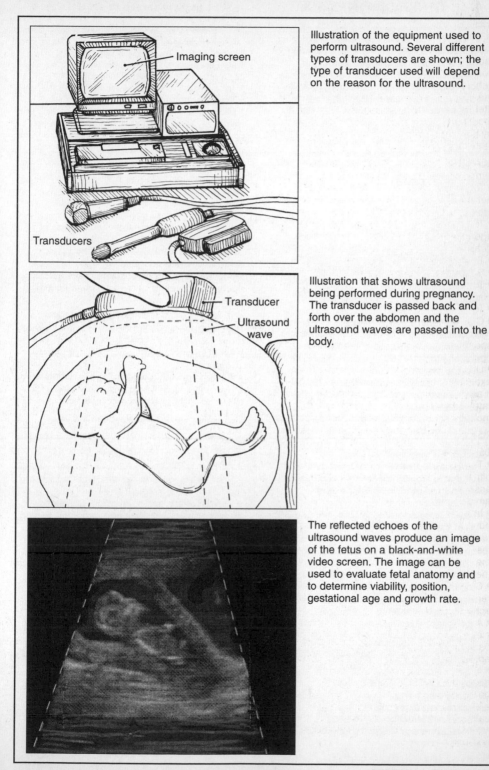

Illustration of the equipment used to perform ultrasound. Several different types of transducers are shown; the type of transducer used will depend on the reason for the ultrasound.

Imaging screen

Transducers

Illustration that shows ultrasound being performed during pregnancy. The transducer is passed back and forth over the abdomen and the ultrasound waves are passed into the body.

Transducer

Ultrasound wave

The reflected echoes of the ultrasound waves produce an image of the fetus on a black-and-white video screen. The image can be used to evaluate fetal anatomy and to determine viability, position, gestational age and growth rate.

Vesico-Vaginal-Fistula Repair

GENERAL INFORMATION

DEFINITION—Repair of a vesico-vaginal fistula, an abnormal tract between the bladder and the vagina that usually results from tearing in childbirth, as a complication of cervical uterine surgery (e.g., vaginal hysterectomy), or as a complication of cervical cancer (particularly when radiation therapy is used).

REASONS FOR PROCEDURE
• Control of urine flow from the bladder.
• Prevention of vaginal and urinary tract infections.

RISK INCREASES WITH
• Adults over 60.
• Obesity; smoking; stress.
• Poor nutrition.
• Recent or chronic illness.
• Alcoholism.
• Previous pelvic surgery.
• Use of drugs such as antihypertensives, muscle relaxants, tranquilizers, sleep inducers, insulin, sedatives, beta-adrenergic blockers or cortisone.

DESCRIPTION OF PROCEDURE
• Laboratory blood and urine studies, pelvic examination and cystoscopy (see Glossary) with biopsy (sometimes) are usually performed prior to surgery.
• Surgery is usually performed in a hospital, by an obstetrician-gynecologist, urologist or a general surgeon.
• Anesthesia is administered: either a spinal anesthesia by injection or a general anesthesia by injection and inhalation with an airway tube placed in the windpipe.
• A speculum is used to hold the vagina open.
• Scar tissue around the fistula is cut free and removed; this tissue will often be sent to the laboratory for examination.
• Healthy tissue is interposed between the 2 layers of the fistula.
• The bladder wall and vaginal wall are closed with sutures that will be absorbed by the body.
• The bladder is filled with blue-colored sterile water or sterile milk to search for leaks. If leaks exist, further repairs are made. If no leaks are found, a catheter is placed in the bladder.
• The catheter usually can be removed about 5 to 7 days after surgery.

PROBABLE OUTCOME
Expect complete healing without complications. Allow about 6 weeks for recovery from surgery.

POSSIBLE COMPLICATIONS
• Excessive bleeding.
• Surgical-wound infection.
• Urinary tract infection.
• Continued urine leakage through fistula.

FOLLOW-UP CARE

GENERAL MEASURES
• Hospital stay averages 6 days.
• Use an electric heating pad or a warm compress to relieve surgical-wound pain.
• Take warm baths several times a day to relieve discomfort.
• Move and elevate legs often while resting in bed to decrease the likelihood of deep-vein blood clots.

MEDICATION
• Prescription pain medication should generally be required for no longer than 4 to 7 days. Use only as much as you need.
• Stool softeners to prevent constipation.
• Antibiotics to fight or prevent infection. Antibiotics may reduce the effectiveness of some oral contraceptives. If you are currently using oral contraceptives for birth control, discuss this with your doctor.
• You may use nonprescription drugs, such as acetaminophen, for minor pain. Avoid aspirin.

ACTIVITY
• To help recovery and aid your well-being, resume daily activities, including work, as soon as you are able.
• Avoid vigorous exercise for 6 weeks after surgery.
• Resume driving 3 weeks after returning home.
• Resume sexual relations when your doctor determines that healing is complete.

DIET—Your doctor will prescribe a diet.

CALL YOUR DOCTOR IF

• Pain, swelling, redness, drainage or bleeding increases in the surgical area.
• You develop signs of infection: headache, muscle aches, dizziness or a general ill feeling and fever.
• You experience nausea, vomiting or constipation.
• You develop urinary frequency and stinging or burning on urination.
• New, unexplained symptoms develop. Drugs used in treatment may produce side effects.

Women's Health Examinations & Immunizations

GENERAL INFORMATION

DEFINITION
• An annual overall physical examination for healthy adults of all ages is no longer recommended by most medical experts. However, there are certain periodic screening tests recommended for healthy women based on risk factors and preventive services. Counseling about lifestyle and health is an important part of a periodic exam. Your doctor will discuss health-related behaviors such as smoking, alcohol use, contraception, eating habits, weight problems, exercise programs, sexual activity (to assess risk of sexually transmitted diseases) and seatbelt use.
• Vaccine-preventable diseases cause needless sickness and death in adults. You can reduce your risks of acquiring these diseases by becoming familiar with the necessary immunizations, and by keeping an accurate record of your immunization history.

PERIODIC SCREENING TESTS FOR HEALTHY WOMEN
Age 18–39 (childbearing years):
• Height and weight.
• Blood pressure.
• Nonfasting total blood cholesterol (every 5 years).
• Clinical breast exam (every 1 to 3 years).
• Pelvic exam and Pap smear (every 1 to 3 years).
• Dental exam (every 6 to 12 months).
Age 40–64 (middle years):
• Height and weight.
• Blood pressure.
• Clinical breast examination (yearly).
• Nonfasting total blood cholesterol level (every 5 years).
• Pelvic exam and Pap smear (annually).
• Digital rectal examination (annually).
• Sigmoidoscopy (every 3 to 5 years after age 50).
• Mammogram (every 1 to 2 years as of age 50).
• Oral cavity examination (every 1 to 3 years).
• Dental exam (every 6 to 12 months).
Age 65 and over (senior years):
• Height and weight.
• Blood pressure.
• Visual acuity and hearing.
• Clinical breast examination (yearly for women until age 75, unless an abnormality is detected).
• Oral cavity examination (every 1 to 3 years).
• Dipstick urinalysis.
• Sigmoidoscopy (every 3 to 5 years).
• Nonfasting total blood cholesterol (every 4 years).
• Mammogram (every 1 to 2 years until age 75, unless abnormality detected).
• Dental exam (every 6 to 12 months).

RECOMMENDED IMMUNIZATIONS
• Tetanus-diphtheria booster—once between ages 14 to 16, then a booster every 10 years.
• Influenza vaccine—below age 65, depends on chronic diseases or occupational exposure; annually if over age 65.
• Pneumococcal vaccine—below age 65, depends on chronic diseases or special conditions; over 65, needed only one time.
• Rubella vaccine—(once) for women of childbearing age without proof of immunity.
• Hepatitis B vaccine—(once) for women in health-care occupations or those working with blood; intravenous drug users; those with multiple sexual partners or who have had sex with a person infected with hepatitis B.
• HIV patients should be evaluated for all immunizations.

OTHER TESTS THAT MAY BE RECOMMENDED FOR WOMEN WITH RISK FACTORS
• Skin exam—for excessive skin exposure to sun or precancerous skin changes.
• Blood test for hemoglobin—heavy menstrual periods; women of Caribbean, Latin American, Asian, Mediterranean or African descent.
• Urine test for infection—diabetes mellitus.
• Sexually transmitted disease (STD) tests—for women having sex with multiple partners or a partner with multiple partners; sexual contact with a person who has or has had an STD.
• Human immunodeficiency virus (HIV)—women being treated for another STD; intravenous drug user; current or past sexual activity with an HIV-positive person or one who injects drugs; women planning a pregnancy or who are currently pregnant.
• Genetic testing—women of reproductive age with risk factors.
• Tuberculosis (TB) skin test—infection with HIV; living or working with someone with TB; other risk factors for TB exposure.
• Blood test for type of lipids (cholesterol)—women with high cholesterol count; diabetes mellitus; smoking; family history of high cholesterol count or heart disease.
• Mammogram—women below age 35 years if mother or sister has had breast cancer.
• Fasting blood glucose (sugar) test—family history of diabetes mellitus; obesity; having had diabetes in pregnancy.
• Thyroid-stimulating hormone test—family history of thyroid disease; having an autoimmune disease (e.g., rheumatoid arthritis).
• Colonoscopy—personal history of inflammatory bowel disease or polyps in the colon; family history of colon cancer.

CALL YOUR DOCTOR IF

You have questions about examinations or immunizations.

Glossary

A

Abdominal Aorta—Section of the aorta that passes through the abdomen to supply blood to the lower part of the body.

Abortion—The premature expulsion from the uterus of the products of conception; can either be induced or can occur spontaneously (miscarriage).

Abscess—Swollen, inflamed, tender area of infection containing pus.

Accident Proneness—Tendency of some persons to have more accidents than normal. It may be due to a risk factor such as poor vision, but unconscious factors are often the cause.

Acetaminophen—Nonprescription medication used to relieve minor pain and to reduce fever. Its analgesic effects are similar to aspirin, but it does not reduce inflammation or swelling. It is less irritating to the stomach than aspirin.

Achalasia—Condition of the esophagus that disrupts normal swallowing.

Acne—A disorder of the skin caused by inflammation of the skin glands and hair follicles, and characterized by the presence of pimples, mostly on the face.

Acquired Immune Deficiency Syndrome (Acquired Immunodeficiency Syndrome; AIDS)—A disease of the human immune system that is caused by infection with HIV (human immunodeficiency virus).

Acupuncture—Method of anesthesia and treatment of pain developed by the Chinese. Needles are inserted through the skin to stimulate precise areas.

Acute—Beginning suddenly; also severe, but of short duration.

Addiction—Intense craving for substances such as alcohol, tobacco or narcotics, or a compulsive behavior such as gambling.

Adenoids—Infection-fighting tissue (part of the lymphatic system) in the upper throat, near the tonsils.

Adenoids, Enlarged—Swollen adenoids that impair speech.

Adenovirus—Group of viruses that cause certain respiratory and eye infections.

Adhesions—Small strands of fibrous tissue that cause organs in the abdomen and pelvis to cling together abnormally, creating a risk of intestinal obstruction.

Adolescence—Time of life from the beginning of puberty until maturity.

Adrenal Glands—Two glands attached to the kidneys. Each has an outer layer (cortex) that produces steroid hormones and an inner layer (medulla) that produces adrenalin.

Adrenalin—Hormone produced by the adrenal glands that increases heart rate and prepares the body for crisis. Also called epinephrine.

After-Birth—The placenta and fetal membranes that are expelled after delivery.

Aging—The normal process of gradual physical and mental decline.

AIDS—See *Acquired Immune Deficiency Syndrome*.

Airways—Tubular passages that air passes through to the lungs: the trachea (windpipe), bronchi and bronchioles.

Alopecia—Loss of hair; baldness.

Alveoli—Lung cells at ends of the airways where oxygen enters the blood and waste gases leave the blood.

Ambulatory Medical Center—A health-care facility for patients who do not require prolonged bed rest or hospitalization.

Amenorrhea—Abnormal absence or suppression of menstruation.

Amniocentesis—The extraction and examination of a small amount of amniotic fluid in order to determine genetic and other disorders in the unborn child.

Amniography—Radiographic visualization of the outlines of the uterine cavity, placenta and fetus after injection of a radiopaque substance into the amniotic sac.

Amnioscope—An endoscope for observation of the amniotic sac and its contents.

Amniotic Cavity—The fluid-filled space between the amniotic sac and the fetus.

Amniotic Fluid—The serous fluid in which the embryo is suspended within the amniotic sac.

Amniotic Sac—The thin, transparent membrane forming a closed sac and filled with fluid in which the embryo is immersed.

Amniotomy—Intentional rupture of the fetal membranes to facilitate or induce labor.

Amphetamine Drugs—Habit-forming drugs that stimulate the brain and central nervous system, increase blood pressure, reduce nasal stuffiness or suppress appetite.

Amyloid Deposits—Abnormal protein material deposited in tissues, usually caused by diseases. These deposits cause impairment of certain organs.

Analgesics—Medications that relieve pain.

Anemia—Condition in which red blood cells or hemoglobin (oxygen-carrying substance in blood) is inadequate.

Anesthesia, Epidural—Temporary prevention of pain by injecting medication (a local anesthetic) into the peridural space of the spinal cord.

Anesthesia, General—Causing temporary loss of consciousness and inability to feel pain by use of inhaled gases or injected anesthetics.

Anesthesia, Local—Temporary prevention of pain in a limited and usually superficial area of the body by injecting medication (local anesthetic).

Anesthesia, Local (Nerve Block)—Injection of the local anesthetic near the nerves of the surgical area.

Anesthesia, Pudendal (Pudendal Block)—Temporary prevention of pain by injecting medication (local anesthetic) into the pudendal nerves that supply the lower vagina and perineum.

Anesthesia, Spinal—Temporary prevention of pain by injecting medication (local anesthetic) into the subarachnoid space of the spine.

Anesthesiologist—A physician specializing in anesthesiology.

Anesthesiology—A branch of medical science dealing with anesthetics and anesthesia.

Aneurysm—Abnormal swelling or ballooning of a blood vessel.

Angina—Pain or pressure beneath the breastbone caused by inadequate blood supply to the heart.

Angiogram, Angiography—Study of arteries and veins by injecting material into them that x-rays can outline.

Anomaly—A deviation from normal, especially of a bodily part.

Anoscopy—Visual examination of the anus by means of a short tube called an anoscope, an optical instrument with lenses and a lighted tip.

Anovulation—Failure or absence of ovulation.

Antacid—Medicine taken orally that reduces or neutralizes stomach acid.

Antiarrhythmics—Medications used to treat heartbeat irregularities (arrhythmias).

Antibiotics—Medications that attack germs and fight infection.

Antibiotics, Cephalosporin—Class of antibiotics related to penicillin, capable of destroying more kinds of germs than penicillin.

Antibiotics, Erythromycin—Class of antibiotics that destroys germs similar to those destroyed by penicillin. Often used to treat infections in patients who are allergic to penicillin.

Antibodies—Proteins created in blood and body tissue by the immune system to neutralize or destroy sources of disease.

Anticancer Drugs—Medications that weaken or destroy cancerous tissues without harming healthy tissues.

Anticholinergic Drugs—Medications that reduce nerve impulses in the parasym pathetic nervous system. They control some activities of the gastrointestinal system, heart, bladder and other organs.

Anticoagulants—Medications that slow or delay blood clotting.

Anticonvulsants—Medications that control seizures (convulsions), pain or conditions in which the brain or nerves are overly sensitive.

Antidepressants—Medications that help control depression.

Antiemetic Drugs—Medications that prevent or stop nausea and vomiting.

Antifungal Drugs—Medications used to treat fungus diseases.

Antigens—Germs or other sources of disease that antibodies (produced by the immune system) neutralize or destroy.

Antihelmintic Drugs—Medications used to treat worms in the intestines.

Antihistamines—Medications used to treat allergies.

Antihyperlipidemic Drugs—Medications that reduce fat (cholesterol) in the blood. They help prevent blood-vessel disease.

Antihypertensives—Medications used to reduce blood pressure.

Anti-inflammatory Drugs—Medications

used to control inflammation not caused by infection.

Antimalarial Drugs—Medications used to prevent or treat malaria.

Antimetabolite Drugs—Medications that are used to treat some cancers and autoimmune diseases.

Antimicrobial Drugs—Same as *Antibiotics*.

Antinuclear Antibody—Substance that appears in the blood, indicating presence of an autoimmune disease.

Antiparkinsonian Drugs—Medications used to treat Parkinson's disease.

Antiprotozoal Drugs—Medications used in treatment of single-celled parasites (protozoa).

Antipruritic Drugs—Medications that reduce itching.

Antispasmodic Drugs—Medications that improve digestion and relieve intestinal cramps.

Antistreptococcal Titer—Blood test that measures body's response to infection by streptococcal bacteria.

Antithyroid Drugs—Medications used to counter the effects of an overactive thyroid gland.

Antiviral Drugs—Medications used to treat infections caused by viruses.

Anus—A muscular band at the end of the rectum that opens and expands to allow passage of feces.

Anus, Imperforate—Congenital abnormality of newborn infants in which the anus cannot pass feces.

Anxiety—Uncomfortable feeling that something unpleasant or dangerous will happen.

Aorta—Body's largest blood vessel, arising from the top of the heart. It carries blood from the heart to all parts of the body.

Aphrodisiac—Substance claimed to increase sexual arousal or pleasure.

Appendage—Body part that has a minor role (or no role at all) in normal body function. For example, the appendix is an appendage to the colon that seems to have no function.

Appendicitis—Inflammation of the appendix.

Appendix—A 3- to 6-inch appendage to the colon that seems to have no function.

Areola—The colored ring around the nipple.

Arteriogram, Arteriography—Studying arteries by injecting material into them that x-rays can outline.

Arteriosclerosis—Hardening of the arteries.

Artery—Blood vessels that carry blood from the heart to the body.

Arthrograms—X-rays of the joints taken with an arthroscope.

Arthroscope—Slender optical instrument with a lighted tip that allows direct visual examination of some joints. It can also be used to correct some defects in joints.

Artificial Insemination—The transfer of semen into the vagina by artificial means, for the purpose of conception.

Artificial Limbs—Mechanical substitutions for amputated arms or legs.

Ascending Colon—First part of the large colon (intestine) extending from the lower end of the small intestine.

Aspiration—1) Removal of accumulated pus or fluid with a needle. 2) Accidental inhalation of objects or fluids into the lungs.

Astigmatism—Visual impairment caused by abnormal eye shape.

Asymmetrical—Uneven in size, shape or position.

Atriums—Small chambers in the heart that pump blood into the ventricles. Also called auricles.

Atropine—Medication used to treat diseases of the eye, heart, gastrointestinal system and nervous system.

Audiogram, Audiometry—Test of hearing ability.

Autism—Mental illness of children in which they seem unaware of their surroundings.

Autoimmune Assays (ANA Tests)—Blood tests to identify autoimmune disease.

Autoimmune, Autoimmunity—Disease in which a person's immune system attacks its own tissues.

Autoimmune Disorder—Disease in which the immune system produces antibodies that attack the body's own tissues.

Autonomic Nervous System—Part of the nervous system that controls organs that function involuntarily, such as the heart, lungs, digestive system and blood vessels.

B

Bacteria—One-celled micro-organisms that can sometimes cause disease.

Balloon Angioplasty—Treatment for obstructed arteries, especially those supplying blood to the heart and brain. A small uninflated balloon is passed up the artery to the obstruction, and then expanded to release the obstruction.

Barium Enema—See *Barium X-rays*.

Barium X-rays—Examining the gastrointestinal system by filling it with a barium solution that is detected by x-rays. Common barium tests are the barium swallow (upper GI series) and the barium enema (lower GI series).

Bartholin's Glands—Small glands in the lips of the vagina that secrete a lubricating fluid, especially during sexual arousal.

Behavior Therapy—Psychotherapy that focuses on ways to change the undesired behavior.

Belladonna—Medication derived from a plant used to treat some diseases of the gastrointestinal system. It is similar to atropine.

Benign—1) Tumor or growth that is neither cancerous nor located where it might impair normal function. 2) Harmless.

Beta-adrenergic Blockers (Beta-blockers)—Medications that reduce heart or blood-vessel overactivity to improve blood circulation. Also used to prevent migraine headaches, high blood pressure and angina.

BhCG—Beta-human chorionic gonadotropin; a hormone produced during pregnancy.

Bile—A digestive juice produced in the liver and stored in the gallbladder. Bile empties into the small intestine for digestive processes.

Bile Duct—A small tube that allows bile to pass from the gallbladder into the intestines.

Bilirubin—A yellowish, red-blood-cell waste product in bile that the blood carries to the liver. It contributes to urine's yellowish color and can cause jaundice if it builds up in the blood.

Biopsy—Removal of a small amount of tissue or cells (such as fluid from a cyst) for laboratory examination that aids in diagnosis. The tissue sample may be removed by a variety of methods depending on the site to be biopsied.

Biopsy Needle—Instrument often used to perform a biopsy.

Biopsy, Skin—Removal of a sample of skin tissue for laboratory examination that aids in diagnosis. Skin biopsy is often required to confirm a clinical (visual) diagnosis. Removal techniques include shave excision, punch excision and elliptical excision.

Birth Canal—Passageway through the cervix and the vagina through which the baby passes during childbirth.

Bladder—An organ that holds fluids such as urine (urinary bladder) or bile (gallbladder).

Blood Cells, Red—Microscopic cells in the blood that carry oxygen to tissues of the body. One drop of blood contains about 200 million red cells.

Blood Cells, White—Microscopic cells in the blood that help fight infection by destroying germs. One drop of blood contains about 400,000 white cells.

Blood Chemistries—Tests that measure chemicals in the blood.

Blood Count—Counting red and white blood cells to aid in diagnosis of many diseases.

Blood Platelets—See *Platelet Count*.

Blood Pressure—The amount of pressure exerted on the walls of the blood vessels and arteries when the heart contracts and when it relaxes between beats.

Blood Studies—Examination of a blood sample to measure white blood cells, red blood cells, hemoglobin, hematocrit and chemical substances. See *Blood Chemistries*.

Blood Test—Laboratory analysis of the blood that provides information for the diagnosis of a disorder or disease.

Blood Transfusion—The infusion of blood into the veins of a patient from an outside source.

Blood Vessels—Arteries, veins and capillaries; the tubes in which blood circulates through the body.

Bone Bank—Facility where human bone is stored and made available for transplantation.

Bone Scan—Method of studying the bone structure or function by injecting into the bloodstream a medication that can be detected by a special scanning camera.

Bone Spurs—Abnormal and sometimes painful protrusions of bone with sharp points near joints or tendons.

Breast—Either of the pair of mammary glands protruding from the upper, front part of a woman's body.

Breech Presentation (Breech)—Presentation of the fetus in which the hind end of the body is the first part to appear at the uterine cervix.

Bronchial Tubes (Bronchi)—Hollow air passageways that branch from the windpipe (trachea) into the lungs. They carry oxygen into the lungs and pass waste gases (mostly carbon dioxide) out of the body.

Bronchioles—Small air passageways that serve the same purpose as bronchial tubes. Bronchioles are the smallest parts of the respiratory system.

Bronchodilator Drugs—Medications used to treat diseases of the bronchi that cause shortness of breath, such as asthma. The medicines help constricted tubes to relax.

Bronchogram—Diagnosing lung diseases by placing a material in the lung that x-rays can outline.

Bronchoscope—An optical instrument with a lighted tip that is passed into the windpipe, then into the bronchi.

Bruising—Discoloration under the skin caused by injury or bleeding.

Bulimia Nervosa—A serious eating disorder that occurs chiefly in females, characterized by compulsive overeating, usually followed by self-induced vomiting or laxative or diuretic abuse. Often accompanied by guilt and depression.

Bulimic—Relating to, or affected with, bulimia.

C

Calcification—A process in which calcium from the blood is deposited abnormally into tissues due to injury, infection or aging. Often it is part of healing and not a sign of active disease.

Calcium-Channel Blocker Drugs—Medication used to treat angina, hypertension and heartbeat irregularities.

Cancerous Growths—Extensions of cancerous tissues that invade nearby healthy tissues.

Cancers—Destructive tumors that can arise in almost all parts of the body. Cancer can destroy nearby healthy tissue and may spread to distant organs.

Capillaries—Microscopic vessels that supply all body cells and tissues with blood.

Carbohydrates, Complex—Starches, sugars, cellulose and gums. Complex carbohydrates are those contained in whole grains, fresh fruits and fresh vegetables. These are considered more nutritious than simple carbohydrates.

Carbohydrates, Simple—Refined carbohydrates (sugars) that have lower molecular weights than complex carbohydrates. They produce a quick rise in blood-sugar levels. Most nutrition counselors recommend that daily diets contain minimal amounts of refined sugars. So-called "junk foods" are frequently very high in simple carbohydrates.

Cardiac Catheter—A slender tube that is inserted into an artery or vein and then passed into the heart. It is used to examine the heart and nearby blood vessels by injecting material into the heart that x-rays can detect.

Cardiac Catheterization—Studying heart function with a cardiac catheter.

Cardiopulmonary Resuscitation (CPR)—Emergency treatment for a patient whose heart has stopped (cardiac arrest).

Cardiovascular—Relating to the heart and blood vessels.

Cardiovascular Surgeon—Doctor specially trained to operate on the heart and blood vessels.

Cardiovascular System—System that supplies the body with blood. It consists of the heart and blood vessels (arteries, capillaries, veins).

Carotid Arteries—Large arteries that supply much of the blood to the brain.

Cartilage—Rubbery, dense connective tissue that permits smooth movement of joints. It also helps shape flexible parts of the nose and external ear.

Caruncle—Small, red protrusion of tissue

near a body opening. The most common caruncles arise from the urethra or cervix.

CAT Scan—See *CT Scan*.

Catheter—A hollow tube used to introduce fluids into the body or to drain fluids away.

Catheterization—Any procedure in which a small flexible tube is inserted into the body for the purpose of withdrawing or introducing substances. It most often involves the passage of a small catheter through a vein in the arm or leg or the neck and into the heart for securing blood samples or to detect problems.

Caudal Anesthesia—Form of local (low spinal) anesthesia used to reduce pain during childbirth and surgery on pelvic areas.

Cauterant—Chemical used to destroy abnormal or diseased cells on the skin.

Cauterization—Destruction of tissue by burning or searing it with a red-hot instrument, caustic chemicals or electricity.

Cautery—Destroying small areas of diseased tissue by burning with an electric needle or laser beam, freezing with low temperature instruments or using a chemical that destroys tissue.

Cecum—The part of the intestinal tract at the beginning of the large colon (intestine).

Central Nervous System—System that controls the body's voluntary acts. It consists of the brain and spinal cord.

Cerclage—Any of several procedures for increasing tissue resistance in an incompetent cervix, usually in the form of stitches or sutures near the internal opening.

Cervical Cancer—Cancer of the cervix.

Cervical Spine—Bones in the neck at the top of the spinal column.

Cervical Stenosis—A narrowing or constriction of the cervix.

Cervix—Lower third of the uterus, which protrudes into the vagina.

Cesarean Section—Delivery of a baby through incisions in the mother's abdomen and uterus. It is performed when normal vaginal delivery would be dangerous for the mother or baby.

Chancre—Hard, slightly ulcerated, painless lesion that forms where syphilis enters the body, usually on the genital lips.

Chemocautery—Destruction of abnormal tissue by means of acids, caustics or poisons.

Chemotherapy—Treatment of cancer by injecting medications that kill cancer cells without harming healthy tissue. It is used to treat cancers that cannot be completely cured or treated with surgery or radiation.

Chiggers—Small red biting insects. Also called "red bugs."

Child—Person in the first 10 years of life.

Chiropractor—Practitioner of chiropractic treatment of disease, which involves massage and manipulations to restore normal body functions.

Chokes—Severe breathing difficulty experienced by scuba divers and others who go from high to normal air pressure too rapidly. Bubbles of nitrogen develop in the blood stream and obstruct blood supply to vital organs, sometimes resulting in severe injury or death.

Cholangiogram, Cholangiography—X-ray procedures to diagnose diseases of the bile system (liver, gallbladder, bile ducts). Special medications are used to make the bile system visible on x-rays.

Cholecystectomy—Surgical removal of the gallbladder.

Cholecystography—An x-ray of the gallbladder.

Cholera—Acute, severe, infectious disease causing extreme diarrhea and dehydration.

Chorionic Villi Sampling (Chorionic Villus Sampling; CVS)—A prenatal diagnostic test that detects chromosomal abnormalities in a fetus, and which can be performed between the 9th and 12th weeks of pregnancy.

Choroiditis—Inflammation of the part of the eye that supports the retina and supplies blood to it.

Chromosome—Structures inside the nucleus of living cells that contain hereditary information. Defects in chromosomes cause many birth defects and inherited diseases.

Chronic—Long term, continuing. Chronic illnesses are usually not curable, but they can often be prevented from worsening. Symptoms usually can be controlled.

Cinematography—Form of motion-picture photography used to record a fast-moving series of x-ray images.

Circulatory System—The system that provides blood to the body, consisting of the heart, arteries, veins and lymphatic system.

Clinician—Health-care professional who has direct contact with patients. The word literally means "someone who is at the patient's bedside."

Clips—See *Skin Clips.*

Clitoris—The small female genital organ located at the upper end of the vulva which is a direct source of orgasm for most women.

Clot Retraction Test—Measurement of the time necessary for a tube of blood to form a clot. Abnormal results often indicate a defect in blood platelets, cells important in blood coagulation.

Clotting—Activity of the blood and blood vessels that cause blood to form a jellylike clot, usually near an injury. Clotting helps stop bleeding. The body's clotting mechanism is slowed or reduced ("thinning the blood") with anticoagulants to treat certain diseases.

Coagulation—Same as *Clotting.*

Cocaine—Medication applied directly to mucous membranes to control pain in the nose and throat. Used illegally as a mind-altering drug, it is addicting and dangerous.

Cognitive Therapy—Psychotherapy that is based on the idea that the way we think about the world and ourselves affects our emotions and behavior.

Colic, Colicky—A pain that recurs in a regular pattern every few seconds or minutes.

Collagen—A gelatinous protein from which body tissues are formed.

Colon—The last major portion of the gastrointestinal tract, where waste material is formed into feces and held for elimination. It is also known as the large intestine.

Colonoscopy—Method of diagnosing diseases of the colon by visual examination of the inside of the colon through a flexible colonoscope, a fiber-optic instrument with a lighted tip.

Color Blindness—Inability to recognize red and green, which appear to be gray. It is usually hereditary.

Colostomy—Surgical formation of an artificial anus by connecting the colon to an opening in the abdominal wall.

Colpectomy—Partial or complete surgical excision of the vagina; also called vaginectomy.

Colposcopy—Visual examination of the cervix by means of a colposcope, a slender optical instrument with a lighted tip.

Combined Immunodeficiency Disease—Serious inherited disease in which the immune system of infants is unable to defend against disease.

Complication—Undesirable event during disease or treatment that causes further symptoms and delay in recovery.

Compress—Cloth, sometimes soaked in warm water or coated with medication. It is applied to the skin to relieve discomfort.

Compression—Applying pressure to the surface of the body, usually to stop bleeding.

Compulsion, Compulsive—Intense, irrational urge to perform some action.

Conception—The process of becoming pregnant, involving fertilization of an egg by a sperm and implantation of the fertilized egg in the uterine wall.

Condom, Female—A thin sheath, usually made of polyurethane, inserted into the vagina before sexual intercourse. It is used as a contraceptive and offers some protection against sexually transmitted diseases.

Condom, Male—A thin sheath, usually of latex, applied to the penis before sexual intercourse. It is used to help prevent disease of the genitals and as a contraceptive.

Congenital—Abnormality of the body, present at birth, usually meaning a defect. Congenital defects may be inherited or caused by conditions occurring while the fetus grows in the uterus.

Congenital Hypoplastic Anemia—See *Hypoplastic Anemia.*

Conization of the Cervix—Removal of a cone of tissue from the cervix. Laboratory examination of the removed tissue identifies possible cancer.

Conjunctiva—The mucous membrane lining the outermost surface of the eye (white of the eye).

Connective Tissue—Body's supporting framework of tissue consisting of strands of collagen, elastic fibers and simple cells.

Contact Lenses—Small plastic lenses worn on the eyes to correct nearsightedness, farsightedness or astigmatism.

Contagious—Disease or condition that spreads from one person to another.

Contraception—Deliberate prevention of conception or impregnation.

Contraindication—A symptom or condition that makes a particular procedure, treatment or medication inadvisable.

Convalescence—Recovery from an illness or surgery.

Copious—Large in amount.

Cornea—Clear thickened surface of the eye through which light passes. It has no blood supply and can be transplanted without danger of rejection.

Coronary—Referring to the blood vessels supplying the heart. Sometimes, it refers to a heart attack resulting from coronary-artery obstruction.

Coronary Care Unit (CCU)—Area of a hospital equipped to care for patients who have suffered a heart attack or other life-threatening heart conditions.

Cortisone Drugs—Medications similar to natural hormones produced by the central core of the adrenal glands.

Cosmetic Surgery—Surgery to improve appearance.

Coxsackie Viruses—Group of viruses causing infections such as poliomyelitis, aseptic meningitis, herpangina and myocarditis.

CPR—See *Cardiopulmonary Resuscitation.*

Crabs—Sexually transmitted parasites, also known as pubic lice, that infest the genital and anal areas, causing extreme itching and discomfort.

Cramps—1) Persistent and sometimes intense lower abdominal pain often associated with menstruation. 2) A painful, involuntary contraction of a muscle.

Cranium—Bones that make up the skull.

Crib Death—Same as *Sudden Infant Death Syndrome.*

Cryosurgery—Destruction of abnormal tissue by applying freezing temperatures, usually with liquid nitrogen.

Cryotherapy—The use of cold (below -200F) temperatures in treatment.

CT Scan, CAT Scan (Computerized Axial Tomography)—A computerized x-ray procedure that provides exceptionally clear images of parts of the body. It aids in diagnosis of diseases that cannot be diagnosed by ordinary x-ray methods.

Culdocentesis—Piercing of the space deep in the vagina under the cervix, to obtain fluid. Laboratory examination of the removed fluid aids in diagnosis of ectopic pregnancy and other disorders.

Culdoscopy—Visual examination of the female pelvic organs by means of a slender instrument brought into the pelvic cavity by penetrating through the space deep in the vagina under the cervix.

Culture—Identification of bacteria, fungi and viruses. Material (pus, blood or urine) from an infected area is collected, placed on nutrient material and kept warm (usually in an incubator) until the infecting agent has grown. The resulting growth is examined with a microscope.

Curettage—Scraping process frequently used to obtain tissue from the lining of the uterus for laboratory examination that aids in diagnosis.

Curette—Instrument with a sharp end used to scrape tissue from the inner lining of the uterus and to scrape away skin lesions.

Cyst—Sac or cavity filled with fluid or diseased matter.

Cyst Aspiration—Removal of cyst contents for examination, or drainage for relief of symptoms.

Cystocele—A hernia in which part of the bladder protrudes into the vagina.

Cystography—An x-ray of the urinary bladder that is obtained by injecting a solution visible on x-rays into the bladder.

Cystoscopy—Visual examination of the inside of the urinary bladder by means of a cystoscope, a slender optical instrument with a lighted tip.

Cytotoxic Drugs—Medications used to destroy cancerous cells with minimal harm to healthy cells.

D

D & C—Same as *Dilatation and Curettage.*

DC Cardioversion—The restoration of normal rhythm of the heart by a brief electrical shock via two metal plates placed on the wall of the chest.

Debilitating—Causing a general weakening or deterioration in health.

Defibrillation, Cardiac—Applying an electric current to the chest over the heart to interrupt fibrillation, a disturbance of heartbeat.

Dehydration—Loss of essential fluids from the tissues and blood of the body.

Dependence—Condition in which a person requires substances such as narcotics or alcohol to remain comfortable. If the substances are not used, withdrawal symptoms develop.

Dermatome—Area of the skin to which feeling (sensation) is provided by a nerve to the spinal cord.

Descending Colon—The part of the colon in the left side of the abdomen that stores feces until they are passed from the body.

Desensitization—1) Reduction or prevention of allergic (hypersensitivity) reactions by administration of graded doses of allergen. 2) Treatment for phobias and other psychological disorders. A patient gradually increases the exposure to the source of fear while simultaneously learning to relax.

Diabetic Retinopathy—Degeneration of the retina that develops in patients with diabetes mellitus. It may cause vision impairment or blindness.

Diagnosis—Identifying disease. A complete diagnosis names the part of the body affected, the disease process (such as inflammation, cancer or allergy) and the cause of disease.

Dialysis—Removal of natural wastes from the bloodstream. It is used to treat patients with kidney failure.

Diaphragm—1) Thin, broad sheet of muscle separating the chest cavity from the abdominal cavity. 2) A flexible, soft rubber cup or dome-shaped device which is inserted into the vagina to cover the cervix to provide a barrier method of contraception.

Diarrhea—Abnormally frequent and watery bowel movements.

Diathermy—Treatment in which mild heat is generated within the body by high-frequency radio waves.

DIC—See *Disseminated Intravascular Coagulation*.

Digestive System—Organs in which food is processed for absorption into the blood stream. The major digestive organs are the mouth, esophagus, stomach, duodenum, small bowel (small intestine), colon (large intestine) and rectum. The liver, gallbladder and pancreas are also considered parts of the digestive system.

Digitalis—A drug used to treat congestive heart failure and some other heart diseases.

Dilatation and Curettage (D&C)—A gynecological treatment or diagnostic procedure that involves the stretching (dilatation) of the cervix so that a spoon-shaped instrument (curette) can be inserted into the uterus to scrape away the lining (endometrium). The scrapings may be examined under a microscope to assess the condition of the uterus.

Dilate, Dilation—To widen, expand or open up.

Dilator—Instrument used to widen organs that have narrowed because of disease.

Discolored Teeth—A yellowish-brown discoloration of the teeth frequently occurring in infants whose mothers took tetracycline while pregnant. Children may also be affected if they take tetracycline before they have their permanent teeth.

Discomfort—Unpleasant physical or mental sensation.

Disease—Adverse change in health; sickness or ailment. A disease can be defined by the body part involved (for example, the heart or liver), by the abnormality present (cancer, infection, allergy, degeneration, etc.) or by its cause (bacteria, poisons, injury, etc.).

Disk—Same as *Intervertebral Disk*.

Disorder—Same as *Disease*.

Disseminated Intravascular Coagulation (DIC)—A pathologic condition associated with inappropriate activation of coagulation systems; can occur as a complication of pregnancy, or as a result of infection or malignancy.

Diuretics—Medications that force the kidneys to excrete more urine, sodium and potassium than normal, which helps eliminate excessive body fluid.

Diverticulum—Small pouch or sac that develops in the wall of tubular organs such as the esophagus or colon.

Dizziness—Sensation of faintness, lightheadedness or spinning (vertigo).

Donor—Person who gives to someone else. In transplantation surgery, the donor gives up an organ (such as a kidney) to be transplanted into the recipient.

Doppler Ultrasound—See *Ultrasound*; this is one of several methods of ultrasound.

Dormant—Sleeping or inactive state of living things. Also, an inactive state of a disease.

Drainage—Passage of fluids out of the body through an opening or incision.

Ductus Arteriosus—Small blood vessel connecting the aorta and the pulmonary artery, which is the main artery to the lung. The vessel is open during the time the fetus is in the uterus, but normally closes at birth.

Duodenum—First 12 inches of the small intestine.

Dupuytren's Contracture—Chronic condition in which scar tissue forms on the palms. In severe cases, it can impair use of the fingers.

Dwarfism—Condition of being undersized for one's age. It may be due to endocrine disorders, malnutrition or an inherited defect.

Dysentery—A disease characterized by severe diarrhea with passage of mucus and blood, usually caused by infection.

Dysmenorrhea—Painful menstruation.

Dyspareunia—Painful sexual intercourse.

Dyspepsia—Indigestion.

Dysplasia—Abnormal growth or development of organs or cells.

Dyspnea—Difficult or painful breathing.

Dysuria—Difficult or painful urination.

E

Ear Canal—Passageway extending from the outer ear inward to the eardrum.

Ear, Nose and Throat (ENT) Specialist—A physician specially trained to treat diseases of the ears, nose and throat.

ECG (Electrocardiography)—Method of diagnosing heart diseases by measuring electrical activity of the heart with an electrocardiograph. The record produced is called an electrocardiogram.

Echocardiogram, Echocardiography—Studying the heart by examining sound waves created by an instrument placed on the chest. The waves reflected from the heart form an image (echocardiogram) on a monitor, aiding in diagnosis of heart diseases.

Echography—The use of ultrasound as a diagnostic aid.

Eclampsia—Convulsions or coma late in pregnancy in an individual affected with preeclampsia.

Ectopic Pregnancy—A gestation which occurs elsewhere than in the uterus, usually in a fallopian tube or the peritoneal cavity.

Edema—Accumulation of fluid under the skin, in the lungs or elsewhere.

EEG (Electroencephalography)—Studying the brain by measuring electric activity ("brain waves") with an electro-encephalograph. The record produced is the electroencephalogram.

EKG—See *ECG*.

Electrocardiography—See *ECG*.

Electrocautery—Destruction of tissue by heat applied with a controlled electric current.

Electroencephalography—See *EEG*.

Electrolyte—A chemical that is dissolved in the blood and all other body fluids. Electrolytes play an essential role in all body functions. The major electrolytes are sodium, potassium, chloride, calcium, phosphorus, magnesium and carbon dioxide. Electrolytes come from food. They are regulated mostly by the kidneys and lungs.

Electrolyte Measurement—Laboratory test on blood or urine to identify and measure the electrolytes present.

Electrolyte Supplements—Electrolytes taken to correct or to prevent body-fluid or electrolyte imbalance.

Electromyography—Studying nerve and muscle disorders by recording electrical activity of muscles with an electromyograph. The record produced is the electromyogram.

Electroneuronography—A diagnostic procedure in which the nerve of a muscle under study is stimulated by application of an electric current.

Embolism—The sudden blockage of an artery by a clot or abnormal particle (such as an air bubble) circulating in the blood.

Embryo—The developing human individual from the time of implantation to the end of the eighth week after conception.

Endemic—Disease that is constantly present in a community or group of people. Endemic disease may affect only a few people at any one time.

Endocrine System—System of organs that secrete hormones into the blood to regulate basic functions of cells and tissues. The endocrine organs are the anterior and posterior pituitary glands, thyroid and parathyroid glands, pancreas, adrenal glands, ovaries (in women) and testicles (in men).

Endocrinologist—Doctor specially trained in diagnosis and treatment of endocrine disorders.

Endometrial Biopsy—A biopsy of the endometrium.

Endometrial Cancer—Cancer of the endometrium.

Endometriosis—A condition in which functioning endometrial tissue occurs in places within the pelvic cavity other than the uterus, and often results in severe pain and infertility.

Endometritis—Inflammation of the endometrium.

Endometrium—The mucous membrane lining of the uterus.

Endomyometritis—Inflammation of the muscular substance (or myometrium) of the uterus.

Endoscopy—Method of diagnosing diseases in hollow organs. An endoscope (an optical instrument with a lighted tip) is inserted into the organ, which allows visual examination of the cavity. Used in the abdomen, pelvis, lumen of the bronchial tubes or intestines.

Endotracheal Tube—Tube temporarily placed in the trachea (windpipe) of patients who are unable to breathe normally because of disease or surgery.

Enteric—Relating to the small intestine. Enteric-coated medicine is coated with a hard shell that dissolves when it reaches the small intestine.

Enteroscopy—Examination of the inside of the intestines with an endoscope, an optical instrument.

Enterostomy—Surgically created artificial opening for elimination of feces. An enterostomy nurse or enterostomy specialist is a professional who teaches patients how to care for the artificial opening.

Enzymes—Proteins manufactured by the body that regulate the rate of essential life processes (metabolism).

Epinephrine—Same as *Adrenalin*.

Episcleritis—Inflammation of tissues on the sclera (the white of the eye).

Episiotomy—Surgical enlargement of the vulvar orifice for obstetrical purposes, usually during childbirth.

Epithelial Horn—Thick, rough lesion protruding from the skin. It may become cancerous if not removed.

Equine Virus—Virus that causes a serious form of encephalitis in horses and humans.

Ergot—Medication derived from a fungus that grows on rye plant. It is used to treat migraine headache and to increase strength of uterine contractions during and immediately after childbirth.

Esophageal Varices—Enlarged veins on the lining of the esophagus. They are subject to severe bleeding and often appear in patients with severe liver disease.

Esophagoscopy—Method of diagnosing diseases of the esophagus by means of an esophagoscope, an optical instrument with lenses and a lighted tip.

Esophagus—Muscular tube connecting the throat and stomach.

Estrogen—Female sex hormone, primarily secreted by the ovaries. It can also be produced synthetically for use in estrogen replacement therapy.

Estrogen Receptor Value—Used in the study of breast-cancer cells to determine the best treatment.

Etiology—Cause or causes of a disease.

Eustachian Tubes—Slender passages between the throat and the middle ear that maintain normal air pressure in the middle ear.

Excise—To remove by excision.

Excision—Surgical removal or resection of

a diseased part.

Exploratory Laparotomy—Diagnosing abdominal disease by surgically opening the abdomen and examining its contents.

Extremities—Arms and legs.

Eye Bank—Facility where living corneas are stored and made available for transplantation.

Eyes, Crossed—Condition in which muscles controlling the eyes are unbalanced. The eyes point in different directions. Also called squint or strabismus.

F

Fallopian Tubes—Organs of the female reproductive tract through which an egg (ovum) passes from the ovary to the uterus. Tying these tubes (tubal ligation) accomplishes sterility.

Familial Polyposis—Inherited condition in which the lining of the intestines contains many polyps, some of which may become cancerous.

Family History—Information about illnesses that tend to occur within a family. This information is used to determine the likelihood of diseases occurring in other members of the family.

Farsightedness—Same as *Hypermetropia.*

Fascia—Sheet or band of tough, fibrous tissue that covers muscles and other body organs.

Fecal—Relating to feces, waste products eliminated through the lower intestinal tract.

Fecal-Oral—Pathway by which some fecal germs gain entry into the bloodstream. Sewage in drinking water, hand-to-mouth transmission after bowel movements or sexual contact can cause infection.

Feces—Body waste formed of undigested food that has passed through the gastrointestinal system to the colon. Feces are produced and stored in the colon until eliminated.

Fertilization—An act or process of insemination or impregnation, as when a sperm penetrates an egg.

Fetal—Of, relating to or being a fetus.

Fetal Monitoring—Measuring the heart rate of the fetus during labor.

Fetal-Scalp Electrodes—Fine wires attached to the scalp of a fetus to measure heart rate and rhythm during labor.

Fetal-Scalp Monitoring—Measuring the well-being of the fetus during labor by obtaining blood from the scalp or by measuring the heart rate of the fetus or contraction strength of the uterus.

Fetus—A developing human from usually three months after conception to birth.

Fever—Above-normal body temperature. Normal mouth temperature is 98.6F (37C). Normal rectal temperature is 99.6F (37.6C).

Fiber—A non-nutritious ingredient of many complex carbohydrates. Fiber increases bulk in the diet. Many nutritionists recommend including ample fiber in the diet. Experimental studies and clinical studies show that people who eat high-fiber diets are less likely to develop colon cancer, diverticulitis, atherosclerosis and gallbladder disease.

Fiber Optics—System of transmitting light and images through thread-like strands of glass. Fiber-optic instruments make some examinations and surgical procedures simple, safe and effective.

Fibrin—Protein formed by the action of blood clotting on fibrinogen.

Fibrinogen—Protein in the blood needed for blood clotting.

Fibrositis—Inflammatory conditions affecting connective tissue of muscles, joints, ligaments and tendons.

First Molars—First permanent flat teeth, used for grinding food, which appear at about age 6 to 7.

Fissure—Break in the skin or inner lining of organs.

Fistula—Abnormal passage between two organs or between the body and the outside.

Flank—Area on the side of the body below the ribs and above the hip.

Fleas—Tiny biting insects. Most cause minor skin irritation; some carry and transmit serious diseases such as plague and typhus.

Flooding—A drastic form of psychotherapy used for treatment of phobias. A patient is suddenly confronted with the feared object or placed in the feared situation with no chance of escape. Having experienced the phobia at its fullest intensity, a person comes to realize that the dreaded thing is not dangerous. Only a competent therapist should subject a phobic person to it.

Fluorescein-dye Test—Method of diagnosis using fluorescein, a dye, to study tissues and germs. When these dyed tissues are exposed to ultraviolet light, they glow. Substances to which the dye does not cling do not glow.

Fluorescent Antibody Studies—Tests used to study some allergic and infectious conditions. When antibodies created by these conditions are present in the blood, they can be made to glow by using a dye and a microscope with ultraviolet light.

Fluoroscopy—Method of x-ray diagnosis in which moving organs (such as the heart or intestinal tract) can be studied in action.

Foley Catheter—Slender, flexible tube used to drain urine from the bladder of patients who are unable to urinate normally.

Forceps—Instrument with two blades and handles. It is used to grasp tissue, body parts or sterile materials. Also used to deliver babies when progress of labor is slow.

Fracture—Break; usually used to refer to a bone or tooth.

Frei Test—Test used to make a precise diagnosis of lymphogranuloma, a sexually transmitted disease.

Friedreich's Ataxia—Rare, inherited nervous-system disease that causes loss of balance and coordination, awkward walking, speech difficulty and tremors.

Frozen Section—A study in a pathology laboratory of fresh tissue that was removed during surgery. The purpose is to determine if a suspicious area is or is not cancerous.

Fungus—Mold or yeast that may infect skin, internal surfaces (mouth, vagina) or tissues.

Fungus Infection—Infection caused by fungus.

Fusiform Bacteria—Bacteria shaped like slender rods.

G

Galactorrhea—1) Continued breast-milk flow after weaning. 2) Excess breast-milk flow during nursing.

Galactosemia—Inherited disease of infants in which milk cannot be digested. Milk should be eliminated from the infant's diet to prevent malnutrition, liver and kidney disease and mental retardation.

Gallbladder—Small organ under the liver that stores bile. For digestion, the gallbladder contracts to empty bile into the intestines.

Gamete Intrafallopian Transfer (GIFT)—An alternative to in-vitro fertilization that allows fertilization to occur in a woman's fallopian tubes, rather than in the lab. One or more eggs, which have been stimulated by ovulation-inducing drugs, are removed from the woman's ovary, transferred to a tiny catheter along with a sperm sample, and then the eggs and sperm are injected into the open end of one or both of the woman's fallopian tubes where fertilization occurs.

Gamma Globulin—Protein in the blood manufactured by the immune system to help destroy or neutralize infection-causing germs. Gamma globulin derived and concentrated from blood of other humans is used to help create temporary immunity to some diseases.

Gammaglobulinemia—Extremely low levels in the blood of gamma globulin brought about by a disease of the immune system. The deficiency causes increased susceptibility to many infections by bacteria, viruses and fungi. Also called hypogammaglobulinemia.

Gangrene—Death of tissue, usually due to partial or total loss of blood supply.

Gastrectomy—Removal of part or all of the stomach.

Gastroenterologist—Doctor who specializes in the diagnosis and treatment of diseases of the gastrointestinal system.

Gastrointestinal Series (Upper GI Series)—X-rays of the upper digestive system (esophagus, stomach and duodenum).

Gastrointestinal Tract—See *Digestive System.*

Gastroscopy—Visual examination of the inside of the stomach by means of a gastroscope, an optical instrument with a lighted tip.

Gene—Basic unit of protein molecules in